OPERATIVE SURGERY

Fundamental International Techniques

Colon, Rectum and Anus

OPERATIVE SURGERY

Fundamental International Techniques

Third Edition

Under the General Editorship of

Charles Rob
M.C., M.D., M.Chir., F.R.C.S.

Professor and Chairman of the Department of Surgery,
University of Rochester School of Medicine and Dentistry,
Rochester, New York

and

Sir Rodney Smith
K.B.E., Hon.D.Sc., M.S., F.R.C.S., Hon.F.R.A.C.S.,
Hon.F.R.C.S.(Ed.), Hon.F.A.C.S., Hon.F.R.C.S. (Can.),
Hon.F.R.C.S.(I.)

Surgeon, St. George's Hospital, London

Associate Editor

Hugh Dudley
Ch.M., F.R.C.S., F.R.C.S.(Ed.), F.R.A.C.S.

Professor of Surgery,
St. Mary's Hospital, London

OPERATIVE SURGERY

Fundamental International Techniques

Colon, Rectum and Anus

Edited by

Ian P. Todd
M.S., M.D.(Tor.), F.R.C.S., D.C.H.

Consultant Surgeon, St. Bartholomew's Hospital, St. Mark's Hospital
and King Edward VII Hospital for Officers, London

BUTTERWORTHS
LONDON - BOSTON
Sydney - Wellington - Durban - Toronto

THE BUTTERWORTH GROUP

ENGLAND

Butterworth & Co (Publishers) Ltd
London: 88 Kingsway, WC2B 6AB

AUSTRALIA

Butterworths Pty Ltd
Sydney: 586 Pacific Highway, Chatswood, NSW 2067
Also at Melbourne, Brisbane, Adelaide and Perth

SOUTH AFRICA

Butterworth & Co (South Africa) (Pty) Ltd
Durban: 152–154 Gale Street

NEW ZEALAND

Butterworths of New Zealand Ltd
Wellington: 26–28 Waring Taylor Street, 1

CANADA

Butterworth & Co (Canada) Ltd
Toronto: 2265 Midland Avenue,
    Scarborough, Ontario, M1P 4S1

USA

Butterworths (Publishers) Inc
Boston: 19 Cummings Park, Woburn, Mass. 01801

First Edition Published in Eight Volumes, 1956–1958
Second Edition Published in Fourteen Volumes, 1968–1971
Third Edition Published in Eighteen Volumes, 1976–1978

©
Butterworth & Co (Publishers) Ltd
1977

ISBN 0 407 00606 0

Library of Congress Cataloging in Publication Data (Revised)

Main entry under title:
Operative surgery.

    Includes bibliography and index.
    CONTENTS: [1] Ear, edited by John Ballantyne.

[5] Gynaecology and obstetrics, edited by D. W. T. Roberts.
—[6] Colon, rectum and anus, edited by I. P. Todd.
    1. Surgery, Operative. I. Rob, Charles. II. Smith,
Rodney, Sir. III. Dudley, Hugh Arnold Freeman.
[DNLM: 1. Nose—Surgery. 2. Pharynx—Surgery. W0500
061 v. 2
RD32.06   1977   617'.91   75-42330
ISBN 0-407-00606 (v.1)

Typeset by Butterworths Litho Preparation Department
Printed in England by The Whitefriars Press Ltd., London and Tonbridge
Bound by The Newdigate Press Ltd., Dorking, Surrey

OPERATIVE SURGERY

Volumes and Editors

ABDOMEN	Charles Rob, *M.C.,* M.D., M.Chir., F.R.C.S. Sir Rodney Smith, K.B.E., M.S., F.R.C.S. Hugh Dudley, Ch.M., F.R.C.S., F.R.C.S.(Ed.), F.R.A.C.S.
ACCIDENT SURGERY	P. S. London, M.B.E., F.R.C.S.
CARDIOTHORACIC SURGERY	John W. Jackson, M.Ch., F.R.C.S.
COLON, RECTUM AND ANUS	Ian P. Todd, M.S., M.D.(Tor.), F.R.C.S., D.C.H.
EAR	John Ballantyne, F.R.C.S., Hon.F.R.C.S.(I.)
EYES	Stephen J. H. Miller, M.D., F.R.C.S.
GENERAL PRINCIPLES, BREAST AND HERNIA	Charles Rob, *M.C.,* M.Chir., F.R.C.S. Sir Rodney Smith, K.B.E., M.S., F.R.C.S. Hugh Dudley, Ch.M., F.R.C.S., F.R.C.S.(Ed.), F.R.A.C.S.
GYNAECOLOGY AND OBSTETRICS	D. W. T. Roberts, M.A., M.Chir., F.R.C.S., F.R.C.O.G.

THE HAND	R. Guy Pulvertaft, C.B.E., Hon.M.D., M.Chir., F.R.C.S.
HEAD AND NECK	John S. P. Wilson, F.R.C.S.(Eng.), F.R.C.S.(Ed.)
NEUROSURGERY	Lindsay Symon, T.D., F.R.C.S.
NOSE AND THROAT	John Ballantyne, F.R.C.S., Hon.F.R.C.S.(I.)
ORTHOPAEDICS [in 2 volumes]	Charles W. S. F. Manning, F.R.C.S.
PAEDIATRIC SURGERY	H. H. Nixon, F.R.C.S., Hon.F.A.A.P.
PLASTIC SURGERY	Robert M. McCormack, M.D. John Watson, F.R.C.S.
UROLOGY	D. Innes Williams, M.D., M.Chir., F.R.C.S.
VASCULAR SURGERY	Charles Rob, *M.C.,* M.D., M.Chir., F.R.C.S.

OPERATIVE SURGERY

Contributors to this Volume

J. ALEXANDER-WILLIAMS
M.D., Ch.M., F.R.C.S., F.A.C.S.

Consultant Surgeon, United Birmingham Hospitals;
External Scientific Officer, Medical Research Council;
Honorary Clinical Senior Lecturer, University of Birmingham

JOHN F. R. BENTLEY
F.R.C.S., F.R.C.S.(Ed.),
F.R.C.S.(Glas.)

Consultant Surgeon, Royal Hospital for Sick Children, Glasgow

ALEXANDER H. BILL, JR.
M.D., F.A.C.S.

Chief of Surgical Services, The Children's Orthopedic Hospital, and
Medical Center, Seattle, Washington and Clinical Professor of Surgery,
University of Washington School of Medicine

ROBERT BRITTEN-JONES
M.B., B.S., F.R.C.S., F.R.A.C.S.

Senior Visiting Surgeon, Royal Adelaide Hospital, South Australia

B. N. BROOKE
M.D., M.Chir., F.R.C.S.

Emeritus Professor of Surgery, St. George's Hospital, London

DAHER E. CUTAIT
M.D., F.A.C.S.

Associate Professor of Surgery, Medical School of the University of
Sao Paulo, Department of Surgery, Head of the Group in Charge of
Colorectal Surgery

STANLEY M. GOLDBERG
M.D.

Clinical Professor of Surgery and Director, Division of Colon and Rectal
Surgery, University of Minnesota Medical School, Minneapolis, Minnesota

J. C. GOLIGHER
Ch.M., F.R.C.S., Hon.F.A.C.S.

Professor of Surgery, University of Leeds;
Surgeon, General Infirmary at Leeds

J. D. GRIFFITHS
M.S., F.R.C.S.

Consultant Surgeon, St. Bartholomew's Hospital and
The Royal Marsden Hospital, London

P. R. HAWLEY
M.S., F.R.C.S.

Consultant Surgeon, St. Mark's Hospital, London

C. N. HUDSON
M.Chir., F.R.C.S., F.R.C.O.G.

Reader in Obstetrics and Gynaecology, Medical College of
St. Bartholomew's Hospital, London

DAVID G. JAGELMAN
M.S., F.R.C.S.(Eng.)

Department of Colon and Rectal Surgery,
The Cleveland Clinic Foundation, Cleveland, Ohio

MARK KILLINGBACK
F.R.C.S., F.R.C.S.(Ed.), F.R.A.C.S.

Surgeon, Edward Wilson Colon and Rectum Unit, Sydney Hospital,
Sydney

K. LLOYD WILLIAMS
M.D., M.Chir., F.R.C.S.

Consultant Surgeon, Royal United Hospital, Bath

H. E. LOCKHART-
MUMMERY
M.D., M.Chir., F.R.C.S.

Consultant Surgeon, St. Thomas's and St. Mark's Hospitals,
and King Edward VII Hospital for Officers, London

PETER H. LORD
M.Chir., F.R.C.S.

Consultant Surgeon, Wycombe General Hospital, High Wycombe and The Chalfonts and Gerrards Cross Hospital

JOHN L. MADDEN
M.D.

Clinical Professor of Surgery, New York Medical College

M. R. MADIGAN
B.Sc., F.R.C.S.(Ed.), F.R.C.S.

Consultant Surgeon to the Herts and Essex Hospital, Bishop's Stortford, and the Hertford County Hospital

C. V. MANN
M.Ch., F.R.C.S.

Consultant Surgeon, St. Mark's Hospital, London and The London Hospital

A. YORK MASON
B.Sc., F.R.C.S.(Ed.),
F.R.C.S.(Eng.)

Surgeon, St. Anthony's Hospital (Medical, Educational and Research Trust); Honorary Consulting Surgeon, St. Helier Hospital and Associated Hospitals; Late Honorary Consultant Surgeon, Royal Marsden Hospital, London

J. F. McPARTLIN
F.R.C.S.

Consultant Surgeon, Ashford General Hospital, Royal Victoria Hospital, Folkestone and Buckland General Hospital, Dover

DOUGLAS M. MILLAR
M.B., F.R.C.S., F.R.C.S.(Ed.)

Consultant Surgeon, Essex County Hospital, Colchester

H. HOMEWOOD NIXON
M.A., M.B., B.Chir.,
F.R.C.S.(Eng.), Hon.F.A.A.P.

Consultant Paediatric Surgeon, The Hospital for Sick Children, Great Ormond Street, London; Paddington Green Children's Hospital, London, and St. Mary's Hospital Group, London

M. J. NOTARAS
F.R.C.S., F.R.C.S.(Ed.)

Consultant Surgeon, Barnet General Hospital; Honorary Senior Lecturer and Consultant Surgeon, University College Hospital, London

A. G. PARKS
M.Ch., F.R.C.S., F.R.C.P.

Consultant Surgeon, St. Mark's Hospital, London and The London Hospital

MAX PEMBERTON
M.B.E., T.D., F.R.C.S.

Consultant Surgeon, Chase Farm Hospital, and Enfield War Memorial Hospital

MURRAY T. PHEILS
M.Chir., F.R.C.S., F.R.A.C.S.

Professor of Surgery, University of Sydney; Surgeon, Repatriation General Hospital, Concord, New South Wales

NIGEL H. PORTER
F.R.C.S.

Consultant Surgeon, Brighton and Lewes Group of Hospitals

MICHAEL REILLY
M.S., F.R.C.S.

Consultant Surgeon, Plymouth General Hospital

W. W. SLACK
M.Ch., F.R.C.S.

Consultant Surgeon, The Middlesex Hospital, London

JAMES P. S. THOMSON
M.S., F.R.C.S.

Consultant Surgeon, St. Mark's Hospital, London

IAN P. TODD
M.S., M.D.(Tor.), F.R.C.S.,
D.C.H.

Consultant Surgeon, St. Bartholomew's Hospital, St. Mark's Hospital and King Edward VII Hospital for Officers, London

RUPERT B.
TURNBULL, JR.
M.D., C.M., F.A.C.S.

Department of Colon and Rectal Surgery, The Cleveland Clinic Foundation, Cleveland, Ohio

MALCOLM C.
VEIDENHEIMER
M.D.

Section of Colon and Rectal Surgery, Lahey Clinic Foundation, Boston, Massachusetts

CHRISTOPHER B.
WILLIAMS
M.R.C.P.

Consultant Physician, St. Mark's and St. Bartholomew's Hospitals, London

OPERATIVE SURGERY

Contents of this Volume

Introduction

In this, the Third Edition of Operative Surgery, a volume devoted for the first time to the surgery of Colon, Rectum and Anus attempts to describe the accepted and the controversial procedures in use today. It cannot cover all eventualities but where several methods exist to treat the same condition, the Editor has allowed contributors more scope in discussing the selection of the procedure. This is so in relation to the treatment of haemorrhoids, a commonplace enough disease where unfortunately personal preference rather than controlled study plays such a large part. However, the principles in the management of cancer are fairly well accepted. Methods of dealing with cancer in the lower rectum and the extension of restorative anastomosis to avoid a colostomy are excercising the profession greatly—the trans-sphincteric, the per-anal or the older modified trans-sacral approaches probably all have a place and all have their advocates. The pros and cons are mentioned as far as possible but this is a book of operative technique so bibliography is included in some sections so that further reading can be undertaken. Maybe some believe in fulguration of cancer in some situations. These techniques have all been described by the accepted experts in these procedures, with many eminent contributors from other countries.

Pelvic floor problems: prolapse, incontinence and insufficiency have achieved greater prominence recently and this section of the book has been greatly expanded and combined fistulae are included for the first time.

It is anticipated that these new sections will prove to be of great value for the less experienced surgeon in this field, faced with these most difficult of problems.

I would like to thank all the distinguished surgeons who have given of their time to make this book, I am sure, a success, particularly my colleagues at St. Mark's Hospital for Diseases of the Rectum and Colon, London, and distinguished surgeons in the U.S.A., Australia and South America. Once again our medical artists have done a superb job and I thank them most sincerely.

IAN P. TODD

Proctoscopy

H. E. Lockhart-Mummery, M.D., M.Chir., F.R.C.S.
Consultant Surgeon, St. Thomas's and St. Mark's Hospitals, and
King Edward VII Hospital for Officers, London

PRE-OPERATIVE

Indications

Proctoscopy is most useful in the examination of the anal canal and the region of the anorectal ring, and particularly in the detection of haemorrhoids. For satisfactory examination of the rectum and its mucosa, sigmoidoscopy is necessary.

Injection of haemorrhoids, and other minor manipulations in the same area, can be carried out with ease through a well-lighted proctoscope of adequate size.

Contra-indications

The anus must be carefully inspected and a finger passed before any instrument is inserted. In this way the presence of any painful lesion such as a fissure or thrombosed haemorrhoids will be detected; proctoscopy is, under these circumstances, usually contra-indicated unless adequate local anaesthesia can be produced.

In children, or in patients with anal stenosis, a proctoscope of smaller size should be used.

Pre-operative preparation

No special preparation is necessary. Enemas are undesirable, but the patient should be encouraged to empty the bowel naturally before coming for examination. If the bowel is very loaded, the examination is best deferred.

Anaesthesia

No anaesthetic is necessary for most patients. Satisfactory local anaesthesia of painful fissures can usually be obtained by application for 5 min of 2 per cent amethocaine in solution or of lignocaine ointment.

Position of patient

The Sims position as described for Sigmoidoscopy, page 5, is very satisfactory. The knee-chest position may sometimes be preferred for male patients.

THE PROCEDURE

1

Instruments

Proctoscopes of many types and sizes are available. The one illustrated is a tubular proctoscope incorporating a lighting system (internal diameter 2 cm). This is the most useful type for most purposes, and will be found more satisfactory than slotted or conical instruments. It is made in several sizes.

Long forceps for swabbing through the proctoscope are invaluable. Illustrated are Emmett's 20 cm forceps.

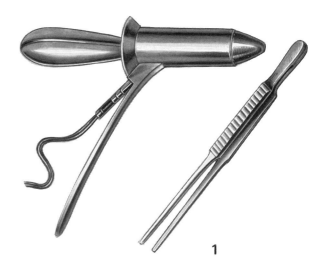

2

Insertion

The proctoscope, well lubricated, is passed slowly and gently into the anal canal, pointing towards the umbilicus. The rectum and anal canal join at an angle, so that once the tip of the proctoscope has entered the rectum, the instrument should be gradually directed backwards towards the sacrum.

The obturator is removed and the light attached.

The pink mucosa of the rectum is now visible and as the instrument is slowly withdrawn the mucosa becomes darker in colour and the lumen narrows at the level of the anorectal ring. Internal haemorrhoids prolapse into the lumen of the proctoscope and are best seen if the patient is asked to strain. Below this line the lining of the anal canal is visualized.

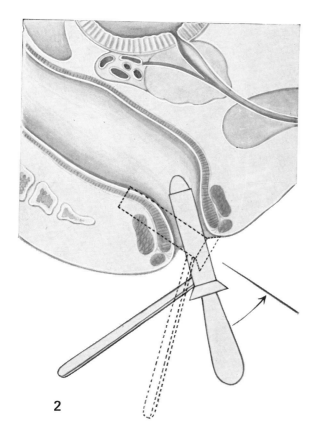

3

Examination

The handle of the instrument is held in the left hand so that the right is free for manipulations. It is often helpful to use the left index finger as shown to hold the upper buttock out of the line of vision.

Before finally withdrawing the instrument, the obturator should be replaced, as discomfort is thereby lessened.

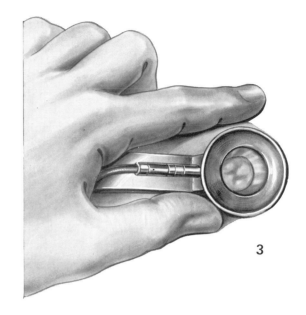

3

POSTOPERATIVE

No special care or treatment is necessary. The patient may leave the hospital as soon as the examination is completed.

[*The illustrations for this Chapter on Proctoscopy were drawn by Mr. R. N. Lane.*]

Sigmoidoscopy

H. E. Lockhart-Mummery, M.D., M.Chir., F.R.C.S.
Consultant Surgeon, St. Thomas's and St. Mark's Hospitals, and
King Edward VII Hospital for Officers, London

PRE-OPERATIVE

Indications

The passage of a sigmoidoscope should be a routine part of any complete rectal examination. It becomes essential if the patient's symptoms suggest the possibility of a neoplasm of rectum or colon. No operation on the anal region should be undertaken without preliminary sigmoidoscopy.

There are no contra-indications.

Sigmoidoscopy in children

Sigmoidoscopy may be carried out in children without anaesthesia if a small sigmoidoscope is used and handled with great gentleness. If a large instrument needs to be passed, for removal of a polyp, for example, then general anaesthesia is necessary.

Preparation

Sigmoidoscopy is best done as an out-patient procedure without any special preparation, after a normal evacuation. In such circumstances flecks of blood and mucus may be seen on the mucosa if there is a lesion higher in the colon, evidence that is removed if a washout is given. Moreover any enema or washout produces some congestion of the rectal mucosa, closely resembling the changes of mild proctocolitis, and errors in diagnosis may thereby follow. In a patient whose bowel is persistently loaded, an enema or even a colonic washout may be necessary before a clear view is obtained.

Anaesthesia

The procedure should be painless and no anaesthetic is necessary. A general anaesthetic is occasionally necessary in the examination of a patient who has persistent spasm or rigidity at the rectosigmoid junction and in whom examination to a higher level is essential. In a patient with anal pain and spasm, as from the presence of a fissure, surface local anaesthesia with lignocaine ointment applied to the anal area is of value.

Position of patient

The patient should lie on a couch on his left side, with head and shoulders on the far side of the couch and buttocks on the near edge; the hips may be raised on a small sandbag.

Alternatively, the knee-chest position may be used, but this is more uncomfortable and embarrassing for the patient. To avoid embarrassment, the patient should be warned that the examination produces a desire to defaecate. This may often be reduced by slow deep breathing.

THE PROCEDURE

1

Instruments

Sigmoidoscopes of many types and sizes are available. The one illustrated is a Lloyd-Davies sigmoidoscope with proximal lighting, and is extremely satisfactory for routine examinations. The instrument of larger bore which fits the same lighting system is valuable if a biopsy has to be taken.

Long biopsy forceps may be needed, and a similar instrument with alligator jaws for swabbing.

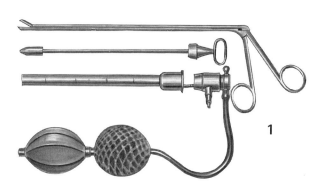

1

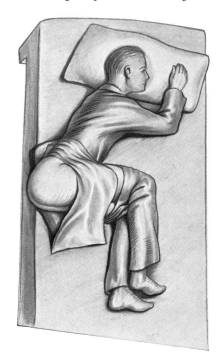

2

2

Position of patient

The Sims position is comfortable for the patient and satisfactory for the surgeon. Note that the patient lies obliquely across the couch, with the buttocks over the edge and raised on a sandbag. The knees are semiflexed, and the patient's feet are forward and out of the surgeon's way.

3

Insertion

A finger should always be passed before any instrument is inserted into the rectum. The sigmoidoscope, well lubricated and with obturator in position, is then gently passed into the anus, in the direction of the umbilicus. As soon as the tip is felt to enter the rectal ampulla, the obturator is withdrawn, and the lighting system and window attached.

Further passage of the instrument is done entirely under vision, with gentle air insufflation. The rectum follows the sacral curve, so the proximal end of the sigmoidoscope is moved ventrally as it is inserted farther. In the region of the rectosigmoid (13–15 cm usually) the proximal end usually needs to be moved again dorsally and somewhat to the patient's right, as the lower sigmoid leaves the sacral hollow and lies ventrally and to the left.

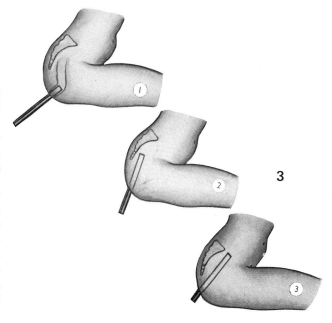

3

4

Holding the instrument

Throughout the examination, the instrument is held lightly with the left hand. The right hand holds the bulbs as shown; the lower bulb can be squeezed between the fourth and fifth fingers and the hypothenar eminence, and the upper one between thumb and index finger.

The amount of air inflation should be the minimum necessary to pass the instrument safely under vision as excessive air inflation causes much discomfort.

Withdrawal of the instrument should also be done under vision, with careful inspection of all quadrants as the instrument is slowly removed.

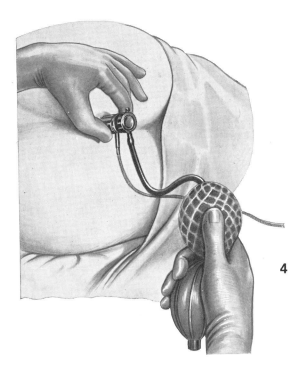

4

5

Biopsy of neoplasm

The sigmoidoscope is manipulated so that the lesion from which a biopsy is needed lies at the end of the instrument, and the biopsy forceps are placed near the right hand. The sigmoidoscope is held firmly, the glass window removed, and the biopsy forceps passed. The biopsy is taken under vision, and never blindly. Any bleeding usually stops quickly with pressure from a cotton-wool swab.

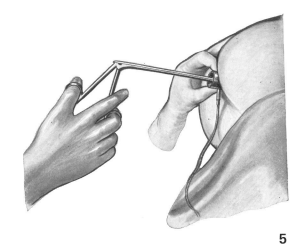

5

POSTOPERATIVE CARE

No special observation is necessary. The patient may leave the hospital as soon as the examination is completed.

Reference

Gabriel, W. B. (1963). *The Principles and Practice of Rectal Surgery,* 5th Edition, Chap. II. London: Lewis

[*The illustrations for this Chapter on Sigmoidoscopy were drawn by Mr. R. N. Lane.*]

Colonoscopy

Christopher B. Williams, M.R.C.P.
Consultant Physician, St. Mark's
and St. Bartholomew's Hospitals, London

PRE - OPERATIVE

Indications

Colonoscopy is normally a second-line procedure performed after clinical assessment, sigmoidoscopy and barium enema, especially if x-ray does not resolve the clinical problem or demonstrates a possible or definite lesion requiring biopsy. Limited colonoscopy or fibresigmoidoscopy is more difficult than procto-sigmoidoscopy with the rigid instrument but it may be a justifiable out-patient screening examination in special centres or for selected patients. Colonoscopy should replace diagnostic laparotomy for most patients with suspected disease of the colon or the terminal ileum and colonoscopic snare polypectomy is the procedure of choice for almost all colonic polyps. Examination through a colostomy is technically relatively easy and may be indicated if x-rays are unsatisfactory.

Contra-indications and problems

There are few contra-indications to colonoscopy, especially if surgery is the alternative, but there are occasional serious complications and mortality so that the procedure should not be undertaken or vigorously persisted in without good clinical reasons. Colonoscopy can cause cardiac arrhythmias and should not be undertaken after a recent myocardial infarction. The most frequent complication of colonoscopy is bowel perforation and colonoscopy is therefore contra-indicated in any form of acute colonic disease where perforation is more likely, including severe ulcerative, Crohn's colitis or acute ischaemic colitis and must be undertaken with care in irradiation colitis. Since the instruments can only be sterilized with ethylene oxide, colonoscopy is usually inadvisable in known infective conditions. In severe diverticular disease or strictures colonoscopy may be particularly difficult and liable to weaken the instrument but the results of a successful examination can be so useful that it is often worth attempting. Postoperative adhesions may make a flexure fixed and impassable.

Bowel preparation

For limited colonoscopy or fibresigmoidoscopy a disposable phosphate enema without dietary preparation may give an adequate view. Otherwise bowel preparation for colonoscopy has to be agressive and the reasons for this should be explained to the patient to obtain full co-operation. Iron tablets and constipating agents are stopped 4–5 days beforehand but other medication may be continued. A high volume liquid (preferably clear liquid) diet is started 24–48 hr before colonoscopy and a drastic purge given 12–18 hr beforehand. A 30 ml dose of castor oil or 140 mg of Sennosides normally gives adequate results but must be followed by two large cleansing enemas 1–2 hr before starting colonoscopy.

Medication

Premedication is unnecessary before colonoscopy and if good and gentle technique is used sedation is often not needed. General anaesthesia is contra-indicated because pain supplies the only warning if the bowel or mesentery is being overstretched. In many patients a 5–15 mg intravenous dose of diazepam (Valium) at the beginning makes a tedious and uncomfortable procedure tolerable though addition of 25–75 mg pethidine intravenously is sometimes necessary. Antispasmodics are not routinely used but intravenous hyoscine (Buscopan) 40 mg will help examination on withdrawal if there is spasm or severe diverticular disease.

TECHNIQUE

Choice of instrument

The shorter fibre-optic colonoscopes (110 cm) are at a slight mechanical advantage over the longer instruments (165–185 cm) and are, therefore, easier to keep in good condition and have a longer life. Except in very expert hands the shorter instruments will not reach beyond the transverse colon and a long colon will make things more difficult. Thus, although a shorter instrument should be used routinely, if total colonoscopy is important and x-ray shows a redundant bowel the longer colonoscope is indicated.

A two-channel instrument is convenient but not essential for colonoscopic polypectomy. Most two-channel instruments are stiffer and may be unsuitable for some elderly (or juvenile) patients.

Is x-ray control needed?

Very limited examinations do not require x-ray screening control and some expert colonoscopists can perform total colonoscopy without x-ray. For the less experienced, however, the extra information given is invaluable and if the facilities are available x-ray will tend to make the procedure quicker, safer and less traumatic. Several of the manoeuvres which are described subsequently are difficult or impossible to perform without screening. Screening time is kept to a minimum because of irradiation danger to patient and instrument. An occasional brief image is sufficient to demonstrate the position or any looping of the instrument and to help in straightening it.

Position of patient

Most endoscopists start with the patient in the left lateral position and it is often possible to complete the examination without a change. If x-ray screening is to be used the patient has to be turned supine or prone. At any stage of the examination if things are going badly a change of the patient's position may be worthwhile to alter the position of the bowel.

1

Insertion and passage through the rectosigmoid

The colonoscope tip and peri-anal region are lubricated with jelly, a digital examination of the rectum performed and the instrument gently inserted. At this point there will be no view because the tip is against the wall of the rectum and the instrument must be *withdrawn* to free the tip before a view can be obtained by angling the tip or rotating the instrument as necessary.

In passing the sequential bends of the rectosigmoid the object is to distend or stretch the bowel as little as possible so as to keep it short and to pass almost straight to the descending colon. This is easier to suggest than to achieve but is made more likely by observing the following points:

(*1*) Insufflate as little air as possible.

(*2*) Follow the bowel lumen accurately.

(*3*) If the view is poor *withdraw* and re-assess.

(*4*) Avoid totally blind passage of the instrument but do not expect a perfect view of all areas on the way in.

(*5*) If angling the tip is ineffective, try twisting the shaft.

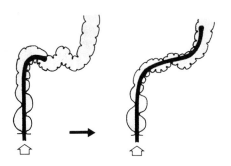

1

2

Sigmoid loop — hook and torque manoeuvre

In spite of all care the commonest situation on reaching the junction of the sigmoid and descending colon is for there to be a sigmoid loop, forming a bend which makes direct passage difficult or impossible. If the tip can be passed only a short way round the bend into the retroperitoneal part of the descending colon it can be held there (without consciously hooking) while the instrument is withdrawn 20—50 cm to reduce and straighten out the loop. Putting a strong clockwise torque or twisting force on to the shaft of the colonoscope will help to straighten the loop, to keep it straight and then to advance the tip up the descending colon. Accurate steering is also important so that the tip does not catch in the haustra of the descending colon and result in the sigmoid loop re-forming.

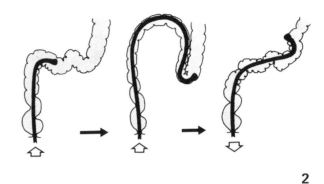

2

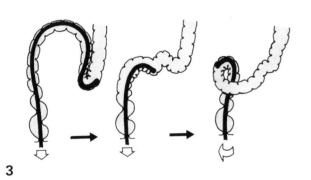

3

Sigmoid loop — the 'alpha manoeuvre'

3

Sometimes the tip cannot be hooked into the descending colon or slips back when the sigmoid loop is reduced. It is then useful to be able to make an 'alpha loop' in the sigmoid colon by performing the 'alpha manoeuvre'. In this manoeuvre an intentional sigmoid volvulus is caused which results in a smooth contoured loop without any acute bend at the junction of the sigmoid and descending colon.

To perform the alpha manoeuvre first withdraw the angled tip of the colonoscope back to 25—30 cm from the anus and then rotate it 180° counter-clockwise so that the tip changes from pointing in the direction of the descending colon towards that of the caecum.

4

Keeping the counter-clockwise torque applied, and keeping the tip angled gently, slide the instrument in round the loop, checking on x-ray from time to time to see that the loop is forming correctly. It may take some time and patience to steer the tip into the descending colon, but this is always possible.

Sometimes an alpha loop will form spontaneously during insertion of the colonoscope or a partially-formed alpha loop is seen on the x-ray screen, which means that the descending colon will be easily reached by pushing in further.

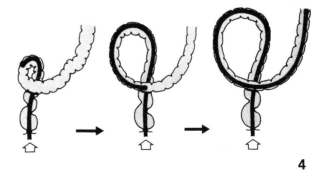

4

5

Straightening out an alpha loop

Having reached the upper descending colon an alpha loop should be removed, since the loop is a disadvantage when trying to angle around and pass the splenic flexure. To remove the loop withdraw the colonoscope 50 cm or more whilst simultaneously rotating the colonoscope *clockwise,* which holds the tip high in the descending colon and makes it unnecessary to hook round the splenic flexure. Even without screening if a redundant loop has obviously formed in the distal colon the likelihood is that it will be an alpha loop and the same derotational manoeuvre can be applied 'blindly'.

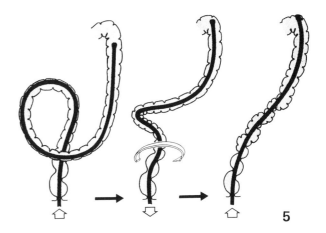

5

6

Straightening or stiffening the sigmoid colon

Once the colonoscope is straightened, with its tip in the descending colon and the sigmoid colon shortened over it, it may be necessary to prevent the sigmoid loop re-forming. Continued clockwise torque on the shaft is often enough to keep it straight during insertion but with a redundant sigmoid loop the 'stiffening tube' or 'over-tube' may be needed. This is a wire-reinforced plastic tube which has to be in position on the colonoscope at the start of the examination but can, after lubrication with jelly, be passed up over the *straightened* instrument to stop it from flexing. It is important that no angle forms in the colonoscope to catch the stiffening tube or damage may result. It is desirable only to insert the stiffener under x-ray control. There is also a possibility of catching redundant mucosa in the advancing lip of the tube, but this can be prevented with a to and fro rotatory movement of the tube as it is pushed in.

Once the stiffening tube is in position there is no possibility of the sigmoid loop re-forming, but the tube has to be firmly held by an assistant to allow the lubricated colonoscope to pass through it.

6

7

The redundant transverse colon

If no sigmoid loop is allowed to form, the splenic flexure, although acutely angled, usually presents little difficulty in passage. The transverse colon, however, may be pushed down into such a deep loop that it is difficult and painful to reach the hepatic flexure. Once again the correct procedure is to *withdraw* the instrument 30—50 cm to shorten the transverse loop. This withdrawal may have to be repeated several times, with the tip actually advancing a few centimetres each time until the loop is straightened. If the hepatic flexure is still not reached the patient is turned on to the left side, and the withdrawals repeated; excess air is sucked out and pressure is applied in the left hypochondrial region to raise the loop.

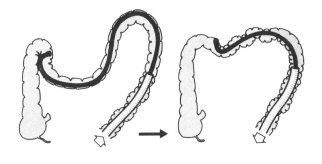

7

8

Passing the hepatic flexure

Having reached the hepatic flexure and angled the tip just around it to the ascending colon, the transverse loop often remains and makes it difficult to pass the rest of the instrument around the flexure. By withdrawing the colonoscope and straightening out the loop the flexure may become easy to pass or, since the hepatic flexure passes posteriorly into the paravertebral space, clockwise torque can be applied to 'corkscrew' the tip into the ascending colon. When the ascending colon is seen deflate the right colon by aspiration whilst steering carefully to avoid the bowel wall and the colonoscope tip will spontaneously descend into the caecum.

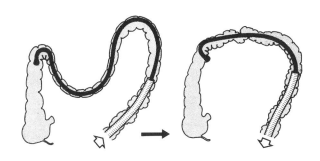

8

Examination

Having inserted the colonoscope as far as necessary and having observed the colon during insertion but not actively examined it, fastidious care is required on withdrawal. It is usually best for the endoscopist to control the instrument himself during the examination, even if he has used an assistant to help in the insertion. Very active manoeuvring of the controls, with rotation and to and fro movements of the shaft may be necessary to avoid 'blind spots' and the examination during withdrawal may sometimes take as long as the insertion. The straightened and shortened colon may be difficult to view completely because of the resulting convolutions of the mucosa; the sigmoid colon can for this reason, sometimes be best examined keeping an alpha loop in position rather than after having straightened it.

POSTOPERATIVE

In most cases no particular care is needed apart from a short period of rest and some food. If sedation has been used the patient must be warned not to drive a vehicle for 24 hr. A few instances of delayed perforation have been reported but if the patient appears and feels well after colonoscopy he can be safely discharged and most examinations are performed on a day-case basis.

COLONOSCOPIC POLYPECTOMY

The principles of colonoscopic polypectomy are identical to those for proctosigmoidoscopic polypectomy but it is particularly important that full coagulation of the stalk vessels is caused before cutting through, since haemorrhage is difficult to control endoscopically. A thick snare wire is used to guard against too fast cutting and a low-power (25—50 watts) coagulating current applied until there is visible electrocoagulation. If bleeding does occur local recoagulation or the application of iced-water or adrenaline are usually effective remedies. Very broad-based or sessile polyps (over 2 cm in diameter) are normally unsuitable for colonoscopic polypectomy because of the dangers of bowel perforation or incomplete removal.

[*The illustrations for this Chapter on Colonoscopy were drawn by Mrs. G. Lee.*]

Total Colectomy

B. N. Brooke, M.D., M.Chir., F.R.C.S.
Emeritus Professor of Surgery, St. George's Hospital,
London

PRE-OPERATIVE

Colectomy may be performed as a primary procedure to be followed by rectal excision, the ileostomy being instituted at the same time, or after ileostomy has been performed. Alternatively it may be combined with excision of the rectum (panproctocolectomy), also as a primary operation or secondary to pre-existing ileostomy.

Indications

Total colectomy is indicated for ulcerative and Crohn's colitis, familial polyposis coli and multifocal carcinoma.

It is quite proper to remove all the large bowel and perform an ileostomy or ileorectal anastomosis in one stage for patients with polyposis coli, since their general condition will permit this; electrolyte depletion is occasionally encountered due to an excessive number of fluid stools but this is readily corrected by pre-operative intravenous infusions. For chronic and subacute ulcerative colitis primary panproctocolectomy is also ideal. Multiple operations increase the possibility of complications and, furthermore, certain technical procedures necessary to colectomy alone, such as the exteriorization of the distal colonic stoma (*see Illustration 9*), introduce additional hazards from wound infection and intestinal obstruction, which may be avoided by total extirpation in one stage. The general condition of patients severely ill with ulcerative colitis may preclude the one-stage operation; colectomy alone with ileostomy should be performed for the predilatation disintegrative phase, and when dilation has developed.

In making the decision it is helpful to pose the question—will this patient withstand an abdomino-perineal dissection? Little general disturbance is caused by colectomy alone in experienced hands; it is dissection within the pelvis which may cause serious deterioration in a debilitated and toxic patient. Primary colectomy done with gentleness and expedition is no more shocking than ileostomy alone and has the advantage of removing diseased bowel and rendering ileostomy technically easier to perform and more satisfactory in its completion, since the ileal 'loop' is then terminal.

In summary the choice for ulcerative colitis lies between (*1*) primary panproctocolectomy for patients who can withstand the pelvic dissection entailed thereby; and (*2*) primary colectomy followed by abdominoperineal excision when the patient's general condition has improved, as it almost invariably does after removal of the colon. For complications such as haemorrhage and perforation, the two-stage routine should be undertaken with primary colectomy as the initial operation, though in the case of haemorrhage bleeding may persist or recur from the rectal stump necessitating emergency abdominoperineal excision.

Contra-indications, pre-operative care and anaesthesia

These are the same as for ileostomy (*see* page 30).

Position of patient

The patient is placed as for laparotomy, or in the lithotomy (St. Mark's) position which allows either procedure to be carried out without moving the patient.

THE OPERATION

1

Liver biopsy

In all cases of inflammatory bowel disease a liver biopsy should be taken. A long left paramedian incision is undertaken to allow access to the whole of the large bowel and the liver. A wedge of liver is excised from the anterior edge; this is closed and haemostasis achieved with one or two through-and-through sutures of 1/0 catgut lying transversely to the wedge excision.

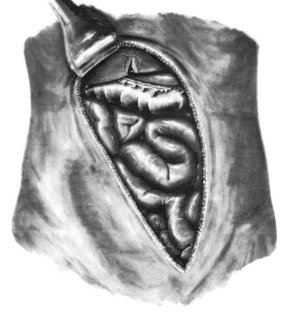

1

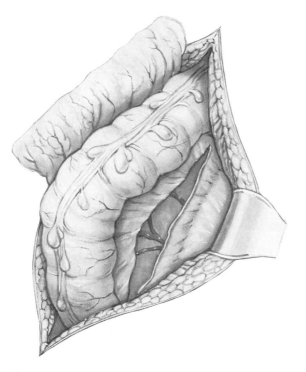

2

2

Mobilization of descending and sigmoid colon

The sigmoid and descending colon are mobilized from the lateral side and drawn into the wound; access to both ascending and descending colon is facilitated by enclosing the small intestine in a plastic bag. For panproctocolectomy a synchronous combined operation is begun after the manner usual for abdominoperineal excision of the rectum. The surgeon working *per abdomen* starts by ligating the inferior mesenteric vessels, opening the retrorectal space and cutting the reflection of peritoneum from rectum on to pelvic parietes; he then leaves further dissection in the pelvis to his partner and proceeds to colonic mobilization but to avoid infertility in the male through damage to the nervi erigentes it is important that the whole of the rectum should be mobilized from above.

3

Stretching of phrenocolic ligament

The omentum is detached from the left half of the transverse colon. The mobilized descending colon and the transverse colon are drawn into the wound so that the phrenocolic ligament is put on the stretch. This is the most difficult part of the operation since the splenic flexure is often situated high up and close to the spleen, and thus may be somewhat inaccessible. The strands of the ligament can be divided without direct vision since no vessel of magnitude is situated there; if, however, the edge of the omentum encroaches upon the ligament, vessels will be encountered which must be clamped and tied.

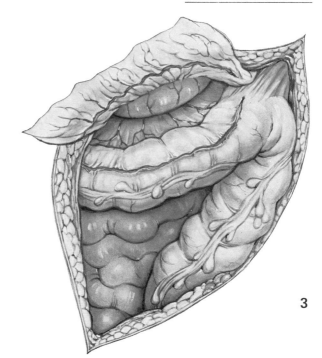

3

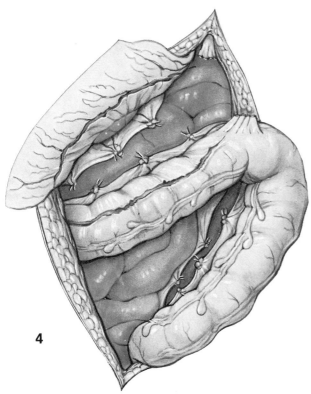

4

4

Freeing of the colon

This ligament is cut and the splenic flexure delivered. With the mesentery to the left half of the colon now free and accessible in the wound the vessels are clamped and ligated in turn. Except where malignant change is suspected, ligation should be undertaken as close to the bowel as convenience will allow so that the mobilized mesocolon may fall back and partially cover the exposed raw retrocolic area. The ramifications of the vessels are best displayed by transmitted light; the vessels are therefore seen most easily when the surgeon operates facing a spot-light. Artery forceps should all be applied from one side to reduce manipulation of the bowel when ligating—an important point when the bowel is friable.

5

Mobilization of the right side

The surgeon now moves to the left side of the patient and proceeds to mobilize the caecum, ascending colon and hepatic flexure. Care must be taken here to avoid damage to the duodenum. The right half of the omentum is detached from its adjacent transverse colon. When mobilization is complete, the middle and right colic vessels are ligated.

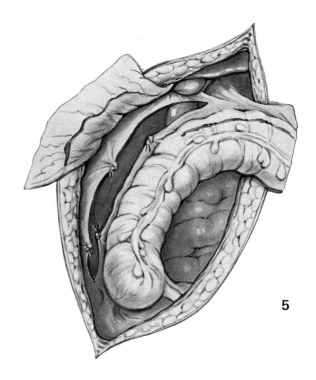

5

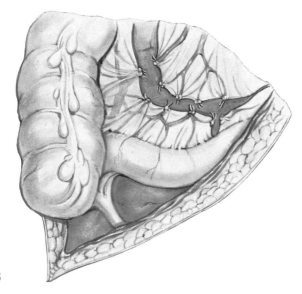

6

6

Freeing the ileocaecal region

On approaching the ileocaecal region a site is chosen in the ileum having sufficient length of mesentery for adequate exteriorization. The ileocolic artery and the vascular arcades are divided, care being taken not to endanger the blood supply to the site chosen for ileostomy. A sizeable artery is frequently present running from the ileocolic to the lowermost ileal vessels; it is helpful to preserve this by dividing the mesentery distal to it.

7

Making the ileostomy

A stab incision is made in the right iliac fossa to accommodate the ileostomy, relating its position to the needs of the adherent bag to be worn subsequently (*see* Chapter on 'Ileostomy', pages 30–37). The ileum is then divided and the proximal end withdrawn through the stab incision to a length of 5 cm. Its position must then be fixed with a stitch placed through the mesentery and the parietal peritoneum where the two meet at the stab wound.

Editorial comment. Many surgeons prefer a Trephined hole through the abdominal wall for an ileostomy (*see* Chapter on 'Colostomy', pages 209–215).

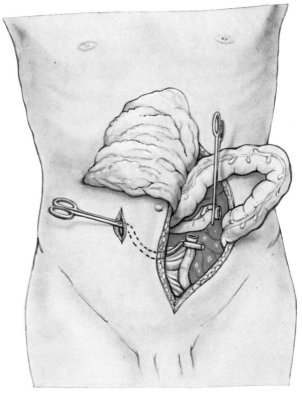

7

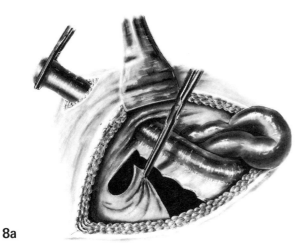

8a

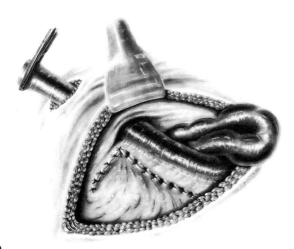

8b

8a & b

Closure of the para-ileal gutter

Retraction can now be applied to expose the para-ileal gutter without fear of displacing the exteriorized portion of ileum. Without previous fixation wound retraction may cause the ileum to recede unnoticed into the abdomen; if the para-ileal gutter is then closed the stoma will subsequently be found to be too short.

The para-ileal gutter is closed by suturing the cut edge of mesentery to a fold of parietal peritoneum, drawn across from the right iliac fossa. This obviates internal strangulation and ileostomy prolapse. The raw areas in each flank are again inspected to ensure haemostasis; no attempt at reperitonealization should be made.

The pelvic floor

In panproctocolectomy the author believes that the peritoneum of the pelvic floor should remain un-sutured to avoid the dead space between this level and the levator ani muscles, one cause of persistent perineal sinus. The levators should be sutured together by the perineal surgeon. As with the paracolic gutters, raw epithelium will cover the raw area. The skin is not sutured. A vacuum drain is placed up to the pelvis through the levators from the perineum.

9

Closure of wound in colectomy without rectal excision

The pelvic colon is placed in the lower end of the incision and the gutter lateral to this obliterated by a purse-string or interrupted sutures. The wound is closed in layers and the colon divided about 2·5 cm beyond skin level. Finally the ileostomy is fashioned by eversion as described previously.

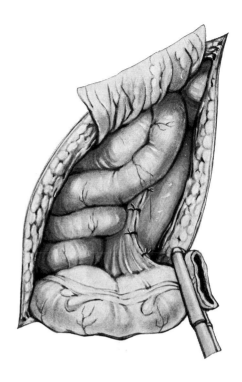

9

10

Second-stage colectomy

In second-stage colectomy the large bowel is finally freed by excision of the distal stoma and closure of that wound. The ileostomy remains undisturbed, though the previous closure of the para-ileal gutter can be further re-inforced using the cut edge of the mesentery. If the ileostomy is inefficient this is an appropriate moment for its revision.

POSTOPERATIVE CARE

The postoperative management of the patient and the complications which may arise following surgical intervention are dealt with at the end of the Chapter on 'Ileostomy' (*see* page 36). If steroid cover has been given, especial care is required as regards postoperative infection, which may develop in the colic gutters. When the rectum has been removed antibiotic cover is routinely given to reduce infection in the pelvis.

Catheter drainage is instituted after colectomy and panproctocolectomy.

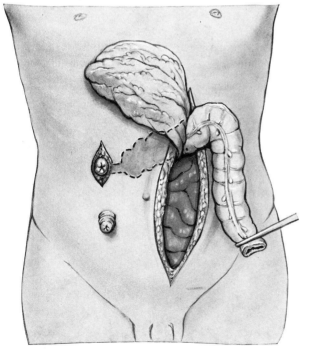

10

[The illustrations for this Chapter on Total Colectomy were drawn by Miss C.M. Lamb and Mr. A.R. Jones.]

Ileorectal Anastomosis for Inflammatory Bowel Disease

J. Alexander-Williams, M.D., Ch.M., F.R.C.S., F.A.C.S.
Consultant Surgeon, United Birmingham Hospitals;
External Scientific Officer, Medical Research Council;
Honorary Clinical Senior Lecturer, University of
Birmingham

PRE-OPERATIVE

Indications

The indications for surgical treatment of chronic mucosal ulcerative colitis of Crohn's disease of the colon are: (*1*) a fulminating attack of profound diarrhoea, not responding to medical treatment, particularly if associated with dilatation of the colon; (*2*) chronic loss of blood and protein (particularly in ulcerative colitis); (*3*) fistulae to the small bowel, bladder or exterior (confined to Crohn's disease); (*4*) intractable complicating diseases such as pyoderma, arthritis or liver disease (particularly in ulcerative colitis); (*5*) a high risk of malignant degeneration (particularly in ulcerative colitis); and (*6*) severe stenosis (almost exclusively in Crohn's disease).

When these indications are present, it is common for the chronic inflammatory bowel disease to affect the rectum and in Crohn's disease also the anal canal. Under these circumstances surgical excision of the disease usually has to be combined with a proctectomy. However, there are instances both in ulcerative colitis and Crohn's disease when the rectum is relatively uninvolved and excision of the large bowel can be considered without having to remove the rectum. Under these circumstances the most commonly employed operation is a total colectomy with ileorectal reconstruction. In Crohn's disease the terminal ileum and caecum are very often involved so that total colectomy is also associated with removal of part of the terminal ileum. In ulcerative colitis, however, where the disease tends to affect the left side of the colon, it is not uncommon to find the caecum and terminal ileum relatively normal and a caecorectal anastomosis can be used as an alternative. Caecorectal anastomosis has the advantage of maintaining a normal ileocaecal valve and theoretically reducing the risk of postoperative diarrhoea and bile salts malabsorption.

Accurate diagnosis

Before contemplating caecorectal or ileorectal anastomosis it is extremely important to make an accurate
assessment both of the type of disease, that is Crohn's
disease or ulcerative colitis, and its extent.

1

Assessment of the distal colon by sigmoidoscopy is
essential, with multiple mucosal biopsies from either
side of the proposed level of anastomosis.

Colonoscopy and multiple biopsies from the
colon is also a valuable investigation to determine
whether or not there is disease of the caecum. Barium
enema can be used to determine the extent of the
disease but it is not as precise as colonoscopy and
tends to under-estimate the involvement.

In Crohn's disease, an accurate assessment of the
state of the small bowel is important; contrast x-ray
is the most practical method.

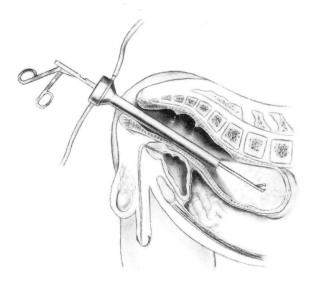

1

THE OPERATION

2

The incision

A mid-line incision is best used, diverging to the left or right of the umbilicus. The incision extends from close to xiphisternum to close to the symphysis pubis. A mid-line incision ensures that, if stomas subsequently have to be performed, there will be no interference from the previous scar.

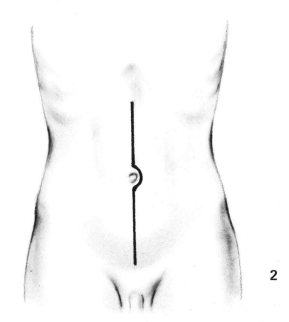

2

3

Colectomy

A total colectomy is performed, the blood vessels are divided at the most convenient site, often close to the bowel; unlike the technique employed in cancer surgery. Similarly the omentum is not removed unless it is so closely bound to the transverse colon as to make dissection dangerous.

It is almost always possible to preserve most of the omentum. Its preservation has the theoretical advantage of retaining a protective capacity if there is postoperative sepsis or anastomotic leakage. The spleen is also preserved.

The rectum is divided at a point determined by the previous sigmoidoscopy and by the external appearance of the bowel. It is not usually necessary to resect below the sacral prominence and so the subsequent anastomosis is not technically difficult or performed under tension.

The terminal ileum is divided well proximal to any macroscopical disease (in Crohn's disease) or close to the ileocaecal valve (in ulcerative colitis). If the caecum is being used in the anastomosis the resection is immediately distal to the ileocaecal valve. The appendix should always be removed.

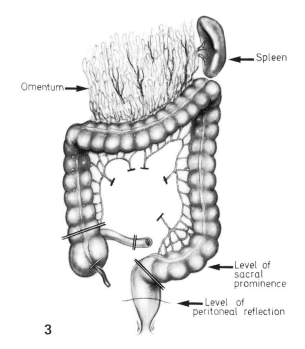

Spleen

Omentum

Level of sacral prominence

Level of peritoneal reflection

3

4,5&6

Caecorectal anastomosis

After dividing the ascending colon just above the ileocaecal valve, the mobilized caecum and terminal ileum is rotated anticlockwise ensuring that there is no twisting of the blood supply to the terminal ileum. The anastomosis can be affected according to the preference of the surgeon. The author prefers to use interrupted non-absorbable external seromuscular and an internal running absorbable suture on a double-ended needle. As the anastomosis is regularly to be inspected by sigmoidoscopy the author prefers not to have the ends of absorbable sutures visible at the suture line where they frequently cause granulomata.

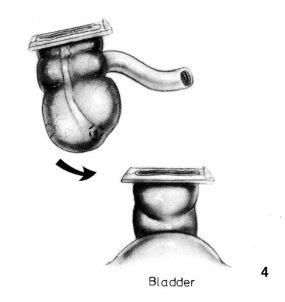

Bladder

4

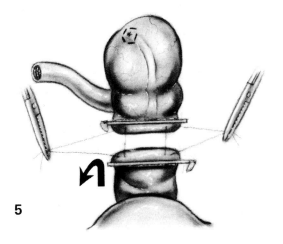

5

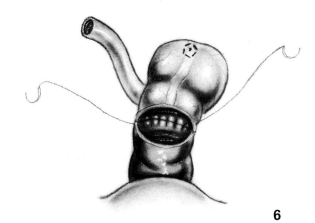

6

7&8

Ileorectal anastomosis

When the section is through the ileum, there is a size discrepancy between ileum and the wider upper rectum. Nevertheless an end-to-end anastomosis can always be performed without difficulty by performing an antimesenteric longitudinal V-shaped incision into the ileum to make a 'fish-mouth' appearance of the terminal ileum.

After either a caecorectal or an ileorectal anastomosis, the gap between the mesentery of the proximal bowel and the posterior peritoneum of the pelvic brim should be closed with interrupted non-absorbable sutures.

Protecting ileostomy

When the patient is in a relatively good nutritional state, when there is no florid disease and when the ends of the bowel to be sutured are free of gross macroscopical disease, the author makes the anastomosis without any protecting proximal diversion. However, it is sometimes necessary to make an anastomosis in the presence of a relatively diseased rectum or in an ill patient on steroids and with hypoproteinaemia. Under these circumstances it may be considered prudent to perform a proximal diverting ileostomy. With increasing experience the author finds that such a protection is done less often.

9

A loop ileostomy is performed at a point mid-way between the umbilicus and the right anterior iliac spine, through the substance of the rectus muscle. A circular disc is cut in the skin, the rectus sheath is divided in a cruciate fashion and a hole big enough to admit the tips of two fingers is made in the abdominal wall. A loop of ileum, approximately 15 cm proximal to the anastomosis is pulled through the hole by a rubber sling inserted through a small hole in the mesentery close to the edge of the ileum. A marking stitch is put distal to the rubber sling to facilitate recognition of the distal end of the loop after the abdomen is closed.

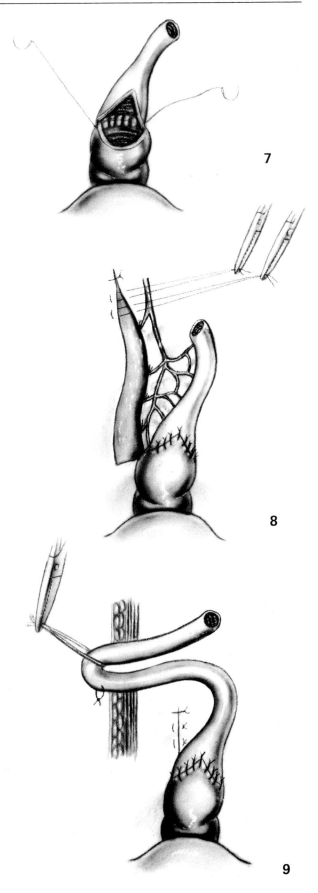

7

8

9

The loop is held out on the abdominal wall by a small vulcanite rod which can be removed on the fifth postoperative day. The rod is short enough to fit within the ring of an ileostomy appliance (*see Illustration 10*).

10

The abdominal wall is closed with a non-absorbable suture and the skin closed by a subcuticular suture, either using an absorbable material or a single mono-filament fine non-absorbable suture that can later be removed. Conventional transverse interrupted skin sutures are avoided in the hope of minimizing the risk of secondary wound infection from the ileo-stomy. The peritoneal cavity is not drained.

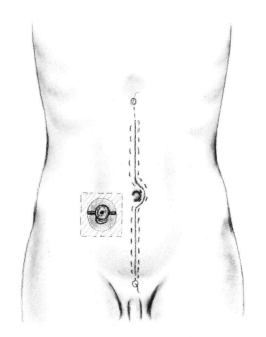

10

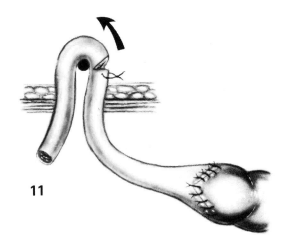

11

11 & 12

After the abdomen is closed, an incision is made in the loop of the ileum at its distal end close to the marking suture. The incision is almost half-way through the bowel. The mucosa is then everted to form an ileostomy which has an appearance very similar to that of a conventional end-ileostomy. Primary mucocutaneous suture is performed and an ileostomy flange applied to the skin.

Ileostomy appliance
flange

12

POSTOPERATIVE CARE

Bowel function does not usually return until the second to fourth postoperative day. During this time the patient is given parenteral fluids and occasionally parenteral nutrition. A nasogastric tube is not normally used unless the patient feels nauseated. As patients are often potassium depleted, parenteral potassium 80–120 mEq/day is given once adequate urinary output is established.

It is our practice to cover the operation with a short course of parenteral antibiotic, effective against anaerobic organisms (lincomycin).

As soon as the ileostomy works or bowel function returns, the patient is allowed to take fluid by mouth. There is almost invariably an initial diarrhoea or ileostomy 'flux' (particularly in those patients suffering from Crohn's disease). If the flux amounts to more than 1·5 litres per day the parenteral fluid and electrolyte regime is maintained. Codeine or Lomotil may be effective in reducing the diarrhoea and are frequently used. If the patient's recovery is uninterrupted the faecal or ileostomy output begins to thicken up by the fifth or seventh day and intravenous feeding is stopped and a light diet begun.

Ileostomy closure

In those patients having a diversion ileostomy, the ileostomy is usually closed approximately 2 months after the first operation. However, in those patients who do particularly well (under these circumstances there was probably no need for the loop ileostomy) it can be closed in 2–3 weeks, before the patient leaves hospital.

The closure is usually a simple procedure that can be accomplished without having to re-open the main abdominal incision. A circumstomal incision is made, freeing the mucosa from the skin. Blunt dissection then permits the loop to be drawn out through the small hole. The mucosa is then peeled forward and the incision closed transversely with two layers of sutures. If it is then difficult to reduce the sutured bowel through the small hole, a vertical incision in the anterior–posterior rectus sheath permits reduction. Closure of the hole is effected with one or two horizontal mattress non-absorbable sutures in the posterior sheath. The rest of the wound is allowed to heal by granulation.

Results

In patients with Crohn's disease, ileorectal anastomosis is successful in approximately 50 per cent of cases; the other 50 per cent eventually having to have a permanent ileostomy and proctectomy. However, in some of those patients who eventually have to have a proctectomy, the ileorectal anastomosis may give a few years of normal intestinal continuity that may be of great importance, particularly to young people.

In those patients with ulcerative colitis in whom the rectum is not particularly severely involved, the prognosis tends to be better than in those with Crohn's disease; only a relatively small proportion eventually have to come to proctectomy. The main indication for subsequent proctectomy is bleeding from disease of the rectum, unacceptably frequent bowel actions or the appearance of premalignant changes in the mucosa on one of the regular follow-up biopsy examinations. Regular follow-up is mandatory in all cases, once yearly is probably sufficient.

[*The illustrations for this Chapter on Ileorectal Anastomosis for Inflammatory Bowel Disease were drawn by Mr. G. Lyth.*]

Conservative Excision of the Rectum in Inflammatory Bowel Disease

P. R. Hawley, M.S., F.R.C.S.
Consultant Surgeon, St. Mark's Hospital, London

PRE-OPERATIVE

Indications

This procedure is advocated for use in patients coming to proctocolectomy for ulcerative colitis in the absence of malignant change involving the rectum. It is also of value in patients with Crohn's disease without extensive destruction of the sphincters or peri-anal region.

This method of excision guarantees the preservation of the pelvic nerves and leaves the patient with a strong pelvic floor. Only a small wound is produced and hospitalization much reduced.

THE OPERATION

1

Position of patient and the incision

The patient is placed in the lithotomy-Trendelenburg position using the Lloyd-Davies stirrups as described in the Chapter on 'Abdominoperineal Excision of the Rectum', page 120. The abdomen is opened through a long left paramedian incision and the site of the ileostomy is shown.

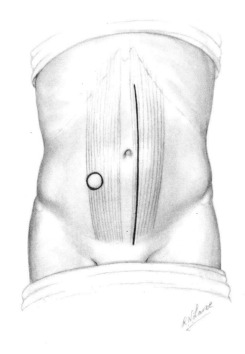

1

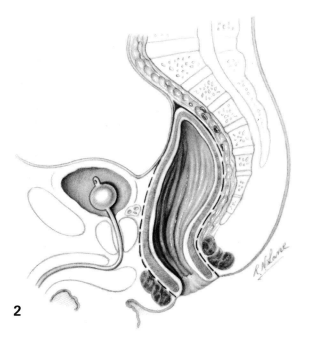

2

2

Extent of excision

This diagram shows the extent of the rectal excision. The perineal operator commences his excision in the intersphincteric plane, leaving the external sphincter and the levator muscles intact. The abdominal operator should preserve the superior mesenteric vessels and as much of the presacral fat as possible. The dissection is at all times close to the rectal wall.

3

Abdominal excision

After the proximal colon has been mobilized the abdominal surgeon commences the excision of the rectum. Incisions are made in the pelvic peritoneum close to each side of the rectum and joined anteriorly at the lowest point of the rectovesical pouch. The sigmoid colon is mobilized, the sigmoid arteries and veins being individually ligated close to the colonic wall. The posterior dissection extends downwards behind the rectum which is mobilized from the underlying mesentery by ligating the vessels as they pass into the rectal wall. The vesicles are dissected and held forwards with a St. Mark's lipped retractor. The fascia of Denonvillier is divided and the dissection is carried down to the apex of the prostate. The lateral ligaments are divided close to the rectal wall. At this stage the operation by the perineal dissector will be complete and the specimen can be removed from the perineal wound. The pelvic peritoneal floor is usually closed by continuous 2/0 catgut without tension and the abdomen is then closed without drainage.

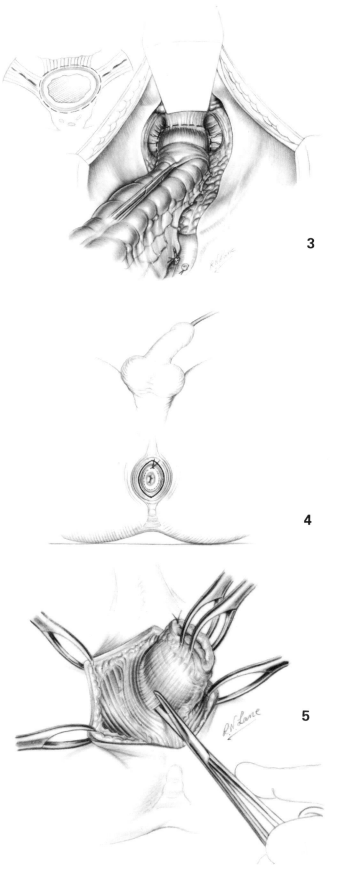

3

4

Perineal dissection

The anus is closed with a strong purse-string suture close to the anal margin. A circumferential incision is made over the intersphincteric groove.

4

5

The intersphincteric plane

The pale fibres of the internal sphincter muscle are identified on each side of the anus and the intersphincteric plane developed by blunt and sharp dissection. The longitudinal fibres passing through to the internal sphincter need to be divided. The plane can thus easily be developed with blunt dissection into the pelvis. Following mobilization of each lateral quadrant the posterior aspect is dissected out.

5

6

Completion of the perineal dissection

Anteriorly the external sphincter decussates in the mid-line and becomes attached to the fibres of the recto-urethralis muscle. Part of the external sphincter is therefore cut in this plane to expose the posterior aspect of the prostate. Because the wound is small a self-retaining retractor cannot be inserted and retraction is carried out by an assistant using a Langenbeck retractor or a lateral retractor of the Lockhart-Mummery type.

The perineal part of the operation is then completed by dividing the visceral pelvic fascia laterally on each side, and anteriorly where it is condensed on to the lateral lobes of the prostate. The vesicles are seen and the lower part of the lateral ligaments divided close to the rectum. At this stage the abdominal and perineal operators will have completed the excision and the whole specimen can be drawn downwards through the perineal wound. In the female dissection is carried out in a similar way in the intersphincteric plane, the vagina being left intact anteriorly.

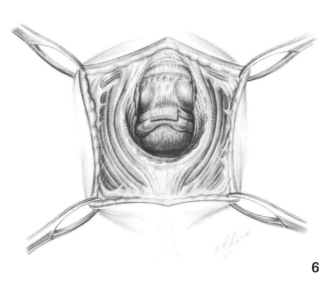

6

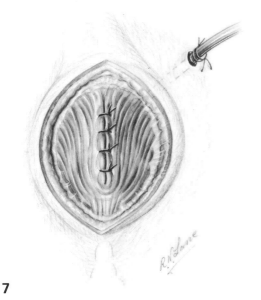

7

7

Wound closure

One or two suction catheters of the Shirley sump type are inserted through a lateral stab wound and placed above the levator muscles. The puborectalis and levators are then approximated loosely with interrupted catgut sutures. The skin is closed with interrupted mattress sutures. Continuous suction drainage is started immediately by connecting the catheter to a vacuum pump. The wound is sealed with Whitehead's varnish and gauze dressings which are left undisturbed until the sutures are removed. When the perineal wound is closed a broad-spectrum antibiotic is administered intravenously at operation and for 48 hr afterwards. The small pelvic wound heals rapidly. Continuous suction drainage is maintained for approximately 5 days and then the catheter is removed. The sutures are kept in place for 10 days.

Complications

The complications of excision of the rectum as part of the proctocolectomy are similar to those described in the Chapter on 'Abdominoperineal Excision of the Rectum', pages 118–132.

[The illustrations for this Chapter on Conservative Excision of the Rectum in Inflammatory Bowel Disease were drawn by Mr. R. N. Lane.]

Ileostomy (without Colectomy)

B. N. Brooke, M.D., M.Chir., F.R.C.S
Emeritus Professor of Surgery, St. George's Hospital,
London

PRE-OPERATIVE

Indications

Ileostomy is seldom undertaken as a sole procedure for ulcerative colitis; it is usually instituted at the time of colectomy, either partial or complete; however, a recent trend has developed for employing ileostomy alone in the management of Crohn's colitis. Temporary ileostomy has been necessary in paediatric cases for the relief of certain types of obstruction.

Contra-indications

Though a diseased ileum, as in Crohn's disease, precludes the institution of an ileostomy, in contradistinction ileostomy may be performed with safety when the ileum is involved secondarily to ulcerative colitis, even at a site where the ileum is inflamed.

Ileostomy is not the operation of choice for the acute complications of ulcerative colitis; haemorrhage is not relieved by simple diversion of the intestinal contents; once perforation has occurred it is liable to recur and massive haemorrhage may also ensue. Removal of the colon by primary colectomy is indicated; despite the poor condition of such patients this gives better results, as it also does for the fulminating disintegrative disease.

Mental deterioration renders the patient incapable of managing an ileostomy.

Pre-operative care

Ileostomy patients are particularly susceptible to electrolyte loss in the immediate postoperative period due to voluminous fluid motions. All the more care is therefore required to ensure that the fluid, chloride, sodium and potassium balance, so markedly disturbed by the severe diarrhoea of ulcerative colitis, is restored before operation. Blood transfusions and protein infusions are usually required.

The site for the functioning stoma should be chosen with care to ensure adequate clearance (4–5 cm) from the anterior-superior iliac spine, the navel and the fold in the groin when the right hip is flexed, for accommodating the adherent flange of the ileostomy bag.

The patient should be visited before operation by another ileostomist to instill confidence and to resolve the fears and problems of an individual facing the prospect of a stoma. An ileostomy association provides this service.

Anaesthesia and position of patient

General anaesthesia with relaxants is given and the patient is placed in the dorsal position. If the patient has been treated with corticosteroids, steroid cover should be given.

THE OPERATION

ILEOSTOMY WITHOUT COLECTOMY

1

The incision and division of ileum and mesentery

An oblique right iliac incision is made in which the stoma is ultimately to be placed. Six to eight centimetres gives adequate access; either the rectus fibres are split or the external and internal oblique, and transversus abdominis muscles are cut in the line of the incision. (The appendix should be removed if the ileostomy is to be permanent and there is no intention of removing the colon subsequently.) A loop of ileum is chosen as close to the ileocaecal valve as possible which will yet permit exteriorization without tension. At an appropriate point where the vascular arcades may be divided without jeopardizing the ileal blood supply, the mesentery and ileum are divided.

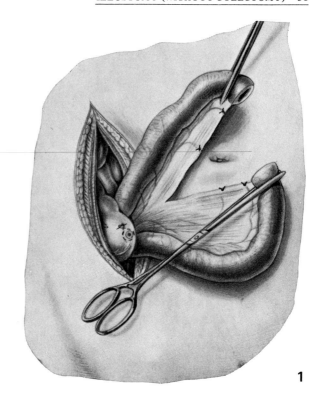

1

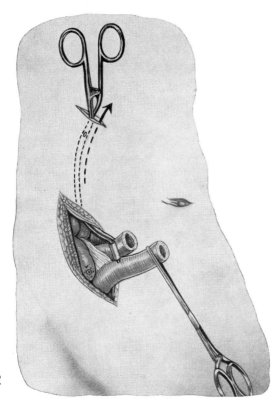

2

2

Procedure for bringing up distal portion of ileum

A stab incision to accommodate the distal end is made at sufficient distance to clear the flange of the adherent bag; a non-crushing clamp is placed on the distal end through this incision.

3

Fixation of mesentery

The distal end is withdrawn through the stab incision. The cut edge of mesentery is then attached to the parietal peritoneum of the anterior abdominal wall to avoid internal herniation; care must be taken to leave 5 cm of proximal ileum exposed for the formation of the functioning stoma.

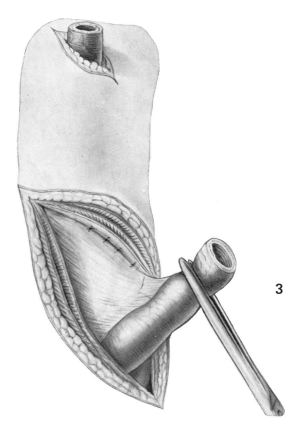

3

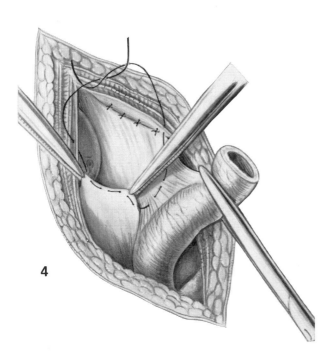

4

4

Closure of para-ileal gutter

A purse-string suture is placed through mesentery and parietal peritoneum of the iliac fossa and that part of the anterior abdominal wall lateral to the incision, in order to close the para-ileal gutter and thus another potential site of internal strangulation. This also prevents ileostomy prolapse by fixing the mesentery.

Closure of abdominal wall around the stoma

5

Inner layers

The abdominal wall is closed in layers around the functioning stoma; relieving incisions are made, if necessary, in the individual layers, at right angles to the direction of the wound, to avoid pinching of the stoma. A Duval lung-holding forcep is inserted into the ileal lumen and the intestinal wall grasped to form a fixed point on which the terminal portion may be everted.

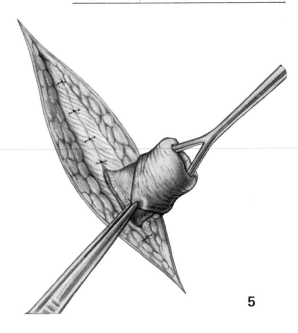

5

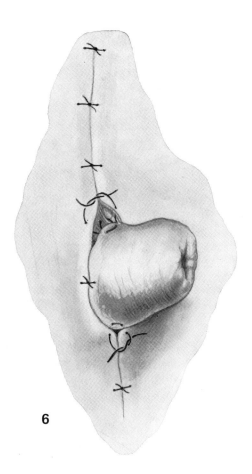

6

6

Outer layer

Finally the skin is sutured; at the stoma the cut edge of mucosa is sewn directly to skin, one suture being placed through skin, mucosa and mesentery so as to fix the position of the everted portion to the underlying ileum. No sutures should be placed in the wall of the underlying ileum since this leads to fistula formation.

ILEOSTOMY WITH LAPAROTOMY

7

Incision left lower paramedian

An alternative method provides an opportunity for examination of the abdominal contents through a paramedian incision, the left side should be chosen to provide sufficient skin surface free of scars to accommodate the flange of the bag. A stab wound site is then chosen with care (*see* Pre-operative care, page 30) in the right iliac fossa to accommodate the functioning stoma. The distal end is placed in the main incision.

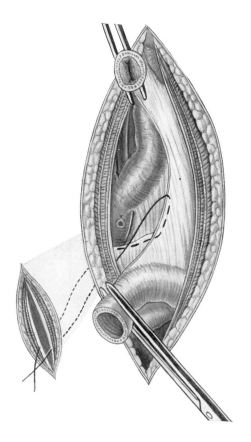

7

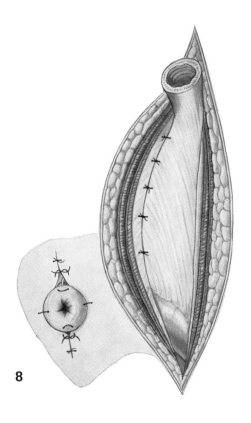

8

8

Obliteration of the para-ileal gutter

The purse-string suture obliterating the para-ileal gutter is passed through the stab wound before the ileostomy is withdrawn, and tied subsequently. The cut edge of mesentery can only be attached to the parietal peritoneum of the anterior abdominal wall after the purse-string has been tied.

The paramedian incision is closed around the distal opening.

ALTERNATIVE METHOD

Incision left lower paramedian

The purpose is to construct an ileostomy with proximal and distal orifices accommodated at one site. It should only be undertaken if colectomy at a later date is not contemplated. Proceed as shown in *Illustration* 7; the loop of terminal ileum is then withdrawn through the stab incision after marking with a suture the proximal limb, which should lie inferiorly.

The mesentery is fixed by closure of the para-ileal gutter and a few stitches at the peritoneal level of the anterior abdominal wall.

The paramedian incision is closed.

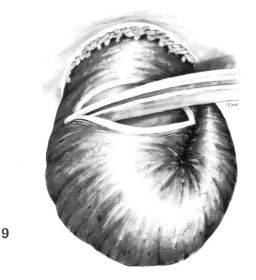

9

9

The distal limb is opened transversely at skin level to $^4/_5$ of its diameter. The mucosa on the proximal side is then everted over the inferior proximal limb; to facilitate this the transverse incision may need to be extended by an incision at the antimesenteric border running towards the apex of the loop.

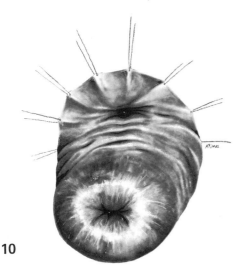

10

10

The mucosa is sutured to the skin around the skin incision leaving the functioning stoma at the apex.

POSTOPERATIVE CARE AND COMPLICATIONS

Fluid and electrolyte balance must be under the immediate control of an intravenous infusion in the first 3–4 days since 1–1·5 litres of fluid may be passed once the stoma starts to evacuate and before the ileal contents thicken. Hourly fluids may be given by mouth after 24–48 hr and the amount increased in the usual way until solids are taken on the third or fourth day. Methyl cellulose or psyllium seeds assist the process of thickening the stool.

No antibiotic nor chemotherapeutic agents need be given.

The adherent bag is applied to the stoma before the patient leaves the theatre, using latex cement, Karaya gum washers, Stomahesive, or double-sided adhesive if the bag is not self-adhesive. In the immediate postoperative period a transparent plastic bag should be used so that the stoma can be inspected without disturbance of the bag. When normal stoma function has been achieved the definitive permanent bag is substituted and the patient should then be instructed in bag management and be encouraged to change the bag himself. Perfect adhesion may not be obtained at the outset on patients with ulcerative colitis as the result of the scaphoid form of the abdominal wall due to emaciation, particularly in the area medial to the anterior superior iliac spine. Reinforcement with adhesive tape, applied to skin and the outer side of the flange of the bag, is helpful. The bag is emptied when full and, in hospital, changed only when the flange is no longer secure. On becoming ambulant the bag is changed as infrequently as hygiene and security of adhesion permit; for some patients this is daily; others find longer periods up to 3 days or more convenient.

The variety of ileostomy bags is numerous, causing difficulty in choice. The matter is simplified if it is borne in mind that bags are either disposable in type or otherwise, and that they are made either in one piece or as a separate flange to be applied to the stoma with a bag which fits over the flange. For the established ileostomy, disposable bags are less convenient than might be supposed; the bags themselves cannot be flushed down a toilet and either have to be burnt or discarded in some other way. Conversely non-disposable bags have to be cleaned carefully and aired between applications in order to avoid odour, which will occur due to bacterial decomposition of stoma effluent. The materials of the non-disposable bag, which include rubber and its bonding agents, sometimes give off a notable odour which is reduced in those bags with carbon incorporated in the material. The two-piece bag was designed to allow the bag to be changed without always disturbing the adhesive face piece, thus minimizing the possibility of skin soreness. In practice no form of bag has to be changed more frequently than 3–7 days, even up to 10 days, according to individual preference; and after this interval it is usually necessary to replace the flange in order to renew the adhesion. However, for those who wish to change the bag daily the two-piece arrangement fulfills its advantage. The two-piece bag is more bulky than the single-piece and protrudes from the surface of the abdomen in a way which may be noticeable through clothing.

As regards adhesives, these are now of three main types: latex, which was used originally and is now almost obsolete, adhesive plasters with adhesive material on both surfaces, (already incorporated in the flange of some bags), and adhesive rings of material which is emollient to skin, such as Karaya gum and Stomahesive. The aim is to avoid skin irritation, soreness and excoriation, all of which result from either contact with ileostomy effluent, sensitivity to latex or other adhesive material, or to too frequent removal of the adhesive face. There is therefore much individual variation and choice in this respect for, in general, Karaya or Stomahesive rings are more satisfactory as regards the maintenance of the skin but have less adhesive power than the adhesive plaster rings.

It is wise for a hospital unit to adopt a uniform basic course of management using the same bag and materials at the outset for all the patients, thus enabling them to accustom themselves to the principles of management. Individual deviation from the basic routine should only be allowed to develop when the patient is fully conversant with bag management and understands his individual and personal needs. In this respect a stomatherapist or an ileostomy association can give much guidance and advice.

Certain complications cause the stoma to become inefficient. Fistula is rare and usually due to siting the stoma too low so that the flange of the bag chafes the lower surface at skin level when the thigh is flexed. Prolapse should not occur with proper fixation of the mesentery. Stomal retraction into the peritoneal cavity may take place if mesenteric fixation is insecure or if the abdominal aperture is too large when it may also be associated with hernia. All these conditions will require operative revision. A complete new stoma is needed in the case of a fistula. Recession within the interstices of the abdominal wall can occur; further laparotomy is not required for this but instead an operation designed to promote adhesion between the two layers. Stenosis at skin level is rare with an eversion stoma; it can be dealt with by simple local excision.

Excoriation of the skin should not occur if the stoma is controlled with a bag from the outset. Too frequent changing of the bag may induce this complication which is usually best treated with Karaya powder, Karaya washers, or Stomahesive.

References

Brooke, B. N. (1952). 'Management of an ileostomy including its complications.' *Lancet* **2,** 102
Brooke, B. N. (1954). *Ulcerative Colitis and its Surgical Treatment.* Edinburgh: Livingstone
Brooke, B. N. and Walker, F. C. (1961). 'A method of external revision of an ileostomy.' *Br. J. Surg.* **49,** 401
Brooke, B. N. (1967). 'Acute adrenal dysfunction.' *Br. J. Surg.* **54,** 489
Counsell, P. B. and Lockhart-Mummery, H. E. (1954). 'Ileostomy, assessment of disability, management.' *Lancet* **1,** 113
Heanley, C. (1954). 'Ileostomy for congenital obstruction of the small intestine.' *Lancet* **2,** 888
Lee, E. G. (1975). 'Split ileostomy in the treatment of Crohn's disease of the colon.' *Ann. R. Coll. Surg. (Eng.)* **56,** 94

[The illustrations for this Chapter on Ileostomy (without Colectomy) were drawn by Mr. W. J. Pardoe.]

Ileostomy (with Colectomy)

James P. S. Thomson, M.S., F.R.C.S.
Consultant Surgeon, St. Mark's Hospital, London

PRE - OPERATIVE

Indications

An ileostomy is made in association with a total colectomy when the distal bowel is either oversewn or brought to the surface as a mucous fistula, or in association with a proctocolectomy. The usual indications are when operative treatment is employed in the management of patients with inflammatory bowel disease, either idiopathic proctocolitis (ulcerative colitis) or Crohn's disease. On rare occasions an ileostomy is needed in patients with multiple neoplasms of the large intestine when a proctocolectomy is undertaken. An ileostomy is also required when a urinary ileal conduit is made as a method of urinary diversion.

Pre-operative preparation

The main aspects of the pre-operative management of the patient will be concerned with the disease for which the ileostomy is to be fashioned. However, an important aspect of this is the correct siting of the ileostomy. This is usually on the right side of the abdomen near the waist-line, lateral to the umbilicus through the outer third of the rectus abdominis muscle. Care must be taken to select the site so that an appliance with its adhesive backing may be applied without impinging on the umbilicus, the anterior superior iliac spine, or the groin crease. If there are previous scars in the vicinity, such as an appendicectomy scar, then these should be taken into account, as they may prevent good fixation of the appliance. It is wise to select the site and fit an appliance pre-operatively, so that the suitability of the chosen position may be established with the patient lying, sitting and standing. When a suitable site has been chosen the skin should be marked so that at operation the surgeon will be in no doubt where to make the trephine.

One other important aspect of the preparation of the patient is an adequate explanation of what an ileostomy is and re-assurance that the patient will receive as much instruction as is required to ensure competence to cope with the stoma. The patient can often be encouraged by meeting an ileostomist of similar age and sex.

Anaesthesia and position of patient

This will be determined by the procedure to be performed and will be referred to in the appropriate section.

THE OPERATION

1

Site of the ileostomy

The ileostomy is placed on the right side of the abdomen near the waist-line, through the outer third of the rectus abdominis muscle. The main laparotomy wound should be on the opposite side of the mid-line, and usually a long left paramedian incision is made.

The trephine

This is performed in an identical manner to that described in the section on terminal colostomy (*see* Chapter on 'Colostomy', page 213).

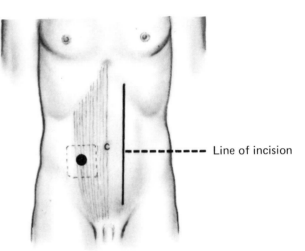

------ Line of incision

1

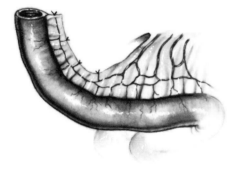

2

2

Preparation of the ileum

The ileum is prepared in such a way that the distal 5 cm may be used in the construction of the ileostomy. It is important that the mesentery is narrowed to allow eversion of the stoma, but great care must be taken to ensure that the distal bowel retains a good blood supply. When this has been done, the mesentery usually adopts an 'L' shape.

3a&b

Fixation of the mesentery

The mesentery of the ileum at the angle of the 'L' is sutured to the parietal peritoneum at the edge of the trephine wound. The remainder of the free edge of the ileal mesentery may be secured by suturing it to the parietal peritoneum laterally with a purse-string suture and by interrupted sutures to the posterior abdominal wall, closing the lateral space. Alternatively,

it may be sutured to the anterior abdominal wall and the falciform ligament. Non-absorbable sutures should be used for the fixation of the mesentery. The former method is to be preferred, however this may be difficult if there is thickening of the mesentery, in which case, the latter method of fixation is justified.

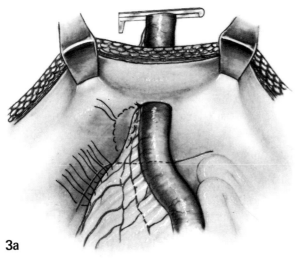

3a

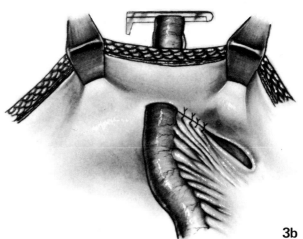

3b

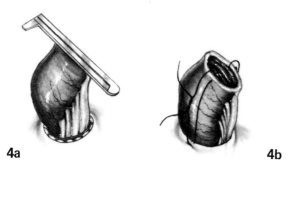

4a   4b

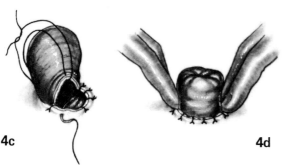

4c   4d

4a-d

Delivery of terminal ileum through the trephine and mucocutaneous suture

After fixation of the mesentery, the distal ileum which is to be used for the ileostomy is delivered through the trephine wound. The operation is then completed and the main incision closed and dressed. The clamp is removed from the distal ileum and a series of mucocutaneous sutures inserted — usually twelve are required. Most surgeons avoid direct suturing of the ileum to the aponeurotic layers of the abdominal wall, as there is a definite risk of sepsis and fistula formation. When the suturing is complete pressure on the abdominal skin around the ileostomy secures full projection of the stoma. A transparent ileostomy appliance is then fitted immediately.

POSTOPERATIVE CARE

The postoperative care of the patient is largely determined by the associated colectomy or procto-colectomy. The following aspects of postoperative management refer to the ileostomy in particular.

(*1*) The stoma should be examined frequently during the first 48 hr to check its viability and to make certain that it has not become detached.

(*2*) The ileostomy does not usually begin to function for 48–72 hr, when it does it is important that the appliance does not become excessively full of effluent as this may lead to leakage — this is very distressing to the patient in the early postoperative period.

(*3*) The patient must be adequately taught about the management of the ileostomy and must be able to cope competently with the appliance before discharge from hospital. He should be re-assured that advice is always available and membership of an ileostomy association should be discussed.

Complications

Loss of viability

This is a rare complication, but if it should occur then a new ileostomy will have to be fashioned urgently.

Skin irritation

This is usually the result of leakage of the ileostomy effluent. However, it may occur as the result of sensitivity to the adhesive used in the appliance.

Leakage of effluent is usually due to faulty application of the appliance, but it may be the consequence of bad siting of the stoma or a failure of the stoma to remain everted. Application of Karaya gum or a preparation such as Stomahesive will improve the condition of the skin in most instances. Administration of medicines such as codeine phosphate or kaolin to render the effluent less liquid also confers some benefit. If these measures fail to help and the stoma has not been well constructed, refashioning may be needed.

If the skin irritation is due to sensitivity a change to a different type of appliance may help, but the use of Stomahesive may be all that is required.

Stenosis

Now that a mucocutaneous suture is employed stenosis of an ileostomy is almost unknown.

Prolapse

This is an unusual problem. It is not satisfactorily treated by amputation as recurrence practically always occurs. Fixation of the ileum and its mesentery to the abdominal wall or resiting of the ileostomy are usually necessary.

Recession

As previously mentioned this is a major cause of skin irritation and is due to a failure of the peritoneal surfaces of the stoma to adhere. It is to encourage this process that Goligher (1975) inserts sutures between the abdominal wall and the seromuscular layer of the ileum. However, many surgeons do not follow this practice as there is a definite incidence of sepsis and fistula formation.

Hernia

To treat a para-ileostomy hernia successfully the ileostomy has to be resited and the original defect closed either with non-absorbable sutures or by the insertion of a synthetic mesh.

Reference

Goligher, J. C. (1975). In *Surgery of the Anus, Rectum and Colon,* 3rd Edition. London: Bailliere Tindall

[*The illustrations for this Chapter on Ileostomy (with Colectomy) were drawn by Mr. G. Lyth.*]

The Continent Ileostomy (Ileal Reservoir)

M. R. Madigan, B.Sc., F.R.C.S. (Ed.), F.R.C.S.
Consultant Surgeon to the Herts and Essex Hospital,
Bishop's Stortford, and The Hertford County Hospital

PRE - OPERATIVE

Introduction

This operation provides an alternative to a conventional ileostomy, and obviates the need for wearing an external appliance. An intra-abdominal reservoir, or pouch, is fashioned from the patient's terminal ileum, with a stoma opening on to the anterior abdominal wall through which the reservoir is emptied with a catheter. The reservoir must have a capacity of over 500 ml to cater for a 24-hr output, must not respond with increasing pressure on filling, must be continent for faeces and gas at all times, and be easily and quickly emptied.

Indications

The operation may be carried out whenever a permanent ileostomy has to be made, e.g. (*1*) conversion of a conventional ileostomy because of complications, or at the patient's request; (*2*) as a primary procedure in conjunction with a total proctocolectomy for ulcerative colitis, familial polyposis coli, multiple carcinoma of the colon, etc; and (*3*) excision of an isolated rectal stump and conversion of the ileostomy, or following an ileorectal anastomosis.

Contra-indications

When the proctocolectomy has to be performed in a debilitated patient where healing is likely to be deficient, as in fulminating ulcerative colitis or in the presence of a perforation of the colon, a conventional ileostomy should then be made, which can be converted to a continent ileostomy later.

Although a perfectly functional reservoir can be made in Crohn's disease, there is a danger that the reservoir may become affected later, necessitating excision. This operation is thus contra-indicated in all cases of Crohn's disease.

Pre-operative preparation

No special preparation of the gut is required.

Anaesthesia

General anaesthesia of choice as for an abdominal or abdominoperineal operation is used.

Position of patient

This will be either in the combined excision of the rectum position (*see* Chapter on 'Abdominoperineal Excision of the Rectum', pages 118—132), or supine, with the operator standing at the patient's *left* side.

THE OPERATION

1

Incision

If a proctocolectomy is to be carried out, an extended mid-line incision is used, and the colon and rectum excised by a synchronous combined or abdomino-perineal approach (*see* Chapter on 'Abdominoperineal Excision of the Rectum', pages 118–132). The pelvic peritoneum is reconstituted and the mesocolon oversewn to cover the raw areas.

If only a reservoir is to be made, a shorter mid-line incision is used, and the conventional ileostomy disconnected by a circular incision.

The site for the reservoir stoma is marked just medial to the lateral edge of the right rectus sheath, below the waist-line, and just above the hair-line in females. This is much lower than the conventional stoma.

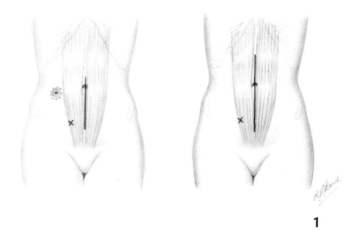

1

FIRST STAGE OF RESERVOIR FORMATION

2

Construction of ileal loop

Fifteen centimetres of terminal ileum is left free for the formation of the valve and stoma.

A fold of the ileum is joined just below the anti-mesenteric border with a continuous 3/0 chromic catgut suture on a fine atraumatic needle as a sero-muscular layer. Each limb of the fold measures 15 cm.

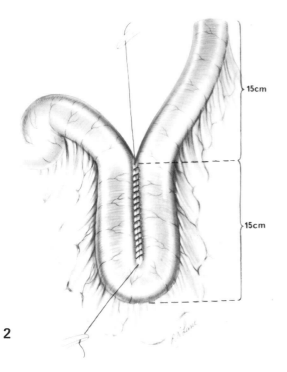

2

3

Conversion to an intestinal flap

While a soft clamp occludes the proximal bowel, the loop of ileum is opened along the antimesenteric border, leaving a margin several millimetres wide from the first suture line. The incision is continued along the proximal ileum for 4 cm.

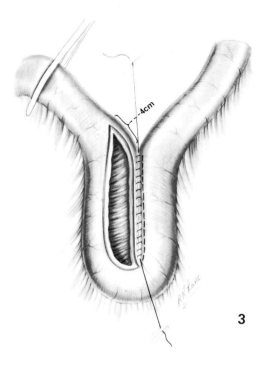

3

4

Completion of flap

An all-coats continuous 3/0 chromic catgut suture unites the free edges of the first suture line as a second layer.

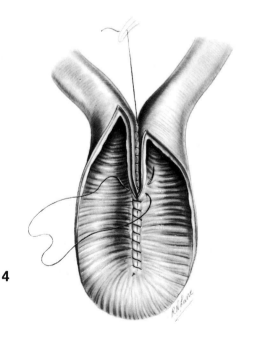

4

FORMATION OF NIPPLE VALVE

5

Preparation of distal mesentery

The visceral peritoneum is stripped for about 8 cm from both sides of the mesentery of the distal ileum.

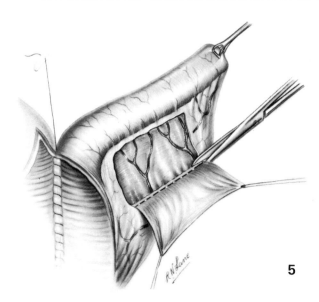

5

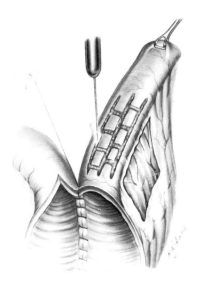

6

6

Division of muscle

Eight centimetres of the distal ileum is scarified carefully with longitudinal and transverse cuts through the muscle coats with a diathermy needle.

7

Making the valve

With a Babcock forceps the distal ileum is intus-suscepted, making a nipple 4 cm long. A catheter is placed through the valve and 8–10 absorbable sutures of catgut or polyglycolic acid are placed through both layers of the ileum and tied firmly.

The distal ileal stump emerging from the reservoir is sutured to the reservoir with interrupted non-absorbable sutures.

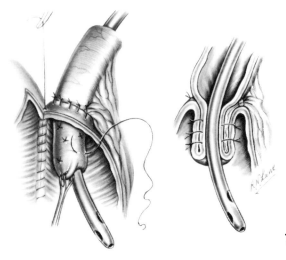

7

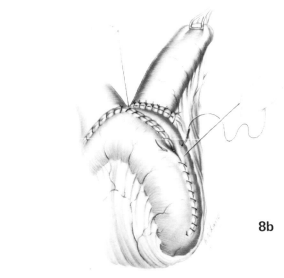

8a

SECOND STAGE OF RESERVOIR FORMATION

8a&b

Suture of intestinal flap

The ileal flap is turned up and sutured with continuous 3/0 chromic catgut sutures in two layers, firstly an all-coats and finally a seromuscular, to complete the reservoir.

8b

9

Testing of valve

The reverse side of the reservoir is brought in to view by inverting the reservoir between the leaves of the mesentery. This allows the reservoir to lie easily in the right iliac fossa. A catheter is inserted into the reservoir and 50 ml of air or saline injected. The soft clamp on the proximal ileum must be in place. The catheter is then withdrawn and no leak should occur. The air or saline is then removed by re-inserting the catheter, which should pass easily into the reservoir.

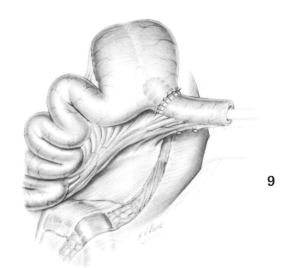

9

10

Stoma formation

A trephine opening 2 cm in diameter is made in the skin and down to and including the anterior rectus sheath. A way is then made with a finger through the rectus muscle in a medial and caudal direction down to the peritoneum, which is incised. The free distal ileal segment is drawn through the opening on to the surface. A special ileostomy catheter (size 28 Ch and made by A. B. Medena, 5–43400 Kungsbacka, Sweden) is inserted from the outside into the reservoir, and is kept in position during subsequent manoeuvres and for drainage.

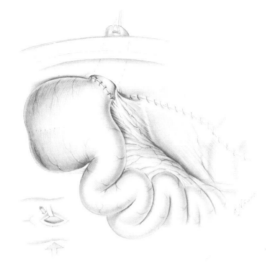

10

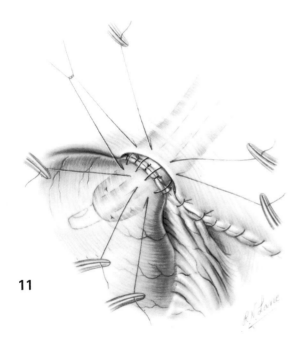

11

11

Closing the lateral space

The free edge of the mesentery is sutured to the parietal peritoneum using a continuous non-absorbable suture. Interrupted stitches attach the reservoir to the peritoneum of the internal opening in the abdominal wall.

12

Finishing the stoma

The emerging distal ileum is cut flush with the surface of the skin and sutured to it with interrupted catgut stitches.

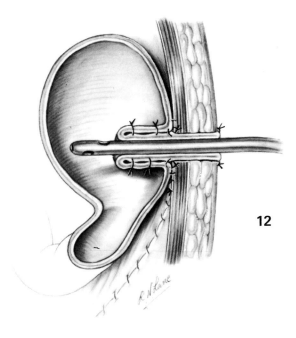

12

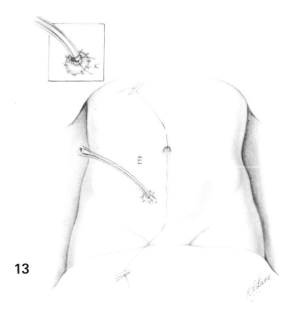

13

13

Closure of abdomen

The abdominal wound is sutured with continuous nylon for the peritoneal and fascial layers, and polyglycolic acid interrupted sutures for the subcutaneous layers, and a similar continuous subcuticular stitch for the skin.

If a conventional ileostomy has been removed, the old stoma site is sutured in layers.

The catheter is anchored to the skin with a non-absorbable stitch, after making sure that it is through the valve and lying comfortably in the reservoir.

14

Final dressing

A waterproof dressing covers the mid-line incision. Tulle gras is placed around the mucosa of the stoma, and a cone of cotton wool is built up to support the catheter, kept in place by waterproof strapping.

The catheter is joined to a collecting bottle, making sure that any connections do not narrow the internal diameter of the drainage system.

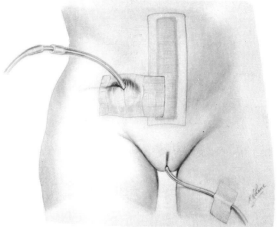

14

EMPTYING THE RESERVOIR AFTER HEALING

15

An ileostomy catheter is inserted into the reservoir through the stoma, and the contents drained into a receiver or lavatory pan. A small waterproof covering is placed over the stoma to prevent moisture from the mucosa coming into contact with the clothing.

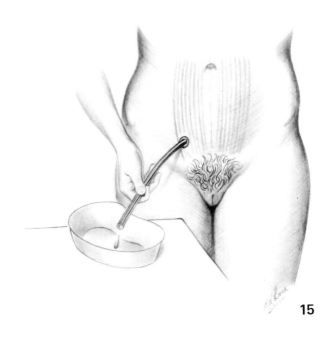

15

POSTOPERATIVE CARE AND COMPLICATIONS

General

Nasogastric suction and intravenous fluid therapy is maintained for several days until intestinal contents drain from the reservoir via the ileostomy catheter, when oral feeding is begun in the normal way. There are no restrictions when a full diet is taken. The dressings are left undisturbed unless they become too wet, when they are carefully changed.

Management of the ileal catheter

Postoperative (days)	Reservoir drainage via ileostomy catheter
1–10	Continuous; catheter tied *in situ.* Ten millilitres of saline are injected into the reservoir daily, via the catheter to keep it clear.
8–10	Catheter occluded for 3–4 hourly periods during the day. Continuous drainage at night.
11	Catheter removed. Intermittent emptying continued, gradually increasing the time between catheterizations until it is only necessary 2–3 times in 24 hr.

This table is a guide only. If the patient feels full or uncomfortable, more frequent emptying can be done. In principle, the catheter should not be left tied in for too long and the number of catheterizations reduced to avoid possible trauma. The reservoir is designed so that one emptying in 24 hr should suffice, which can be achieved in a few weeks. Some patients feel 'safer' with two to three catheterizations daily.

Washout and emptying

If the ileal contents become too viscous to flow easily, 50–100 ml of water can be injected into the catheter using a plastic syringe with a rubber bulb. In practise this is hardly ever necessary. The patient is trained and encouraged in emptying the reservoir from the start, and in how to wash out the reservoir if needed. Indigestible material like fruit skins may block the catheter holes, which are cleared simply by withdrawing, cleaning and re-inserting the catheter.

Immediate complications

Leakage from the reservoir suture line may cause peritonitis, requiring laparotomy. Simple repair of the reservoir may be possible. Otherwise excision of the reservoir and formation of a conventional ileostomy must be performed.

A faecal fistula may develop around the stoma, or through the abdominal or perineal wound. The reservoir should be placed on continuous drainage and the patient fed parenterally. If the fistula persists it will require exploration.

Late complications

Incompetence of the valve

Leaking from the reservoir has occurred after several months, and often begins with the patient having difficulty in inserting the catheter. It is usually due to partial reduction of the nipple between the reservoir and the abdominal wall inside the peritoneal cavity. An internal fistula at the root of the nipple has been described as a cause of incontinence of gas or faeces. There has also been a case of complete external eversion of the nipple. The loss is mostly minimal. Laparotomy with or without opening the reservoir and resuturing of the nipple and further stitching of the reservoir to the abdominal parietes, as described, will restore continence. Otherwise a bag can be worn.

References

Goligher, J. C. and Lintott, D. (1975). *Br. J. Surg.* **62,** 893
Halvorsen, J. F. and Heimann, P. (1975). *Br. J. Surg.* **62,** 52
Kock, N. G. (1971). *Ann. Surg.* **173,** 545
Kock, N. G. (1973). *Prog. Surg.* **12,** 180
Madigan, M. R. (1976). *Ann. R. Coll. Surg.* **58,** 62
Philipson, B. (1975). Ileostomy reservoir; a clinical and experimental study of bacteriology, morphology, and absorption. MD Thesis, Department of Surgery, Sahlgrenska Sjukhuset, Gothenburg, Sweden. Kungsbacka Elanders Boktryckeri Aktiebolag

[The illustrations for this Chapter on The Continent Ileostomy (Ileal Reservoir) were drawn by Mr. R. N. Lane.]

DIVERTICULAR DISEASE: GENERAL INTRODUCTION

There is considerable controversy over the correct surgical management of the complications of diverticular disease. This is inevitable because there is a wide range of choice open in many situations, when the final decision taken rests on small details. Not least among the factors influencing the selection of the operation to be performed are the skill and experience of the surgeon.

In diverticular disease, there is widespread disorder of the wall of the colon. This manifests itself in a tendency to increased muscular spasms with greatly enhanced intraluminal pressures. This is accompanied by considerable muscular hypertrophy. As a result of these abnormalities, the lumen of the bowel becomes reduced in size. Therefore, after any resection for diverticulitis, and its complications, the surgeon is left with considerable problems if he wishes to rejoin the bowel by a primary anastomosis, since he is working with two tubes of narrow diameter circumscribed by thickened rigid walls. Any anastomosis that he achieves will probably be subjected to abnormally increased pressures. When one considers these factors, it is possible to enumerate several general principles that should be taken into account in *all* operations for diverticulitis:

(*1*) The length of the resection should always be greater than the macroscopic evidence of the disease, and as far as possible division of the colon should be carried out through normal bowel wall.

(*2*) When the sigmoid colon is the site of the disease and its complications, the distal limit of the excision must be below the rectosigmoid junction, in order to be certain that the area of pathophysiological change has been removed. This implies that the line of any postresection anastomosis should be through the upper one-third of the rectum, but care should be taken not to open the retrorectal space as this increases the incidence of pelvic abscess and anastomotic disruption.

(*3*) The greatest possible lumen should be preserved by the anastomosis; the 'one-layer' turns in less tissue than the 'two-layer' technique and should be preferred for this reason.

(*4*) Catgut stitches are too weak to be relied on to resist the extra strains imposed by the excessive muscular contractions of diverticular disease, and the anastomosis should always include an unabsorbable layer of suture material.

(*5*) Since the surgeon is required to operate for severe pathological changes that have additionally a background of physiological disorder, in many cases protection of the operation site by a preliminary or accompanying proximal colostomy is to be regarded as a wise precaution rather than an admission of technical inadequacy.

(*6*) If the inflammatory complications are more than usually severe, the colostomy must achieve complete diversion of the faecal stream to be properly effective; since a loop colostomy does not always do this, a Devine-type colostomy may be required under these exceptional circumstances.

(*7*) A caecostomy is not as effective as a loop colostomy, and diverts even less of the bowel contents; for this reason, while some surgeons use a caecostomy as a means of luminal decompression after resections unaccompanied by severe inflammatory changes, it should never be used for diversion after operations for the complications of diverticular disease.

(*8*) Effective intraperitoneal drainage of the anastomosis should accompany all resections, since abscess formation at the operation site is a frequent occurrence, and unless a track is easily available to the surface, anastomotic disruption is inevitable.

The major complications of diverticular disease are acute inflammation (diverticulitis), pericolic abscess formation, peritonitis, obstruction, haemorrhage and vesicocolic fistula. In many patients, inflammatory changes and obstruction are present at the same time.

Acute diverticulitis is managed conservatively wherever possible, but occasionally the inflammation is so severe that a local peritonitis develops, and the patient may manifest the signs of septicaemia. The correct management of this situation is to carry out a laparotomy to assess the situation without preconceived surgical prejudice: usually a proximal loop colostomy is then performed, to rest the distal inflamed portion of bowel, but in many cases it is safe to perform a primary resection with reanastomosis or Hartmann's operation. The decision to carry out an immediate definitive resection should be made only by a surgeon with special skill and experience in this type of surgery, and it is often necessary to protect the anastomosis by a temporary loop colostomy. The alternative procedure, to exteriorize the inflamed colon has now been largely abandoned, because the technical difficulties of mobilizing the grossly inflamed bowel which has a short, fat and adherent mesentery are so great that a primary resection is an easier and safer operation. The same objections apply to the Mikulicz operation.

If a pericolic abscess is present, this should be drained. A stiff tubular drain should not be used, as this can cause pressure necrosis of large vessels against the brim and side-wall of the pelvis; instead, a soft corrugated drain of latex rubber or Portex should be employed, and this should be brought to the surface through a separate stab wound by the shortest available route. Sometimes a pericolic abscess arises without evidence of serious peridiverticulitis or obstruction of the bowel. Under these circumstances, the situation can be managed conservatively until the abscess has localized and pointed to a particular area of the abdominal wall; when this has happened, a small incision over the apical point sufficient to establish effective drainage is all that is required immediately. Although this minor operation may be followed by a faecal fistula, this may close spontaneously and after a suitable period (2–3 months) an elective resection of the diseased bowel will be possible by a one-stage procedure.

Peritonitis can complicate diverticulitis in two ways—either by rupture of a single diverticulum, or as a result of widespread disruption of the colon wall. In the first instance, only a small area of bowel is affected by the inflammatory process, but in the latter case a significant length of bowel is involved. The handling of these two situations is different. If a single point of rupture is present, surrounded by a small area of peridiverticulitis, treatment can be along the same lines as for a perforated duodenal ulcer; the peritoneal cavity should be cleaned up, the perforation sealed by an omental patch and the area drained; no colostomy is required. If a long length of colon is involved by peridiverticulitis and no single point of rupture can be incriminated as solely responsible for the peritonitis, in addition to peritoneal toilet and drainage of the affected zone, a temporary diversion

by a colostomy is essential. It is in this situation that a Devine-type colostomy has its use for long-term *complete* diversion of the faecal stream. Primary resection has little place in the surgical treatment of diverticulitis complicated by peritonitis, but many surgeons would prefer the Hartmann operation in these circumstances as it removes the diseased segment.

Obstruction caused by diverticulitis can be compared with the situation of acute pyloric stenosis associated with active duodenal ulceration. Provided the diagnosis is certain, conservative treatment by intestinal decompression via a nasogastric tube, antibiotics and gentle enemas will almost certainly succeed in relieving the obstruction without recourse to surgical aid. However, if the diagnosis is in doubt (in which case an annular carcinoma may be present) and especially if evidence of abdominal tenderness may suggest the possibility of a stercoral perforation, it may be dangerous to pursue a non-invasive policy. If circumstances dictate that the obstruction must be relieved without a definitive diagnosis being known (and this can still be the situation after a preliminary laparotomy), the obstruction should be decompressed by the simplest available means—a proximal loop colostomy.

Bleeding is not usually an important symptom of diverticulitis, but occasionally a massive and persistent haemorrhage may occur. Although the changes of diverticular disease are seen most frequently in the distal colon, in many cases of severe bleeding the haemorrhage is coming from the caecum or right colon. Localization of the bleeding point can be most difficult even with expert angiographic and colonoscopic assistance. Not infrequently the surgeon is forced to operate without precise knowledge of the source of the haemorrhage. In this situation, where immediate and certain control of the bleeding is essential, a total colectomy and ileorectal anastomosis may be the most safe and effective surgical treatment*. If the actual site of the arterial leak is known, a more limited left- or right-sided colectomy may be possible.

Every type of abdominal fistula can occur in diverticular disease complicated by a pericolic abscess, but a vesicocolic fistula is by far the most common form. In the presence of active inflammation of the urinary bladder—as evidenced by pyrexia, leucocytosis and the appearance of the bladder mucosa at cystoscopy—a preliminary diversion of the faecal stream for a few weeks by a transverse loop colostomy is advisable. However, in many cases, the amount of active infection is surprisingly small and, under these circumstances, a definitive procedure is permissible at once. Usually the bladder and the colon are

---

* This procedure may need to be staged with initial ileostomy and rectostomy if the patient's condition is desperate, and the intestine, which is unprepared, is distended and full of blood.

adherent only over a small area and can be separated safely by combined blunt and sharp dissection. The bladder defect can be closed with absorbable sutures after the edges have been trimmed to remove the oedematous margins, but postoperative closed-system urinary drainage through a self-retaining catheter should be continued for 7–14 days postoperatively. The normal operation to remove the diseased segment of colon is next performed, and the anastomosis completed in the usual way, but when the anastomosis is finished, it should be wrapped around with omentum to keep it completely separated from the bladder. Unless the two wounds are kept apart in this manner, they can adhere to each other during the postoperative period and the fistulous connection can re-form. If the fistula is unusually low in the bladder, or the dissection to separate the colon is particularly difficult, a preliminary colostomy for a few weeks will greatly ease the situation and will make the subsequent definitive operation less risky; in particular, the danger of trauma to one or both ureters will be much reduced.

C. V. MANN

Elective Operation for Sigmoid Diverticular Disease

Mark Killingback, F.R.C.S., F.R.C.S.(Ed.), F.R.A.C.S.
Surgeon, Edward Wilson Colon and Rectum Unit,
Sydney Hospital, Sydney

INTRODUCTION

The recent concept that patients may have clinical and x-ray features of diverticular disease not due to inflammation but associated with functional and colon muscle abnormalities has lead to a better understanding of surgical indications.

There can be a disproportion between the clinical and radiological assessment of diverticular disease and a barium enema can under-estimate or exaggerate the significance of diverticular disease.

Better appreciation of the response of functional symptoms in relation to diet and the effects of increasing faecal residue with unprocessed bran has greatly reduced the number of patients requiring surgery for 'failed medical treatment'.

Caution must always be exercised in attributing abdominal and bowel symptoms to diverticular disease and this applies particularly to those patients whose principal complaint is chronic abdominal pain.

Once disease has become refractory to treatment, early surgery is best performed as repeated attacks of inflammation will cause progressive pericolic fibrosis and lead to more difficult technical aspects.

It is doubtful if prophylactic resection of sigmoid diverticular disease is justified in the early or mild stage to prevent such complications as perforation and fistulae. The development of such complications is largely unpredictable and is often the first manifestation of the disease.

Most elective resections are currently performed for complicated disease such as chronic phlegmonous diverticulitis, chronic pericolic or pelvic abscess and fistulae. Some of these patients will be having a second-stage procedure subsequent to a previous laparotomy for acute diverticulitis and peritonitis.

Indications

(1) Chronic symptoms despite conservative management with a high-residue diet and unprocessed bran, may warrant elective surgery. In this group, patients with an associated irritable colon are difficult to assess for surgical treatment.

(2) Repeated attacks of acute diverticulitis of moderate severity with evidence of peritoneal irritation, fever and systemic effects. Such attacks usually settle with antibiotic therapy in a few days but often leave a focus for subsequent attacks. Two or three such episodes in fit patients are sufficient indication for elective surgery but this may be modified in the elderly and unfit. The recurring type of acute inflammatory disease may be more prone to develop some of the serious complications.

(3) Despite the diagnostic advances of the air contrast barium enema and colonoscopy, the differential diagnosis between diverticular disease and carcinoma of the sigmoid colon remains a problem. The two conditions may be coincidentally associated. It should be realized that the patient may have an associated carcinoma elsewhere in the colon although barium enema demonstrates marked diverticular disease in the sigmoid colon.

1&2

(*4*) A barium enema may show a localized stricture of the sigmoid colon and it may not be possible to exclude the possibility of carcinoma on any other investigation or clinical feature. An important finding on any barium enema is the lines of mucosal pattern which flow through the stricture indicating that the diagnosis is diverticular disease. If a patient has had an acute exacerbation of abdominal or colorectal symptoms it is reasonable to regard this as a 'hot stricture' associated with an acute phlegmonous diverticulitis and a barium enema 4 weeks later will often show almost complete resolution of the deformity in the favourable case obviating the need for the surgery on the basis of the stricture and the risk of cancer that it represents.

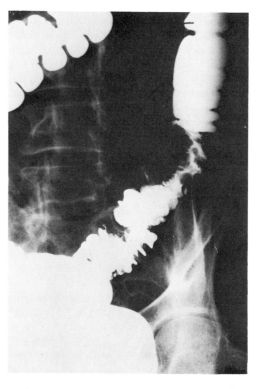

2

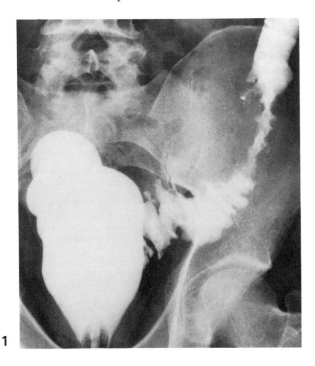

1

(*5*) If a mass is present in the sigmoid colon palpable from the abdomen or the pelvis, usually it is best resected. This mass may be due to thickened muscular changes in the segment of sigmoid colon with palpable faecoliths in diverticula, or it may represent intramural, intramesenteric or paracolic inflammation which has more serious significance. Some attempt should be made clinically to decide which of these pathologies is responsible for a palpable mass. Although the inflammatory mass is best excised in all patients, in the elderly and unfit the mass which is due to muscular, non-inflammatory diverticular disease may be treated conservatively. Of patients treated by resection approximately 30 per cent have a pelvic mass and 10 per cent have an abdominal mass.

(*6*) Colovesical and colocutaneous are the more common fistulae which may complicate sigmoid diverticulitis. The less common fistulae are colo-vaginal, colo-enteric and colofallopian but diverticular disease may form a fistula to any organ and many bizarre fistulae have been described. In fit patients these fistulae are absolute indications for resection of the sigmoid disease but in some elderly patients with a fistula that is not associated with an active, perisigmoid abscess, these fistulae can be quiescent and there may be less risk to the patient by treating them conservatively rather than performing major surgery.

(*7*) Surgery may be necessary as a second stage after the initial surgical management of acute diverticulitis with peritonitis. In some patients treated only with pelvic drainage, the disease will not settle and in a few, a delayed colocutaneous fistula will occur within the first 2 weeks of initial management. Other patients will develop a chronic inflammatory pelvic phlegmon. Of those patients treated initially by excision with closure of the rectal stump or a distal mucous fistula, reconnection of the colon will be necessary.

(*8*) Acute obstruction due to diverticular disease may occur in association with an acute pelvic or paracolic abscess and its management is directed to the treatment of the acute inflammatory disease rather than the obstruction which will settle if adequate control of the acute inflammatory process is achieved. Rarely does acute large bowel obstruction occur due to chronic intramural and pericolic fibrosis. Such patients are best treated by three-stage resection of the sigmoid colon with an initial colostomy. Subsequent to this first stage, a barium enema and endoscopy assessment will be essential to exclude carcinoma of the sigmoid colon which more commonly presents with acute large bowel obstruction.

(9) Profuse bleeding from diverticular disease is not common and almost always ceases spontaneously. It is desirable to exclude sources of haemorrhage in the upper gastro-intestinal tract by barium meal and gastroscopy and if it is concluded that the colon is the source of bleeding it must be realized that the pathology may be one of a number of diseases. It is often assumed that bleeding is arising from a diverticulum when in fact it is due to spontaneous rupture of an arteriosclerotic vessel in the colon, small vascular abnormalities, polyp and carcinoma. In those few patients with continued profuse bleeding after admission to hospital, mesenteric arteriography is essential and such an investigation may indicate the precise site of bleeding which will allow appropriate segmental colon resection to be performed if it should become necessary. A barium enema is desirable but not always possible in such patients who continue to bleed profusely. If no bleeding point can be identified by arteriography it is most unlikely that it will be identified at laparotomy and total colectomy will be necessary. Ileorectal anastomosis (with or without a complementary loop ileostomy) or end-ileostomy (with closure of the rectal stump) should be performed according to the experience of the surgeon and the state of the patient's health.

Pre-operative preparation

The preparation for the patient is that applicable to major colorectal surgery and will include investigations of blood count, blood biochemistry, chest x-ray and ECG. An intravenous pyelogram is an essential investigation before sigmoid resection for diverticular disease. It may reveal incidental urinary tract abnormalities such as ureteric duplication, deviation of the ureter, non-functioning in one kidney and obstruction of the ureter by the inflammatory disease in the pelvis.

The bowel preparation is carried out over a 48-hr period. The patient is given clear fluids each day. Two doses of magnesium sulphate (30 ml) are administered orally each day. One thousand five hundred millilitres saline enemas are administered on each of the two pre-operative days of preparation. Oral Kanamycin is given over a 48-hr period to reduce the intestinal flora. This is given as 1 g/hr for four doses and then 1 g 4-hourly until operation.

It is important to select an appropriate site for a stoma such as a transverse colostomy before the day of operation and this site should be selected with the patient in various postures.

Ureteric catheterization

In those patients in whom a large pelvic inflammatory mass is evident on rectal examination it is likely there will be considerable extraperitoneal pelvic fibrosis. In such patients the introduction of ureteric catheters before operation can be most helpful.

Position of patient

When an uncomplicated resection of the sigmoid colon is anticipated, the patient can be operated upon in the usual laparotomy position. If complicated disease is expected, the Lloyd–Davies position (modified lithotomy-Trendelenburg position) with stirrups is preferable. This not only facilitates ureteric catheterization but allows rectal irrigation and better retraction by an assistant standing between the patient's legs. The assistant can also perform digital examination of the vagina which may assist a difficult anterior pelvic dissection.

THE OPERATION

A mid-line incision is made from pubis to just above the umbilicus and improved access can always be obtained by sufficient extension of the incision in the mid-line. A thorough laparotomy is performed to assess the diverticular disease, its complications and then any other intra-abdominal pathology.

In assessing the diverticular disease the possibility of carcinoma must be considered. If there is doubt about such a diagnosis, the pathology is usually diverticular disease. Any attachment of the diverticular disease to adjacent organs will be noted. The extent of the diverticula along the colon must be assessed as well as any abnormal muscular thickening in the bowel wall.

3, 4 & 5

In deciding the proximal extent of colonic resection, several aspects are important. Obviously, active chronic infection in the colon and mesentery must be included. Muscle-thickening (not usually beyond the sigmoid colon) must be removed and it is preferable to remove colon which contains many diverticula. In the fit patient it is reasonable to include the descending colon and distal transverse colon in order to remove diverticulosis. It is doubtful whether more proximal excision of the colon requiring division of the middle colic and right colic vessels is necessary.

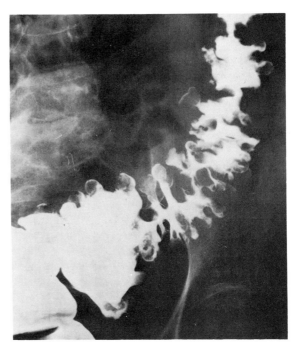

4

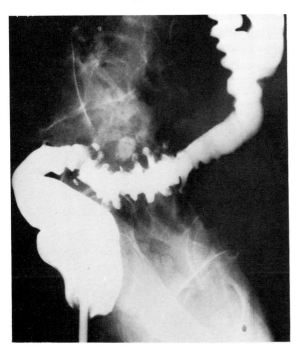

3

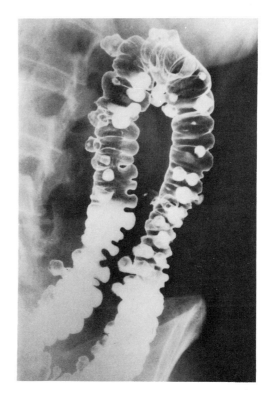

5

In the older patients, compromise is reasonable and residual diverticula in the proximal colon stump are preferable to extending the scope of the surgery.

The distal level of excision is also determined by the site of inflammation in the wall and mesentery of the bowel. It is important to remove distal diverticula which may be obscured in the perirectal fat near and below the rectosigmoid junction. Careful examination of the barium enema may help to localize the distal limit of diverticula formation. The longitudinal muscle is usually thickened in the rectosigmoid and possibly in the upper rectum and it is preferable to remove the muscle abnormality. Therefore, the distal level of resection is *always* below the promontory of the sacrum and frequently through the upper third of the rectum. In addition, those patients with extensive inflammatory disease throughout the pelvis may have the rectal wall secondarily involved by chronic pelvic sepsis and this may need further excision to obtain a low but normal rectal stump for anastomosis.

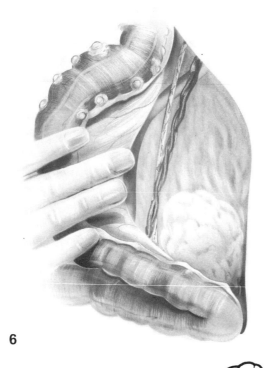

6

6

The sigmoid colon is mobilized from the left paracolic gutter by dividing the lateral peritoneal attachment from pelvic brim to the splenic flexure of the colon. The mesentery is mobilized to the mid-line from the retroperitoneal tissues, avoiding bleeding from the gonadal vessels which lie anterior to the ureter. Both of these structures, carefully identified, are pushed away from the mesentery to lie on the retroperitoneal plane. In this area, blunt digital dissection is helpful. The mesentery must be mobilized anteriorly from the retroperitoneal tissues until caudally it is completely separated from the perinephric fat to the level of the splenic flexure. This plane of dissection is extended laterally to meet the incision previously made in the peritoneum of the left paracolic gutter. Most of the kidney will then be palpable through the perinephric fat at the upper limit of this dissection. The splenic flexure is not usually mobilized further in this resection but the surgeon should not hesitate to do so at this stage if more mobility for anastomosis is required.

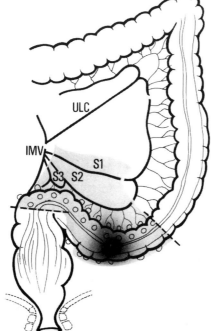

7

7

The extent of mesenteric resection and vascular ligation will depend on the proximal division of the colon and distal division of the rectosigmoid or rectum. If the anastomosis is to be just below the rectosigmoid then the mesentery is dissected to ligate the first, second and third sigmoid vessels from the inferior mesenteric vessel bundle which is then left intact to supply and drain the rectal stump. It should not be necessary to undertake any dissection to protect the lumbar sympathetic nerves in this manoeuvre.

8

Those patients requiring a lower resection removing the upper third or rarely the upper half of the rectum, will require a different mesenteric ligation. The inferior mesenteric vascular bundle is ligated proximally at a convenient point below the upper left colic vessels. Dissection any closer to the inflamed bowel will not be as convenient and more individual vessels will need ligation. In these circumstances greater care is necessary to avoid damaging the lumbar sympathetic nerves in the pre-aortic and presacral areas. These nerves should be carefully identified, lying closely posterior to the inferior mesenteric vascular bundle. The presacral space will need some, if not full, dissection and it may be necessary to divide most or all of the lateral ligaments. Appropriate dissection in the rectovaginal or rectoprostatic plane will be necessary to gain an adequate length of mobile rectal stump for anastomosis. It is in these planes that any perirectal fibrosis will create difficulties in dissection. It is preferable to use absorbable ligature material throughout the operation, particularly in the pelvis to reduce the possibility of chronic sepsis around the ligatures subsequently.

CANCER OR DIVERTICULITIS—EXTENT OF LOCAL EXCISION

If real doubt is present that the lesion being resected is cancer then an adequate cancer operation must be performed. The proximal level of the mesenteric ligation would still be satisfactory below the upper left colic vessel but the extent of the local excision will require a more radical procedure. Adjacent small

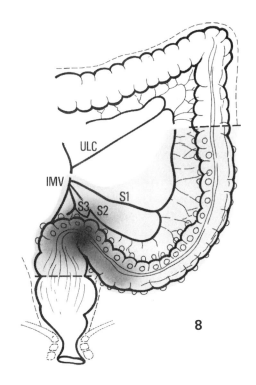

8

bowel, uterus, ovary and fallopian tube may need excision *en bloc* with the specimen. If attachment to the bladder has occurred, then a segment of bladder wall should be excised in continuity. If the attachment to the bladder wall appears to be more posterior and deeper in the pelvis than the usual vault attachment, dissection can be facilitated by instilling saline into the bladder to lift the attached sigmoid colon from the depth of the pelvis.

9

Preparation of the proximal stump for anastomosis

The division of the marginal artery and vein must be meticulously performed to preserve maximum blood supply and venous drainage. The marginal vessel must be ligated and divided square with the proximal level of colon division and the small arcade vessels carefully preserved. Clearing of the pericolic fat is best avoided altogether but one or two obtrusive appendices epiploica may need excision. Minimal clearing of fat from the colon wall is one of the advantages of the single-layer anastomotic technique. If diverticula have unavoidably been left near the divided end of the colon stump, they should be avoided with any anastomotic sutures. They need no further attention. Twenty centimetres from the divided end of the bowel linen tape is tied closely around the wall of the colon (without compression of marginal vessels) and the colon stump then irrigated with saline to obtain a clean segment for anastomosis.

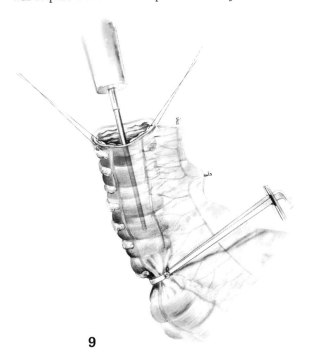

9

10

The preparation of the distal rectal stump

The distal level of division having been selected, it is necessary to prepare the posterior wall of the rectum for anastomosis. If the inferior mesenteric vascular bundle is being preserved, then multiple small vessels entering the posterior wall of the recto-sigmoid region will need individual ligation and a 1 cm width of the posterior wall is cleaned for anastomosis. If a lower anterior resection is being performed then the mesorectum is divided at the selected level similarly to expose no more than 1 cm of 'cleaned' rectal wall. A single Hayes autogrip angled rectal clamp is then applied immediately above the prepared segment of rectal wall, applying the clamp from the right side of the pelvis.

If a short, low rectal stump is being prepared, then it is convenient to irrigate the rectum with normal saline through the anus (the patient being in the Lloyd-Davies position) via a proctoscope to obtain a clean rectal stump for anastomosis.

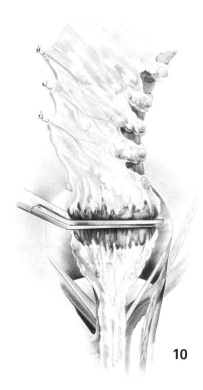

10

It is useful at this stage to place a 4 inch (10 cm) gauze pack into the presacral space in those patients having a low anterior resection which will protect the pelvic tissues from any inadvertent bowel content contamination.

The rectum is divided from right to left immediately below the angled clamp. As it is divided stay sutures are placed through all layers of the rectal wall to hold the rectal stump in a convenient position for the anastomosis. As division takes place it is useful to diathermy arterial bleeders in the submucosa to avoid the development of submucosal haematomas. If irrigation of the rectal stump has not been carried out below, it is convenient at this time to perform irrigation with syringe, cannula and suction until the rectal segment is clean.

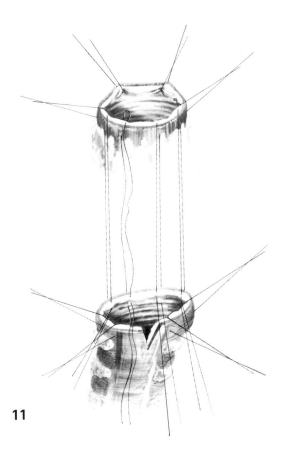

11

11

Set-up for the anastomosis

It is important to arrange the colon and rectal stump conveniently with stay sutures so that anastomotic sutures can be meticulously placed with an even distribution. An open technique of anastomosis is used. 3/0 Atraumatic black silk stay sutures are placed as illustrated. With the set-up of the anastomosis completed, a Cheatle slit in the anterior margin of the proximal colon may be conveniently performed to equalize the circumference of the bowel ends for anastomosis.

12 & 13

The anastomosis

The suture material for the single layer of interrupted sutures can be 3/0 silk, 3/0 green Dexon or 3/0 Vicryl. The posterior layer of the anastomosis is performed first and the initial four sutures placed are mattress sutures commencing on the colon stump. With traction on the mattress sutures the end of the colon can then be approximated to the rectal stump by gently sliding the colon along the mattress sutures which are then tied. With traction in turn on two adjacent mattress sutures, simple all-layer sutures can then be placed through the colon and rectum between the mattress sutures to complete the single layer on the posterior aspect of the anastomosis. To close the corners of the anastomosis, an inverting mattress suture is used. The single layer of interrupted sutures on the anterior aspect of the anastomosis is completed by using an inverted technique with sutures which pass obliquely through the muscle layer and submucosa of the colon wall without passing through the surface of the mucosa. It is important to obtain a definite 'bite' on the submucosal layer. When placing the anterior layer of sutures they are held in position without being tied until all anterior sutures are placed in position. When tied, these sutures satisfactorily invert the anterior layer. Correct tension on the tying of these sutures is important and approximation only is obtained to avoid ischaemic necrosis of the edge of the bowel used in anastomosis. At the conclusion of the anastomotic suture convenient pericolic and perirectal fatty tissue can be placed around the anastomosis but care must be exercised in using sutures in case small, but vital blood vessels are interfered with by such a manoeuvre.

After completion of the anastomosis the presacral gauze pack is removed and the pelvic cavity carefully inspected for small bleeders which are coagulated. The tape occluding the colon stump is removed. The mesenteric peritoneal defect may be closed to the right side of the anastomosis.

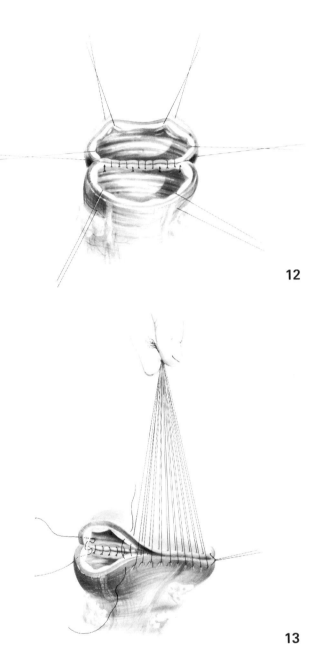

12

13

Drains

In uncomplicated resections of the sigmoid colon with minimal pelvic dissection and a satisfactory anastomosis, no drains will be necessary.

If chronic infective changes are present in the pelvis, the haemostasis may be difficult, delayed sepsis very likely to occur and drains will be required. Two, three or four 1 inch soft Penrose drains are placed into any residual area of inflammatory tissue and such drains brought out through a separate stab incision. If the pelvic dissection has been extensive and bare surfaces remain on to which the small bowel may adhere causing obstruction, then such Penrose drains can be also used to seal off the pelvis and anastomosis from small bowel adhesions.

When the presacral space is fully dissected, the likelihood of presacral haematoma formation is present and two Salem sump catheter drains are placed into this space through separate stab incisions and continuous suction-lavage (normal saline) used for 48 hr.

In the patients where Penrose drains are used to anticipate the delayed development of pelvic sepsis, these drains are removed at 7 days and replaced with a Foley catheter which is then used to irrigate the residual cavity for a prolonged period until the drain sinuses are healed. This manoeuvre prevents sequestration of pelvic pus around the anastomosis which may burst through the suture line after colo-rectal anastomosis.

Indications for proximal defunctioning colostomy

In the management of diverticular disease, the need for a complementary colostomy will vary according to the extent of the pathology requiring treatment and the degree of difficulty in performing an anastomosis with a good blood supply and healthy bowel wall. The author is at present using loop ileostomy more frequently than loop colostomy for proximal defunction of colorectal anastomosis but the indications are indentical.

(1) Difficulty in obtaining rectal wall without abnormality for colorectal anastomosis due to perirectal fibrosis and inflammatory changes.

(2) Any significant submucosal haematoma arising during anastomosis.

(3) In circumstances when the rectal stump has been manipulated to some excess in its mobilization, with minor trauma or intramural haematoma.

(4) Final concern about the blood supply to the colon segment despite the measures adopted to preserve it.

(5) An 'untidy closure' of the suture line due to thickening of the bowel wall despite attempts to use a normal rectal stump.

(6) Extensive chronic pelvic infection with residual inflammatory tissue in the pelvis after completion of the anastomosis.

(7) Inadequate preparation of the colon. If the colon contains formed faeces it may be preferable to stage the operation performing an initial colostomy. If the faecal content is not a contra-indication to resection then the operation may be complemented by a proximal colostomy.

(8) A prolonged operative procedure with excessive blood loss in a patient whose general health is not optimum, is probably best treated with a complementary colostomy.

Colovesical fistula

The management of a colovesical fistula is principally that of the diseased colon with its implications. The fistula in the bladder wall is usually not a difficult technical problem and may not be identifiable. The operation is usually performed in the chronic phase of diverticulitis and a preliminary colostomy followed by second-stage resection is usually unnecessary. Blunt digital dissection will separate the colon from the bladder and if a small defect is noted in the vault of the bladder (usual site) it can be closed with a single layer of 2/0 chromic catgut. On rare occasions a larger defect in the bladder wall is present nearer the trigone than the vault and under these circumstances excision of the defect in the wall of the bladder and a two-layer closure with interrupted 3/0 chromic and then 2/0 chromic sutures is performed. It is important to separate the bladder repair from the colorectal anastomosis and particularly so in the presence of chronic residual pelvic granulation tissue which will suppurate subsequently. The use of Penrose drains in this situation previously referred to will effectively separate these two areas of repair and prevent postoperative development of an anastomotic-vesical fistula should there be any defect in either closure. If omentum is available, it can be placed between the intestinal anastomosis and the bladder.

The indications to use a complementary transverse colostomy are those already referred to in colorectal anastomosis and they are not related specifically to the problem of colovesical fistula.

The bladder is drained with a urethral catheter for 10 days and during this period the urinary drainage is measured 4-hourly to ensure blockage of the catheter does not go undetected.

SPECIAL POSTOPERATIVE CARE

(1) Intravenous therapy continues for 5–7 days.

(2) Re-alimentation with a soft diet is usually commenced on the eighth day but only if the patient's abdomen is soft, not distended, flatus is passing per rectum and there is no nausea or vomiting.

(3) Intragastric aspiration is not used as a routine but is promptly carried out if the patient complains of persistent nausea, develops hiccoughs, vomits significant amounts of fluid or has a persistently distended abdomen.

(4) Attention to adequate breathing exercises and intermittent positive pressure therapy is often important.

(5) Attention to the lower limbs with physiotherapy and exercise is essential because of the risk of venous thrombosis.

(6) The urinary catheter is kept on continuous drainage and usually removed when the patient is well enough to sit on a commode (female) or stand (male) to void.

(7) Proper stomal care is essential for those patients with a defunctioning colostomy or ileostomy and the decision to close such stomas is made after radiological assessment of the anastomosis which is performed as a routine via the rectum on the fourteenth day. In patients with complicated pelvic diverticular disease with residual infection treated by extended surgery, there should be no hurry to close the stoma which is a further major procedure. These patients often benefit from a further few weeks of rest and recovery before the final stage of their procedure is performed.

(8) If a defect has occurred in the anastomosis demonstrated by extravasation of barium, then the stoma is not closed until the defect has healed. Serial barium enemas are performed to assess this at appropriate intervals depending on the size of the defect in the anastomosis. Some patients may develop a chronic small para-anastomotic cavity and if the healing appears to be static it is usually safe to close any defunctioning stoma without waiting for final resolution.

[The illustrations for this Chapter on Elective Operation for Sigmoid Diverticular Disease were drawn by Mr. R. Stokes.]

Acute Sigmoid Diverticular Disease

Mark Killingback, F.R.C.S., F.R.C.S. (Ed.), F.R.A.C.S.,
Surgeon, Edward Wilson Colon and Rectum Unit,
Sydney Hospital, Sydney

INTRODUCTION

Of patients suffering from acute diverticulitis with sufficient signs of peritonitis to warrant emergency surgery, the pathology is one of three groups of equal distribution.

(*1*) *Acute phlegmonous diverticulitis.* In most instances this condition will settle with antibiotics but clinically a precise pre-operative pathological diagnosis is not possible and surgery is undertaken because the clinical signs of peritonitis warrant it.

(*2*) *Localized abscess* around the colon or in the pelvis with peritonitis. This pathology is only appreciated after assessment at laparotomy. Such abscesses may cause a spreading of pus from the pelvis to the abdominal cavity causing generalized peritonitis. Alternatively, they may partially resolve and if not treated surgically during the acute phase, become chronic and require surgery later.

(*3*) *Free perforation* from the lumen of the colon in communication with the peritoneal cavity is the most hazardous of the three groups. The size of the perforation varies considerably. It is in this group that faecal peritonitis may occur (25–30 per cent) leading to more serious sequelae of intra-abdominal infection.

In approximately 75 per cent of all patients, the acute peritonitis is the first sign of diverticular disease and it therefore does not represent a predictable sequence in chronic diverticular disease. The most important considerations in the management of severe acute diverticulitis are saving the patient's life and preventing morbidity from intra-abdominal infection. Definitive surgical treatment of diverticular disease is not the aim of surgical treatment under such circumstances.

Pre-operative preparation

A haemoglobin estimation, blood for the operation and an x-ray of the chest and abdomen are essential. If a perforation has occurred, free gas on the abdominal x-ray will be present in 40 per cent of such patients.

In the seriously ill patient with peritonitis, dehydration and possibly septicaemia, serum electrolytes, blood culture, blood biochemistry, blood gases and electrocardiograph are desirable. After a period of appropriate resuscitation surgery should be undertaken as early as possible. It is not relevant in these patients to attempt bowel preparation. Rectal enemas are contra-indicated. Parenteral antibiotics suitable to treat infection of colonic origin such as a cephalosporin and gentamicin should be commenced before operation.

Assessment of pathology at operation

At operation the pathology should be identified accurately because the surgical management is not the same for all patients.

It should be noted that carcinoma of the colon may produce similar clinicopathological features to acute diverticulitis and at laparotomy it may be difficult to distinguish. If, however, a free perforation of a carcinoma of the colon is present, then excision is necessary. If a carcinoma is associated with a phlegmonous, non-perforated inflammatory lesion, then the patient can also be treated by immediate resection but if the circumstances and facilities are less favourable, this can be managed conservatively by peritoneal toilet and antibiotics.

To diagnose the acute phlegmonous diverticulitis or to find a paracolic or pelvic abscess the surgeon may use gentle digital or sucker dissection of the tissues being careful not to damage the oedematous small bowel or colon and create further problems. The pus must be looked for in the paracolic gutter and in the depths of the pelvis (often obscured by a prolapsed sigmoid loop) and between adjacent loops of bowel. If an abscess is not detected at operation it will become chronic and inevitably require surgical treatment later.

A perforation should be identified if present because the surgical treatment is more radical. It must be searched for gently and no probing of the bowel wall or mesentery should be undertaken lest a near perforation be converted to a free perforation by the surgeon.

Soft, small bowel adhesions may need releasing, some of which may be causing overt small bowel obstruction, an associated complication which is present in 20 per cent of these patients.

THE OPERATION

An adequate lower mid-line incision is made and may be extended to the pubis or above the umbilicus.

The management depends on the pathology found at laparotomy:

1

Laparotomy and drainage

This is recommended for (*1*) Acute phlegmonous diverticulitis where there is no perforation of the wall of the colon is treated by drainage with a soft 2–5 cm Penrose drain placed near the phlegmon and brought out through a separate stab incision. (*2*) An acute paracolic or pelvic abscess should be debrided gently, the pus sucked away and two or three 2 or 5 cm Penrose drains placed into the abscess cavity and brought out through a separate stab incision.

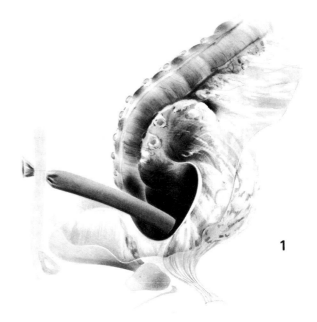

1

A defunctioning transverse colostomy is not recommended in these two pathological groups associated with peritonitis as there is no evidence that it improves the prognosis. The colon distal to the colostomy will always contain faeces and therefore the colostomy will not prevent continuing contamination of the peritoneal cavity when it is most needed, i.e. immediately subsequent to surgery. A further important consideration is the subsequent management of the patient. Acute diverticulitis which warrants emergency surgery, if treated by adequate drainage alone can resolve to a remarkable extent and if the patient is not treated with a proximal loop colostomy, then the option is available for the surgeon to avoid resection of the sigmoid colon. If, however, a colostomy is present, the surgeon is committed to proceed to resection rather than close the colostomy. There are also elderly patients, who, having survived the first stage of such surgery, will be left 'stranded' with a loop colostomy.

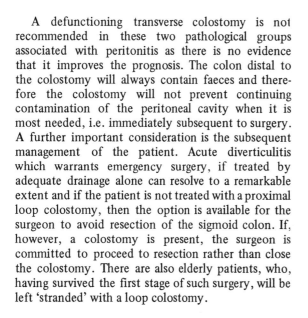

Laparotomy — resection of sigmoid colon

The colon with a free perforation with communication between its lumen and the peritoneal cavity must be removed from the abdomen and this is best achieved by excision without anastomosis. Occasionally a small perforation in the mesocolon fat is present associated with a short 'fistula' leading into a perforated diverticulum and this is best treated by excision also. It is important to complete the operation quickly, particularly, in those patients who have a severe peritoneal infection. This is not the occasion for meticulous attention to anastomotic technique with possible dissection of the splenic flexure and presacral space. In a seriously ill, poorly prepared patient the risk of anastomotic leak is higher than under ideal surgical circumstances.

2

The sigmoid colon is mobilized by dividing the peritoneal attachment in the left paracolic gutter and reflecting the mesentery of the colon medially, identifying the gonadal vessels and ureter. Usually blunt digital dissection is ideal in the oedematous tissue planes and in these circumstances damage to adjacent structures is less likely to occur. First, second and third sigmoid vessels are divided clear of the inferior mesenteric vessel bundle which is preserved usually to nourish the rectosigmoid stump. A conservative excision of the inflamed sigmoid is adequate and a search for proximal and distal diverticula should not be made. The colon proximally and distally needs only to be excised through non-inflamed tissue to cope with the emergency situation. Absorbable ligature material should be used to prevent subsequent infection around ligated vessels.

Proximal colon stump

After division of the proximal colon between clamps, the end of the colon can be brought through a muscle-splitting incision in the left side of the abdomen immediately lateral to the rectus sheath, bearing in mind that it must be a suitable site for stomal appliances. A circle of skin is excised over this incision which must permit the passage of two fingers to avoid a narrow abdominal wall tunnel which might compress the blood supply of the emerging colon. A small glass rod can be placed through the mesentery to hold the colon on the abdominal wall and an immediate mucocutaneous suture performed with 3/0 chromic catgut as an interrupted suture. No attempt is made to close the left paracolic gutter lateral to the emerging colostomy.

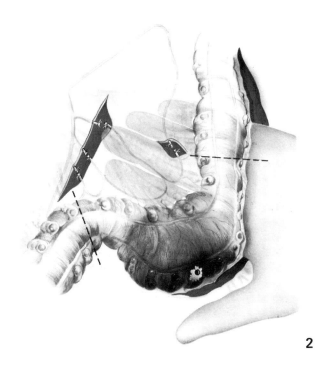

2

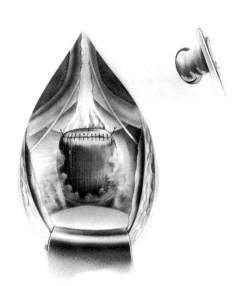

3

Distal rectal or rectosigmoid stump

3

Closure of stump

The distal line of resection is usually too low to bring the rectosigmoid through the lower end of the mid-line wound as a mucous fistula. It is important, however, not to make this stump any shorter than is necessary and only to excise the inflamed area of bowel. In the presence of peritoneal infection it is not desirable to dissect the presacral space. The rectal stump should be oversewn with a single layer of interrupted 3/0 absorbable sutures (green Dexon or Vicryl). The stump can then be hitched to the presacral tissue with an interrupted suture on each side which will avoid prolapse of the stump into the pelvis and subsequently facilitate dissection and anastomosis at the second stage.

4

Distal mucous fistula

A distal mucous fistula can be made in less frequent circumstances when there is sufficient length of distal colon available after excision of the inflamed sigmoid. The colon can be brought through the lower end of the mid-line wound which is closed around the colon leaving at least one finger's clearance to avoid compression of the blood supply. One or two sutures can be used between the linea alba and the mesentery of the colon to prevent recession of the colostomy. A Zachary-Cope clamp is left attached to the bowel for 4 days and subsequently removed in the ward.

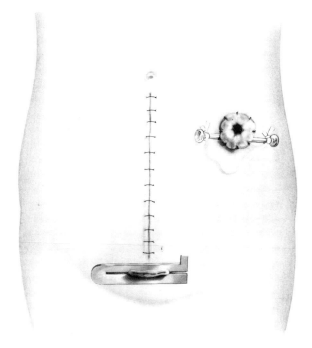

4

An open intrapelvic rectal stump

In some circumstances the patient may have a very short rectal stump and the surgeon may wish to avoid the extra operating time in closing the stump. This should be avoided. The effectiveness of drainage tubes via the rectum into the pelvis is poor because of the action of the anal sphincters and this circumstance inevitably leads to continuing pelvic infection after operation making the subsequent anastomosis a much more difficult undertaking.

Drains

After completion of excision without anastomosis and with adequate peritoneal toilet no drains may be required. If, however, there are any areas in the abdomen or pelvis where the haemostasis is not entirely satisfactory or residual areas of granulation tissue remain, two or more soft 2 or 5 cm Penrose drains should be placed in the abdomen or pelvis and brought out through a separate stab incision. Drains are replaced with a Foley catheter on the seventh day and continued irrigation of these drain sinuses is necessary until they heal.

Peritoneal toilet

In all cases generous intra-operative peritoneal lavage with saline is indicated. If general peritonitis of the abdominal cavity is present the subphrenic spaces should be thoroughly lavaged. Intraperitoneal antibiotics at operation and continuing postoperative lavage of the peritoneal cavity by peritoneal catheter is not practised by the author.

SPECIAL POSTOPERATIVE CARE

Intravenous therapy, parenteral antibiotics and vigorous support of respiratory function are all essential in these patients, particularly the elderly who are also suffering co-existent medical diseases.

A few patients who have been treated with laparotomy and drainage will develop a colocutaneous fistula along the drain site but this will usually not be a serious intra-abdominal or pelvic extension of infection. It will, however, indicate that subsequent resection of the sigmoid colon is necessary.

Excision without anastomosis will require reconnection of the colon at a later time and this is preferably undertaken when the patient is fully recovered from the previous effects of abdominal and pelvic sepsis. If clinical signs of recovery are evident, then anastomosis should be performed 6–12 weeks after the initial laparotomy.

Reference

Killingback, M. J. (1967–1971). 'Emergency surgery for peritonitis due to acute diverticulitis.' *Royal Australasian College of Surgeons Survey*

[*The illustrations for this Chapter on Acute Sigmoid Diverticular Disease were drawn by Mr. R. Stokes.*]

Operations for Complications of Diverticular Disease

C. V. Mann, M.Ch., F.R.C.S.
Consultant Surgeon, St. Mark's Hospital, London
and The London Hospital

COLECTOMY FOR ACUTE DIVERTICULITIS

INTRODUCTION

Many patients have diverticular changes in the colon without suffering more than constipation and mild discomfort in the left iliac fossa. The differential diagnosis from other diseases such as the spastic (irritable) colon syndrome can be very difficult, and some patients have severe symptoms without objective evidence of inflammatory complications being found when operation is performed. The diagnosis of acute inflammatory complications from diverticular disease is open to serious error, both negatively and positively.

For these reasons, surgery has usually been advocated only when there are clear indications of inflammatory complications; such evidence is usually based on radiological findings.

However, diverticular disease is potentially very dangerous, and now that operations are much safer due to good anaesthesia and antibiotics, the patient is being given the benefit of doubt to an increasing extent, even when objective evidence of acute inflammatory complications cannot be obtained by clinical or radiological investigation.

PRE-OPERATIVE

Indications

Colectomy for acute diverticulitis is indicated when the inflammation is localized to a resectable area of the colon (usually the sigmoid colon), and there are no other contra-indications.

Contra-indications

If the area of inflammation is so extensive and severe that the technical problems of resection become so formidable as to make the surgery unreasonably hazardous, the operation should not be performed. Each surgeon must form his own judgment as to where he will draw the line, but generally the decision should err on the side of extreme caution.

If severe complications are present, e.g. obstruction, perforation, peritonitis or vesicocolic fistula, resection should be deferred for several months while other measures, such as a temporary colostomy, allow the diseased area to settle enough for a more favourable local environment to develop for the resection to be performed. (Turnbull has described this as 'allowing the pelvic inflammatory nest to clean itself'.)

Many patients with acute diverticulitis are old, extremely obese or have severe atheromatous disease of the cardiovascular system. More than a few are diabetic. In such patients, a staged operation, starting with a preliminary colostomy, is safer than a one-stage colectomy.

Preparation

If circumstances permit, the colon should be emptied by a low-residue diet and the use of enemas. Laxatives must be avoided when acute inflammatory changes are present.

Antibiotics should be given both systemically (ampicillin 250 mg intramuscularly every 6 hr) and orally (neomycin 1g every 8 hr) over the period of the operation. If possible, this regime should start 24 hr before the operation, and in the case of the neomycin longer than this, if possible.

Position of patient

The operation should be performed using the Lloyd-Davies stirrups, so that the rectum can be washed out prior to performing the anastomosis.

Anaesthesia

General anaesthesia is required. A nasogastric tube should be passed to empty the stomach prior to induction. Intubation to facilitate the use of muscle relaxants is desirable.

Non-operative treatment

Whenever possible, non-operative treatment is employed.

THE OPERATION

1

Special points for resection

If operation is required for acute sigmoid diverticulitis *without* complications (e.g. pericolic abscess or peritonitis), an ideal resection includes the following points:

(*I*) All inflamed or abnormal colon should be removed, leaving a good margin of normal tissue.

(*II*) The lower limit of resection should be below the rectosigmoid junction.

(*III*) The blood vessels can be divided near to the colon for greater safety, in contrast to a resection for carcinoma when the arteries are divided as close to their origin as is feasible to achieve the maximum clearance of possibly involved lymph glands.

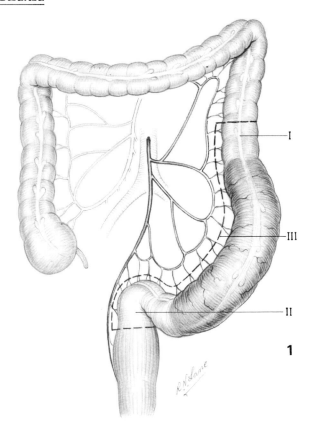

1

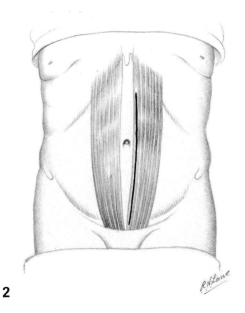

2

2

Preliminary exploration

The approach is through a long left paramedian incision. Since most patients with diverticular disease are obese, the wound should extend well above the umbilicus and down to just above the pubis.

The operation starts with a *limited* examination of the abdomen so as not to spread infection unnecessarily throughout the abdominal cavity. However, the liver should be inspected first in case an unsuspected carcinoma is present in the area of diverticulitis that may have caused hepatic metastases to be present already. After this, the operator can inspect the left colon, and decide whether a resection is indicated.

The decision whether to institute a colostomy to 'cover' the resection is made at this stage.

3

Colostomy cover for resection

If a covering colostomy is required, a loop colostomy in the right half of the transverse colon is the usual procedure (*see* page 211). If, however, prolonged and complete diversion of faecal material appears necessary because of the extensive area and unusual severity of the inflammation, a Devine-type colostomy is indicated (illustrated). If a Devine-style colostomy is required, it is not usually wise to proceed to immediate resection. Note that in the modern method of fashioning this form of stoma, it is not necessary to stitch the adjacent loops of transverse colon together to form a spur that can be crushed subsequently; the mesentery and omentum are divided just sufficiently to allow adequate separation of the divided ends of transverse colon, which are then brought individually to the surface through the rectus on either side of the mid-line.

Editorial comment. This procedure must be very rarely necessary nowadays.

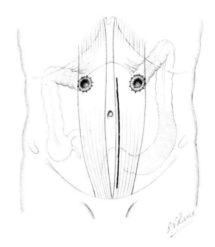

3

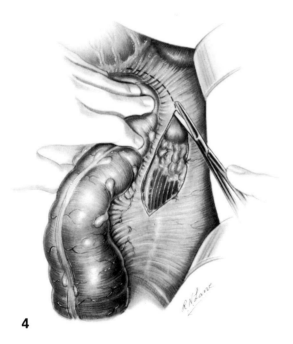

4

4

Mobilization of colon

After the surgeon has satisfied himself about the diagnosis, the extent of the resection to be performed can be decided. This will usually be almost the whole of the left colon, and include the rectosigmoid junction.

The first step in the operation is to free the parietal peritoneum on the lateral aspect of the colon, and this is best started superiorly away from the area of inflammation.

Mobilization of the splenic flexure of the colon by division of the phrenicocolic and colosplenic 'ligaments' is optimally done at the beginning of the operation.

Soon after the commencement of the division of the parietal peritoneum, the ureter should be identified in the upper and medial part of the dissection and its safety ensured during the subsequent colon mobilization as it proceeds in a caudal direction.

5

Vascular ligation

The vessels supplying the colon can be divided where convenient, and close to the bowel. The main trunk of the inferior mesenteric artery need not be divided, so that the full blood supply to the rectum is preserved.

As the mesentery is usually bulky and fat-laden, unabsorbable material (0/0 linen thread) is safer than chromic catgut for the arterial ligatures.

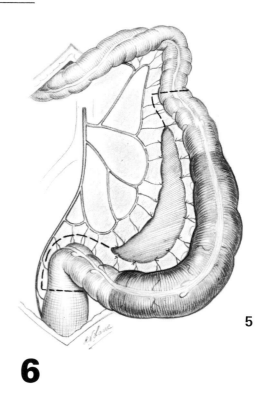

5

6

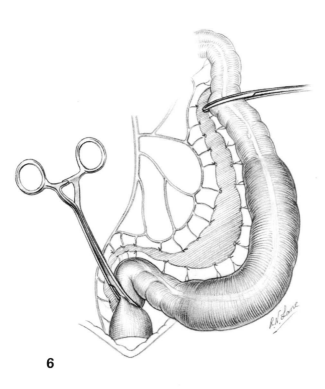

6

Division of colon

As preliminary bowel preparation has been imperfect in the acute case, and the rectum is usually thick-walled as well as wide, light clamps are likely to slip and allow faecal contamination. For this reason, strong crushing clamps should be applied before division of the bowel. Two pairs of Parker-Kerr clamps are ideal.

After the inflamed loop of colon has been removed, the ends of the clamps left on the bowel should be cleaned with an antiseptic solution (1 : 2000 Hibitane) and the surgeon should check that the clamps can be approximated without tension, for the anastomosis, and carefully preserving the correct alignment of the mesentery, i.e. making sure that the colon is not twisted.

It can be helpful in making the anastomosis easier if the clamps are applied prior to division so that when they are approximated the mesenteric edges (which are the most difficult to turn in) are not directly opposite to each other. This can be achieved by applying the rectal clamps in a sagittal plane prior to division, while cross-clamping the colon proximally in the usual transverse manner (*see Illustration 6*).

7

End-to-end anastomosis

Prior to anastomosis, the rectum should be washed out with an antiseptic solution (1 : 2000 Hibitane) until no faecal material remains in the lower stump. The proximal colon should have any faeces or air milked back by the fingers from the area of the anastomosis, and a spring clamp should be applied of a non-crushing type (curved Doyen clamps are very good for this purpose) several inches from the end of the colon; after this, the Parker-Kerr clamp can be cut away and the terminal part of the colon beyond the Doyen clamp is swabbed out with the same antiseptic solution until it is clean. After the lower crushing clamp has been removed with a scalpel, the two clean ends of bowel are ready for an end-to-end anastomosis by a one-layer technique. The absence of clamps makes the anastomosis easier, safer and quicker.

The material used in the anastomosis should be 0/0 silk or linen thread. Interrupted horizontal mattress sutures are used for the posterior layer, leaving the knots on the exterior of the bowel. As the corners are reached, the stitches are changed to Connell-type interrupted (loop on the mucosa) inverting stitches, which are continued on the anterior layer.

After the ends have been united, adjoining appendices epiploicae can be used to re-inforce the suture line by tying them across the anastomosis with the long ends of the stitches.

The edges of the mesentery are then joined by a running stitch of 0/0 chromic catgut.

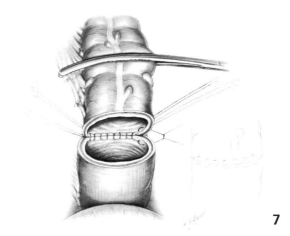

7

8

Drainage and closure

The anastomosis is drained by a soft plastic or corrugated rubber drain brought out retroperitoneally through a separate flank incision. The drain should not abut directly onto the anastomosis, but should repose in the pericolic area. A tube drain should not be used as it can cause erosion of vessels on the pelvic wall and precipitate a serious secondary haemorrhage.

The abdominal wound should be closed in layers in the usual way, but a topical antibiotic applied in the wound is advisable, as many of these wounds become septic.

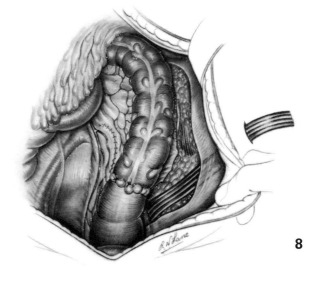

8

9

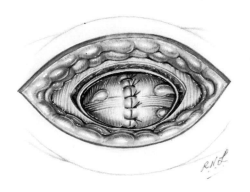

Closure of colostomy

If the operation site has been protected by a temporary covering loop transverse colostomy, this can be closed between 4 and 6 weeks after the resection. Before the colostomy is closed, patency and soundness of the anastomosis should be tested by a barium enema. If a leak is discovered at the join, closure of the stoma should be delayed for a further 4 weeks.

The colostomy should be closed intraperitoneally (*see* page 217).

9

POSTOPERATIVE CARE AND COMPLICATIONS

This is similar to the care of a patient after any major colonic resection. Postoperative ileus may be more prolonged and the tendency to acute postoperative gastric distension may be greater after a resection where the inflammatory changes have been pronounced; for these reasons, nasogastric suction should be maintained during the postoperative period until unequivocal evidence of intestinal activity has been manifested. Because the anastomosis may be subjected to extra strain by reason of the pathophysiological aetiology of the disease, when a primary resection has been performed it may be desirable to control the timing and force of the return of colonic peristalsis; probanthine 5 mg every 6 hr (administered either intravenously or intramuscularly) can be a useful drug for this purpose, but should not be used if there is any history of ophthalmological or cardiac disorder.

Complications

Anastomotic disruption is the complication that is feared most. This usually occurs between the fifth and seventh postoperative days and may be either a small leak or a major breakdown with accompanying peritonitis.

If a small leak has occurred, there is usually little change in the general condition of the patient, although there is usually a moderate rise in the pulse rate and a mild pyrexia, which is followed by the discharge of faecal material from the drain site. Providing the loss of faeces is not excessive and the bowels continue to function *per anum*, the fistula will probably close spontaneously and an expectant conservative policy can be adopted.

If a major disruption has taken place, the patient quickly becomes ill, and there are signs of local peritonitis, which rapidly becomes more general. Urgent surgical re-intervention is required, with the object of peritoneal toilet and the formation of a proximal colostomy. It is not possible to repair the anastomosis at this stage.

Wound sepsis is very common after operation for diverticulitis. This can be reduced by proper preoperative bowel preparation (when this is possible) and meticulous technique. Broad-spectrum antibiotics administered topically and systemically also help to reduce the incidence of wound abscess.

Anastomotic stenosis and recurrence of diverticulitis

Narrowing of the anastomosis and the development of new areas of diverticular disease both occur as late problems after successful operations for diverticulitis. There is evidence that the risks of these late problems developing can be reduced by the regular use of bran (one tablespoonful twice daily) or hydrophyllic colloids (Cologel, Isogel, Normacol—one tablespoonful once or twice daily), which seems to correct the underlying problems of muscular hypertrophy and raised intraluminal pressures.

INCISION OF PERICOLIC ABSCESS

THE OPERATION

10

If the abscess has pointed to the surface of the abdomen, simple incision over the apical point is all that is required. A drain is not usually necessary.

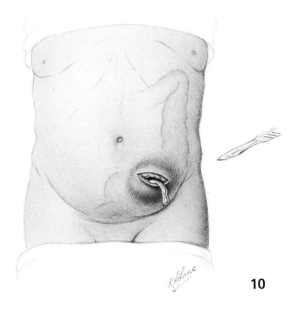

10

11

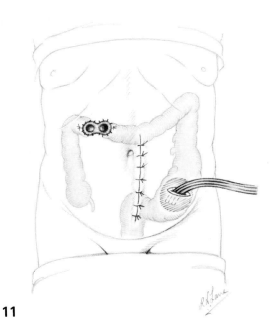

11

If a large collection of pus develops, and neither points to the surface nor discharges spontaneously into the colon or rectum, it may be necessary to institute formal drainage.

The abscess is approached through a left lower paramedian incision. Under direct control, a large drain is introduced into the cavity through a separate stab incision in the left flank; if possible, the general peritoneal cavity is not contaminated. A temporary loop colostomy in the transverse colon is usually required.

OPERATION FOR DIVERTICULITIS WITH PERITONITIS

PRE - OPERATIVE

Indications

This is an acute abdominal emergency which must be operated upon without delay. The typical picture is of an obese middle-aged woman seized with sudden lower abdominal pain—most often in the left lower quadrant, but not invariably so. There is usually fever, vomiting and constipation and the patient is usually much iller than is the case with other lower abdominal inflammations, e.g. appendicitis or salpingitis. On plain x-ray of the abdomen, free gas is demonstrable in the abdominal cavity. Although the other signs of peritonitis are present, ileus may be absent in the early stages (in contrast to the usual findings in perforated peptic ulcer).

Pre-operative treatment

Immediately the diagnosis is surmised, a nasogastric tube should be passed and continuous aspiration started; at the same time, an intravenous infusion is set up (normal saline is usually the best solution to use at this stage). A central venous catheter to monitor the haemodynamic state of the patient is desirable.

Systemic antibiotic treatment is given from the beginning, with the choice of drugs used based on the usual organisms present in the colon: ampicillin (500 mg) plus gentamicin (1 mg/kg body weight) every 6 hr is satisfactory.

Serum should be sent to the laboratory as soon as possible, so that blood loss can be corrected during surgery as it occurs. This can be severe if the diagnosis is proved wrong and a colonic resection becomes necessary (a stercoral perforation behind a carcinoma of the sigmoid colon can present an identical clinical picture).

A catheter should be passed of a self-retaining type, both to empty the bladder prior to operation and to measure the output of urine postoperatively.

Anaesthesia

A general anaesthetic is essential. Since further operations may be required within a short time, certain anaesthetic agents (e.g. halothane) may be contra-indicated if suitable alternatives are available.

Position of patient

No special position is necessary.

THE OPERATION

12

Incision

As it is usually possible to make the diagnosis before surgery, a left lower paramedian incision is used.

When the peritoneum is incised, gas and a thin purulent exudate escape from the hole and are sucked away. A swab for purposes of culture of bacteria is taken and sent to the laboratory immediately. The wound is made sufficiently large to allow adequate and safe exploration of the affected area.

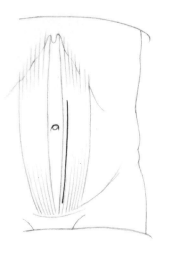

12

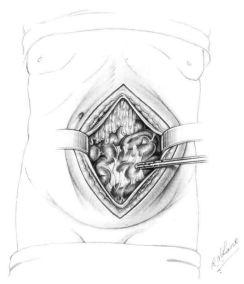

13

Examination of perforation

Omentum and adherent loops of small intestine can be freed and retracted without great difficulty. The inflamed perforated sigmoid colon can then be inspected.

It is not possible usually to close the perforation as the oedematous bowel wall does not hold stitches. Depending on the condition of the patient and the skill and experience of the operator, as well as the local situation, a decision is made as to whether a resection is possible.

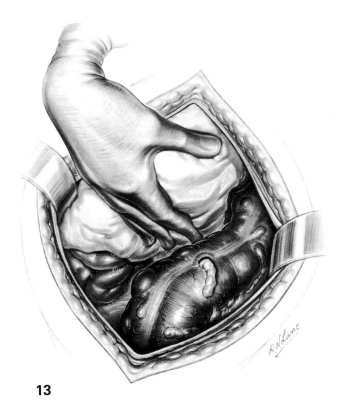

13

14

Excision of inflamed perforated colon

Excision of the colon is carried out in the same way as for diverticulitis uncomplicated by perforation, but a more conservative margin of normal colon is usually made necessary by the need for speed and the undesirability of spreading pus too widely in the peritoneal cavity and retroperitoneal tissues.

Since a primary resection under the circumstances prevailing leaves a minimal margin of normal colon (or relatively normal colon), an immediate re-anastomosis may be very dangerous; under these conditions a Hartmann-type procedure may be the best operation (*see Illustration 14*).

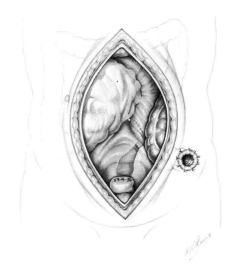

14

15

Drainage of perforation and transverse colostomy

Except under exceptional circumstances, a primary excision will not be chosen for a patient with perforation/peritonitis. Usually, the pus will be sucked out and a drain inserted in the left iliac fossa. Omentum can often be brought down and stitched over the perforation site. The wound is closed in layers, but tension sutures are advisable. A covering temporary transverse colostomy in the right end of the transverse colon is then performed and opened immediately.

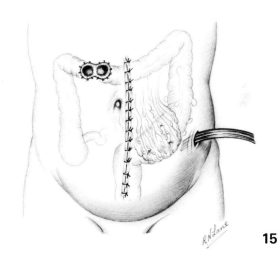

15

POSTOPERATIVE CARE

Early postoperative care

The intravenous infusion and the nasogastric suction are continued until the postoperative ileus has resolved. The drain is removed after 5–8 days.

The antibiotic treatment is continued and altered as the results of the bacterial culture swabs are obtained.

Chest complications, venous thrombosis and embolism are common after this serious emergency; extra precautions should be taken to avert or minimize them. The use of subcutaneous low-dose heparin (calcium heparin 5000 units every 8 hr) can be considered to prevent the danger of pulmonary embolism.

Late postoperative care

Early evaluation (about 6 weeks) of the sigmoid colon by a barium enema is necessary to avoid the risk of overlooking a carcinoma which has been impossible to diagnose at the time of the perforation/peritonitis. Otherwise, early re-operation is not required, and resection of the affected area of colon should not be carried out for at least 3 months. If a Hartmann procedure has been performed, the delay should be even longer so that the best chance is created of primary re-anastomosis without a covering colostomy.

OPERATION FOR DIVERTICULITIS WITH OBSTRUCTION

PRE - OPERATIVE

Introduction

No special operative procedure is required for this situation. After the preliminary laparotomy has confirmed the diagnosis; the obstruction is relieved by a temporary transverse loop colostomy.

Pre-operative treatment

Gastro-intestinal decompression by a nasogastric tube or continuous suction is instituted at once and an intravenous infusion of normal saline started.

Operation should not be unduly delayed, but at least one soap and water enema should be given before surgery, as this can occasionally relieve the obstruction and make immediate operation unnecessary.

Since there is always an element of active diverticulitis accompanying the stenosis responsible for the blockage, a systemic broad-spectrum antibiotic (ampicillin 500 mg every 6 hr) should be given to cover the operation and the first few postoperative days.

Anaesthesia

A general anaesthetic is necessary. A cuffed endo-tracheal tube confers extra safety from the danger of back-flow from the stomach spilling over into the lungs.

Position of patient

No special position is necessary for the operation.

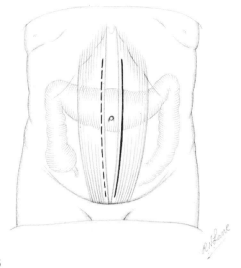

16

THE OPERATION

16

The incision

If there is doubt about the diagnosis, the abdomen is opened through a right paramedian incision. Otherwise a left paramedian incision is employed.

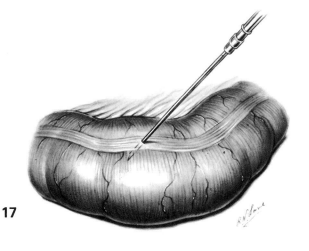

17

17

Colonic decompression

If the colon is grossly distended, suction decompression by a large needle at several points will relieve the gaseous distension of the colon. This makes it easier to draw out a loop of transverse colon through a reasonably short incision without danger of rupturing the thin tense wall of the bowel.

18

Transverse colostomy

This is formed in the transverse colon as far to the right as is possible. A 3 inch transverse incision is made through the rectus above and to the right of the umbilicus. The loop of transverse colon is then drawn through and held by a rod through the mesentery. The colostomy is opened immediately, and the edges of the colonic mucosa are sutured to the surrounding skin on either side of the rod by interrupted 0/0 chromic catgut stitches.

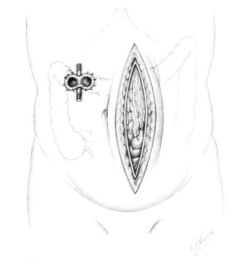

18

19

Wound closure

The incision is closed in layers as usual. As the abdomen has been distended before and during the operation and this condition may persist for some days postoperatively, wound disruption is more likely to occur than normally; re-inforcing tension sutures should be used, therefore, to give additional support to the wound postoperatively.

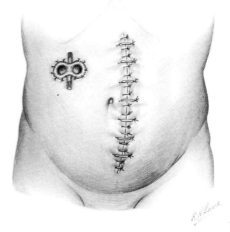

19

POSTOPERATIVE CARE

The rod supporting the colostomy can be removed between the eighth and tenth postoperative days. The definitive operation to remove the diseased area of sigmoid colon containing the stricture can be proceeded with after 2–3 weeks, providing the patient has made a full recovery.

If a right paramedian incision has been used at the first operation to relieve the obstruction, a parallel left paramedian incision should not be made until several months have passed, to avoid devitalizing the intervening mid-line strip of tissue. Alternatively, the formal sigmoid colectomy should be performed through a transverse lower abdominal incision of the Rutherford-Morrison type.

The colostomy should be closed 4–6 weeks after the sigmoid colectomy has been carried out.

Complications

Colostomy prolapse

Prolapse of the transverse colostomy frequently occurs. Since the stoma is temporary, no action for this is required until the time for closure of the colostomy.

OPERATION FOR ACUTE DIVERTICULITIS WITH HAEMORRHAGE

PRE - OPERATIVE

Indications

Unless the bleeding point can be identified with complete certainty, a total colectomy with ileorectal anastomosis is the only sure way to arrest a massive haemorrhage due to diverticulitis and to prevent further (and frequently fatal) bleeds. Every effort must be made to locate the bleeding site, and emergency barium enema studies, mesenteric angiography and colonoscopy can separately and collectively assist in both diagnosis of the cause and localization of the source of the haemorrhage.

Since surgical control of the bleeding is by major colonic resection (often an unprepared bowel), conservative management with replacement of blood losses is always given a good trial before operation is resorted to. In the conservative treatment, the administration of broad-spectrum antibiotics can greatly assist in arresting the bleeding, and prevent further episodes by suppressing the inflammatory changes responsible for the secondary haemorrhage from the artery in the colon wall. There is some evidence that the diagnostic barium enema studies also help to stop the bleeding, but the mechanism is not known.

Anaesthesia and position of patient

These are the same as for total or partial colectomy (*see* pages 118–132). The legs should be raised on Lloyd-Davies' supports so that the rectal stump can be washed out.

THE OPERATION

For details of the operation of total colectomy *see* pages 13–18. Otherwise, a right or left hemicolectomy may be required if the bleeding point is identified in one or other half of the colon (*see* pages 95–105).

POSTOPERATIVE CARE AND COMPLICATIONS

These are the same as after any major colonic resection, except that diarrhoea may be especially troublesome after total colectomy. For severe diarrhoea, codeine phosphate (30–60 mg daily), Lomotil (1–2 tablets every 6 hr) and Isogel (20 ml twice or three times daily) may be effective; occasionally, a bile-acid antagonist (cholestyramine 12 g twice daily) is required to achieve good control.

OPERATION FOR DIVERTICULITIS WITH VESICOCOLIC FISTULA
PRE - OPERATIVE

Indications

Once the diagnosis is established (by the history of pneumaturia, the recurrent or persistent urinary infections, the radiological demonstration of the fistula by barium enema and the cystoscopic appearance) a preliminary temporary right transverse colostomy may be performed and left for 2–3 months to allow the urinary infection to settle and the diverticulitis to subside.

If the patient is fit, the urinary sepsis mild and the diverticular changes on the barium enema are localized to a small area, a definitive operation may be planned without a preliminary colostomy: it is important before deciding on this to pass a cystoscope immediately before the operation and if (unexpectedly) severe cystitis is found, a preliminary colostomy should be done.

Preparation of patient

The urinary infection should be sterilized by the appropriate antibiotics and renal function restored to normal before a definitive procedure is carried out.

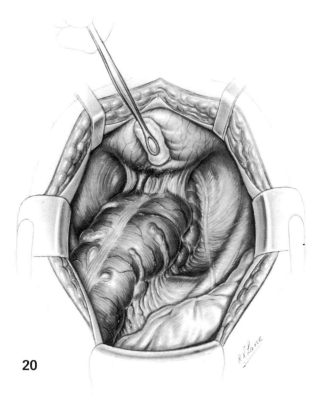

20

This may be impossible without a preliminary colostomy, as indicated above.

If a definitive operation is planned without a preliminary diversion, full preparation of the colon by antibiotics, laxatives and enemas should be carried out before the operation (*see* page 95).

A self-retaining catheter should be passed before the operation.

Anaesthesia

A general anaesthetic is required.

Position of patient

The patient's legs should be raised on Lloyd-Davies' supports so that the preliminary cystoscopy can be performed and the rectum washed out if necessary prior to a colorectal anastomosis.

THE OPERATION

Preliminary cystoscopy

The site of the fistula varies, but is most frequently above and lateral to the left ureteric orifice. Owing to oedema of the surrounding bladder mucosa, the actual opening may be impossible to make out. Sometimes a central depression may be discerned in the middle of the zone of inflammation from which gas bubbles may be expressed by pressure on the descending colon.

If the fistula is very close to the ureteric orifice, a catheter should be left *in situ* to allow identification of the ureter if a colonic resection is embarked upon.

The incision

The fistula is approached through a left paramedian incision.

20

Demonstration of the fistula

After the small bowel has been freed and adhesions divided, the site of the fistula will be evident by the area of attachment of the colon to the bladder. If a preliminary colostomy is not already in place, a decision is made at this stage whether to do this or proceed at once to a formal resection.

If resection is proposed, the patient is placed in a steep Trendelenburg position.

21

Dissection of the fistula

By sharp dissection, and keeping more on the bladder side, the colon is detached from the bladder, and the defects in both viscera displayed. Suction is used to prevent soiling of the peritoneal cavity by urine and faeces.

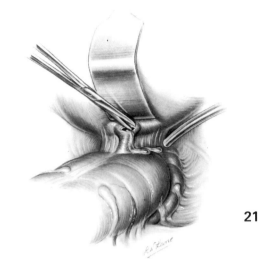

21

22

Repair of bladder defect

The oedematous edges of the bladder opening are trimmed back to normal tissue (taking care not to injure the ureter) and the defect is then closed in two layers—the inner of 0/0 chromic catgut and the outer of 0/0 silk.

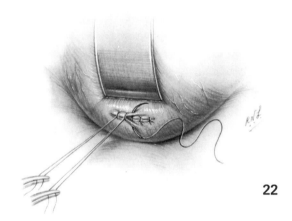

22

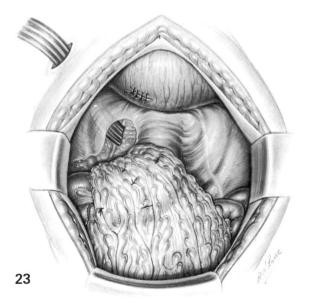

23

23

Removal of diseased colon and placing of omentum

The area of sigmoid colon affected by diverticular changes is resected, including the fistulous defect. The bowel is rejoined end-to-end in the usual way by a one-layer anastomosis of 0/0 linen thread or silk.

Omentum is brought down and sutured in position between the two anastomoses. A drain is introduced to the operation site in the usual way through a separate stab wound in the left iliac fossa.

POSTOPERATIVE CARE

Continuous urinary drainage through a closed system with an antiseptic seal should be continued postoperatively for 7–10 days. After the catheter is removed, normal micturition should be established within 12 hr, or the catheter should be replaced and a further 7 day period of continuous drainage carried out before the catheter is finally discarded.

It may take many months before the urine becomes completely sterile again.

The abdominal drain should be removed after 5 days.

The colostomy, if one has been used, should be closed 4 weeks after the fistula has been repaired.

Complications

If a formal resection is carried out without a covering colostomy, the two anastomoses may adhere and the fistula re-form. Omental interposition may reduce the chances of this happening, but a conservative approach and a willingness to perform a preliminary colostomy are the only certain ways to avoid this catastrophe.

References

Devine, H. (1938). *Surgery* **3**, 165
Goligher, J. C. (1967). *Surgery of the Anus, Rectum and Colon,* p. 1059, 2nd Edition. London: Balliere, Tindall and Cassell
Goligher, J. C. (1967). *Surgery of the Anus, Rectum and Colon,* p. 1026, 2nd Edition. London: Balliere, Tindall and Cassell
Hughes, E. S. R. (1965). *Aust. N. Z. J. Surg.* **34**, 188
Hughes, E. S. R., Cuthbertson, A. M. and Carden, A. B. G. (1963). *Med. J. Aust.* **1**, 780
McLaren, I. F. (1957). *J. R. Coll. Surg. Ed.* **3**, 129
Morson, B. C. (1963). *Br. J. Radiol.* **36**, 385
Painter, N. S. and Truelove, S. C. (1964). *Gut* **5**, 201, 365
Waugh, J. M. and Walt, A. J. (1957). *Surgery, Gynec. Obstet.* **104**, 690

[*The illustrations for this Chapter on Operations for Complications of Diverticular Disease were drawn by Mr. R. N. Lane.*]

Sigmoid Myotomy

Michael Reilly, M.S., F.R.C.S.
Consultant Surgeon, Plymouth General Hospital

PRE-OPERATIVE

Indications

Sigmoid myotomy is indicated primarily for chronic diverticular disease without complications. Suitable cases are those with a long history of troublesome symptoms not responding to correct medical treatment, which includes routine high-residue diet, plus antispasmodics and antibiotics administered during exacerbations. Such cases are usually over 50 years of age and may be up to 90 years old. In these cases a functional and reversible obstruction of the sigmoid colon has become organic and irreversible due to shortening of the longitudinal taeniae and thickening of the circular muscle. The lumen of the bowel is not only narrowed by circular muscle contraction but further by the concertina effect on the mucous membrane of the shortening of the bowel. Cases suitable for myotomy present with a history of frequent small explosive motions, especially in the morning, after which the bowel action may be quiescent for the remainder of the day, though stimulated again by the gastrocolic reflex after meals. Colicky lower abdominal pain, especially in the left iliac fossa, is a feature.

A secondary indication for this operation is in cases which have already undergone emergency laparotomy for complications of diverticular disease, such as perforation and localized paracolic or pelvic abscess, with or without obstruction. Such cases may have been treated by simple drainage, or drainage plus defunctioning colostomy. Myotomy may be carried out at a second operation when the condition is quiescent.

Contra-indications

Sigmoid myotomy should not be carried out in the presence of pus, peritonitis or active inflammation. Neither should it be performed as the sole procedure after separation and closure of colovesical, colocolic, or enterocolic fistulae, even if all inflammation appears to have subsided. Simple suture of the fistulous opening in the colon may break down later owing to poor blood supply in the wall of the colon from fibrosis round the fistula. Fistulae should be excised. Myotomy is not a substitute for excision in all cases, but an alternative treatment in suitable cases.

Bowel preparation

As the colon should not be opened during this operation attempts to reduce the bacterial content are unnecessary, even if they are ever wholly successful. It is more important that the bowel should be as empty as possible of formed faeces. In cases of diverticular disease inspissated faeces may be present as far back as the caecum. These may be softened by the administration of dioctyl sodium-sulphosuccinate orally for 3 days pre-operatively and largely eliminated, even in cases of grossly narrowed lumen, by 30 ml of a saturate solution of magnesium sulphate given every 2 hr, 2 days before operation, until the motions are clear. Massive purgation is to be avoided, as it is both painful and a potential cause of perforation of a diverticulum from raised intraluminal pressure.

Special pre-operative preparation

A nasogastric tube should be passed to keep the stomach empty, and an indwelling catheter inserted in both male and female patients to ensure an empty bladder and good visibility in the depths of the pelvis.

THE OPERATION

Abdominal incision

A low mid-line incision, right down to the symphysis pubis, gives the best view of the important recto-sigmoid junction. The incision is carried up to the umbilicus and 2·5 cm higher: either through the umbilicus if shallow, skirting it if it is deep.

1

Mobilizing the sigmoid colon

The folds of peritoneum binding the sigmoid mesentery to the left pelvic wall should be divided in a bloodless plane without stripping any peritoneum from the mesocolon or the pelvic wall. The sigmoid should be freed until it can be held out of the wound straight and taut down to the rectum.

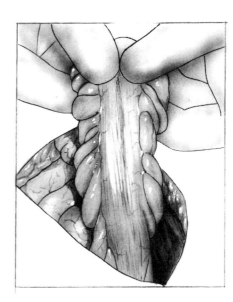

1

The myotomy

A preliminary incision is made with a long-handled scalpel over the upper rectum in the strict mid-line, and carried up in the mid-line over the rectosigmoid junction and as far up over the sigmoid as is necessary. The upper limit is indicated by the divergence of the longitudinal taeniae, and by the softer and thinner feel of the bowel wall, which occurs at about the same point. Normally the uniform longitudinal muscle layer of the rectum is gathered into two separate antimesenteric taeniae a few centimetres above the rectosigmoid junction. In diverticular disease these taeniae are shortened, thickened and widened, leaving only a slit between them. They may not diverge until 20 or 30 cm higher. The incision runs in this slit, though if the slit is not strictly in the mid-line the mid-line incision may be in the medial border of a taenia. The mid-line is relatively avascular, between the terminal blood vessels encircling the bowel on each side.

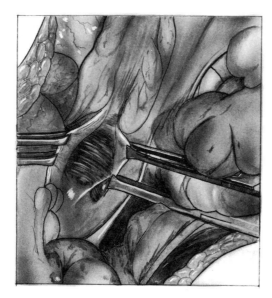

2

2

Division of circular fibres

This is begun over the rectosigmoid junction, the more difficult part of the procedure, so that the site shall not be obscured by any blood running down from inadvertent division of a small vessel above. Two pairs of Stiles' forceps are applied anterolaterally to the bowel wall and held out to display a square of the anterior rectosigmoid about 3 cm × 3 cm. The incision is spread with McIndoe's or Metzenbaum scissors to show the circular fibres, which are then picked up and divided by the scissor tips without puncturing the mucosa. A length of some 5 cm is dealt with, altering the position of the Stiles forceps as necessary.

3

It is then more practicable to begin again at the upper end of the preliminary incision and work down the colon, using two pairs of Allis' forceps to display each short length of bowel to be dealt with in turn, and employing McIndoe's scissors as before.

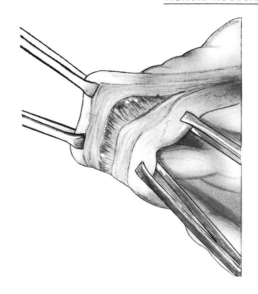

3

4

As each length is completed the upper pair of forceps is removed and replaced below the other pair, until the division of circular fibres is complete down to the rectosigmoid area first dealt with.

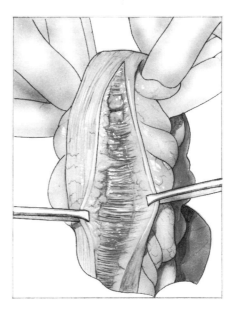

4

Points to note at operation

(*1*) The thick oedematous circular muscle may be slow to retract when first divided. It is difficult then to see if deeper strands are muscle fibres or blood vessels. Proceed to another area of bowel: on return to the first the fibres will have retracted, and any remaining muscle bundles can be seen and divided. It is inadvisable to be too thorough.

(*2*) Bleeding should be minimal in the colonic mid-line. If a small vessel is divided then ligature or cautery should not be used: perforation may occur later. A wet swab should be applied while the operation proceeds elsewhere.

(*3*) If the myotomy has been performed at a second stage after a preliminary colostomy, then the colostomy may be closed with advantage on completion of the myotomy, provided the mucosa has not been damaged. In cases of doubt the colostomy should be closed 2–3 weeks later.

(*4*) If a small portion of colon containing a fistulous opening has been excised and re-anastomosis performed, then myotomy can be carried out above or below the anastomosis, or both, as necessary.

Replacement of colon

No covering of the mucosa bared by myotomy is necessary. The sigmoid colon should be replaced in the pelvis with the myotomized site facing the left pelvic wall. In the rare case where the sigmoid mesentery is so short that the myotomized area faces forwards it is advisable to cover the area with omentum, to prevent adherence of loops of small bowel. Care must be taken that the omentum covers the area widely, or narrow bands may form, with consequent risk of small intestine obstruction.

Closure of abdomen

The peritoneum is closed with continuous catgut. The aponeurotic layer is best closed with continuous monofilament nylon.

Drainage

Drainage is not necessary unless the mucosa of the colon has been inadvertently punctured. Simple suture of the perforation with fine plain catgut is all that is necessary, plus a corrugated drain through a left iliac stab wound down into the pelvis.

POSTOPERATIVE CARE

No special management is needed. The bowels are usually open normally on the second to fourth day, after which normal diet may be resumed, including regular bran for breakfast.

Sedation

Morphine should never be prescribed. It causes plain muscle contraction, and may lead to increased intraluminal pressure, with risk to the myotomy site.

Antibiotics

These should only be used as a precaution in cases where the mucosa has been damaged. In such cases ampicillin is given by injection at the time of operation, and continued postoperatively for 5 days. It is given orally (ampicillin, 500 mg 6 hourly), as soon as the bowels have acted.

References

Reilly, M. (1964). 'Sigmoid myotomy.' *Proc. R. Soc. Med.* **57**, 556
Reilly, M. (1966). 'Sigmoid myotomy.' *Br. J. Surg.* **53**, 859
Reilly, M. (1971). 'Sigmoid myotomy for diverticular disease of the colon.' In *Modern Trends in Surgery*. London: Butterworths

[The illustrations for this Chapter on Sigmoid Myotomy were drawn by Mr. F. Price.]

Polyps and Polyposis

H. E. Lockhart-Mummery, M.D., M.Chir., F.R.C.S.
Consultant Surgeon, St. Thomas's and St. Mark's Hospitals, and
King Edward VII Hospital for Officers, London

PRE-OPERATIVE

Indications; precautions

Since an adenomatous polyp is potentially malignant all rectal polypi should be completely removed and submitted to histological examination. Sigmoidoscopy and opaque double contrast enema should be carried out in every case before removal, as other polypi may be so demonstrated in the colon, or an associated malignant growth detected. In such cases different treatment may be required.

The polyp should be removed *completely*, and the whole sent for microscopic examination. A biopsy of a part of the polyp should *not* be done, because misleading and inadequate information concerning its histology and extent may be obtained by removing only a small part.

A polyp should be suspected of having undergone malignant change if it is unduly hard, ulcerated, or if the stalk or base feels indurated, or if over 2 cm in diameter.

Pre-operative preparation

A clean empty bowel is necessary, and an enema of Veripaque or Clysodrast, given 1 hr prior to the operation, usually ensures this. No other preparation is needed.

Anaesthesia

An anaesthetic is necessary in most patients before the large-bore operating sigmoidoscope can be passed. General anaesthesia is usual, but local anaesthesia to the anal region as described for Haemorrhoidectomy (*see* page 332) may be used if preferred.

Position of patient

The Sims position, but with the buttocks over the edge of the table and raised on a sandbag, is convenient. The surgeon sits behind the patient.

THE OPERATION

1

Instruments required

Operating sigmoidoscope. The one illustrated is the Lloyd-Davies pattern, with an internal diameter of 2·7 cm and lengths of 15 or 20 cm. Wire diathermy snare for use through the sigmoidoscope. Long diathermy button. A large-bore sigmoidoscope is essential for accurate endoscopic excision, though general or local anaesthesia is needed before it can be passed.

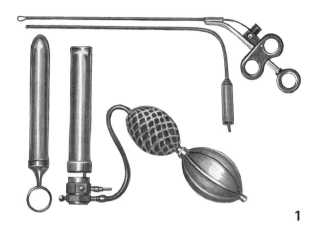

1

2

Use of diathermy snare

The sigmoidoscope is introduced under vision until the polyp and its stalk are clearly seen. The size of the wire loop of the snare is adjusted so that it can be passed over the polyp. The loop is passed through the sigmoidoscope, manipulated over the polyp and then gradually tightened until it is seen to be gripping the stalk near its attachment to the bowel wall. The polyp is then pulled *gently* away from the wall, and a low intensity cutting diathermy current passed through the wire in repeated short (0·25 sec) bursts as the wire is slowly tightened, until the pedicle is cut through. Any oozing of blood is usually very slight and can be arrested with a small swab soaked in liquor adrenaline 1:1000.

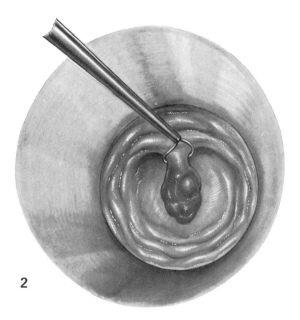

2

3

Use of diathermy button

Small sessile polyps are usually best dealt with by means of the long diathermy button. They are destroyed by short touches with the button, using a low intensity cutting current.

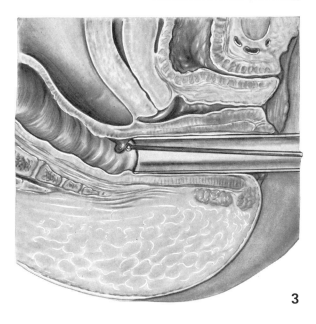

3

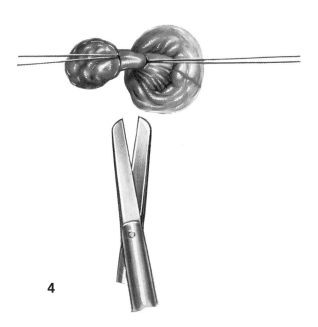

4

4

Ligation of pedicle

Pedunculated polyps in the lower rectum may often be delivered outside the anus when the sphincter is fully relaxed. The pedicle may then be transfixed and ligated, and the polyp removed.

POSTOPERATIVE CARE AND COMPLICATIONS

The patient should be detained in hospital for the night following the operation, but no special treatment is needed.

Perforation of the bowel wall

This complication should not occur; it results from faults in technique, particularly failure to obtain a good view of the polyp, and forcible traction with the wire snare. It is generally unwise to remove, with a snare, a sessile polyp or one which has a short pedicle when it is situated intraperitoneally. The signs of lower abdominal peritonitis, pain, guarding and rigidity, develop within a few hours. Laparotomy is necessary: the hole should be sutured, the peritoneum mopped clean and dry, and the abdomen closed with a drain down to the site. Temporary sigmoid colostomy is advisable if the perforation is large. Antibiotic therapy should be given.

Secondary haemorrhage

This may occur when the slough caused by the diathermy separates, usually between the sixth and tenth days. It is seldom severe, and usually ceases spontaneously. The application of an adrenaline swab through a sigmoidoscope will arrest the bleeding if it should fail to stop on its own.

References

Gabriel, W. B. (1963). *The Principles and Practice of Rectal Surgery,* 5th Edition, Chap. XVII. London: Lewis
Lockhart-Mummery, H. E. and Dukes, C. E. (1952). *Lancet* **2,** 751

[*The illustrations for this Chapter on Polyps and Polyposis were drawn by Mr. R. N. Lane.*]

Colectomy for Malignant Disease

H. E. Lockhart-Mummery, M.D., M.Chir., F.R.C.S.
Consultant Surgeon, St. Thomas's and St. Mark's Hospitals, and
King Edward VII Hospital for Officers, London

PRE - OPERATIVE

A careful assessment of the patient's general condition is essential and conditions such as cardiovascular disease, bronchitis or diabetes mellitus recognized and stabilized. Some degree of anaemia is common among patients with carcinoma of the colon and this, together with evidence of nutritional lack, must receive treatment.

Preparation of bowel

The colon should be preferably as empty as possible and with its bacterial contents diminished. Admission to hospital 4 days before operation is desirable and both physical and antibacterial preparation is given. At present the physical preparation favoured is to give 30 ml Castor oil 3 days before operation and a second similar dose the day before surgery. A low-residue diet is given from the day of admission and clear fluids only after the second dose of Castor oil. No enemas or washouts need be given in addition.

There is much controversy about the need for antibacterial bowel preparation and as to whether there is any advantage in the use of antibiotics. The author's current practice is to use insoluble sulphonamides only, phthalylsulphathiazole 3 G three times daily for 4 days pre-operatively.

Blood transfusion

If the haemoglobin level is below 10 G the patient should receive a transfusion at least 48 hr before operation: 1000 ml of blood should be available for transfusion during and after operation.

THE OPERATIONS

Position of patient and incision

For all growths below the splenic flexure it is an advantage to have the patient in the lithotomy-Trendelenburg position (*see* Chapter on 'Abdomino-perineal Excision of the Rectum' pages 118–132) as this allows access to the anus for washout of the distal bowel when indicated.

A long right or left paramedian incision is usually the best approach when dealing with colonic tumours. Wide access is always an advantage.

Exploration

The actual growth should be handled as little as possible. A thorough exploration of the whole abdomen must first be made to determine the resectability of the growth, the presence of metastases or of another neoplasm in the colon and other associated disease. The condition of the colon above the growth is important, for if the pre-operative preparation has been ineffective and the bowel is loaded with faeces, it may be desirable to carry out a preliminary colostomy and perform the resection at a later date. In discussing the operation of resection at different sites it will be assumed that the condition of the bowel is suitable for elective resection.

General principles of colonic surgery

After removal of that part of the bowel containing the growth with its related lymphatic field, the surgeon should aim to restore continuity by end-to-end anastomosis. In order to do this safely the two ends of bowel must both have a good arterial supply and must come together without any tension, and therefore the remaining colon must be mobilized as necessary in order to achieve this. Before carrying out the actual anastomosis, both ends to be joined together should be mopped out and cleaned carefully with sterile distilled water or cancericidal solution, for this manoeuvre will reduce considerably the risk of implantation recurrence at the suture line.

In those cases in which the growth in the colon has led to complete intestinal obstruction, it is seldom safe or desirable to attempt immediate removal of the tumour with anastomosis. Obstructed carcinomas in the sigmoid or descending colon are best dealt with by establishing a loop colostomy in the right half of the transverse colon, thus allowing adequate bowel distal to the colostomy for resection and anastomosis a few weeks later. If the growth is accessible and not fixed, such cases *may* be treated by immediate removal of the tumour, with closure or exteriorizing the lower end and bringing the upper end out as a terminal colostomy. Continuity can be restored by a further operation some weeks or months later.

Obstructing growths of the ileocaecal region are often suitable for immediate resection and anastomosis, as the small bowel may be emptied by suction, and a safe anastomosis carried out (*see* Chapter on 'Ileocolic Anastomosis', pages 260–261).

RIGHT HEMICOLECTOMY

1

Parts of ileum and colon removed

In dealing with all malignant growths of the colon it is more important to aim at wide removal of the related lymphatic field than at wide clearance of the bowel itself. Probably 7–10 cm clearance within the bowel suffices and unnecessary removal of terminal ileum and right colon should be avoided. For growths of the caecum, adequate lymphatic removal will usually still allow preservation of the hepatic flexure with plentiful blood supply from the middle colic artery; growths of the ascending colon may need a wider removal of the right colon with ligation of the right branch of the middle colic vessels. There is however considerable individual variation in the 'normal' arrangement of the arterial supply to the colon.

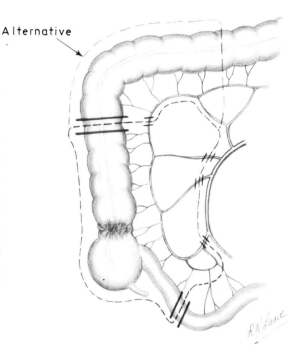

1

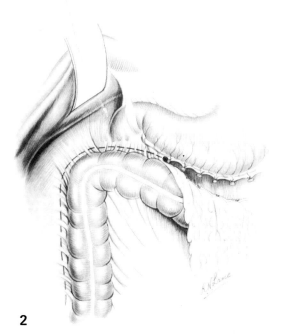

2

2

Mobilization of growth (I)

The operation is best started by entering the lesser sac between the gastro-epiploic vessels along the greater curve of the stomach and the omentum attached to the right transverse colon. Small vessels will need ligating and the dissection is continued round the hepatic flexure and down the right para-colic gutter; here there are usually only small vessels which can be touched with diathermy.

3

Mobilization of growth (II)

The colon containing the growth is mobilized medially, exposing the perinephric fat, the right ureter, the second part of the duodenum and the right testicular or ovarian vessels. The last few inches of terminal ileum are also mobilized. It is usually easier to carry out this dissection from the opposite side of the table, i.e. the patient's left.

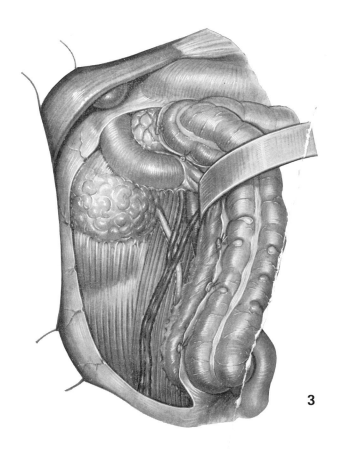

3

4

4

Division of mesentery

After full mobilization, the surgeon should now decide on the exact extent of removal to be carried out. Light forceps of Babcock type are placed on the colon and small bowel at the points of planned division. With good transillumination the mesentery of the right colon and terminal ileum are divided and the main vessels carefully ligated near the superior mesenteric artery and vein. Near the bowel fine forceps are used to pick up the small vessels and the dissection is taken right up to the bowel at the points previously marked. Clamps are applied across the bowel, which is divided and the specimen removed.

5

Closure of mesentery

After ensuring that the mobilization of the two ends of bowel has been adequate to allow them to come together without tension, the next step is to close the mesocolon from its base near the superior mesenteric vessels to within 2·5—5 cm of the bowel ends which remain clamped. A continuous catgut stitch is used.

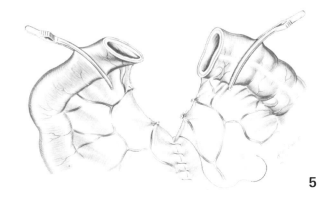

5

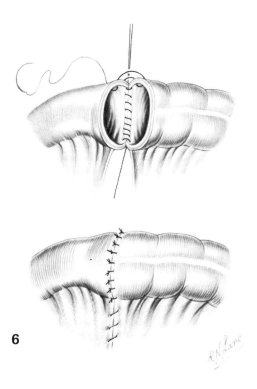

6

6

End-to-end anastomosis

A light clamp may be placed across the bowel about 2·5 cm from the cut ends. The ileum is cut obliquely in order to increase the size of the lumen and ensure a good blood supply on the antimesenteric side. The two ends of bowel are then mopped out as previously described. A series of interrupted non-absorbable sutures are placed through the seromuscular coats to form the posterior layer of the anastomosis. In this way the disparity of size between the ends that often exists is equalized and the subsequent continuous all-coats catgut suture with an inverting Connell suture on the anterior wall allows a satisfactory and safe anastomosis. A final layer of interrupted non-absorbable sutures completes the anastomosis anteriorly. The mesocolic suture is then completed up to the bowel.

After checking for haemostasis the abdomen is closed. A stab drain may be inserted through the right flank if there has been much oozing or soiling, but is not always necessary.

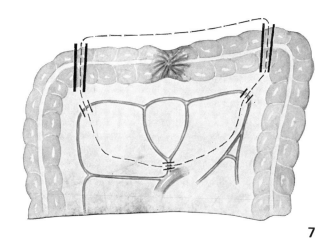

7

CARCINOMA OF TRANSVERSE COLON

7&8

Growths arising near the hepatic flexure are resected by right hemicolectomy; those near the splenic flexure are considered later. For growths of the mid-transverse colon, resection aims at removal of the greater part of the transverse colon, the attached omentum and the lymphatic field lying in the drainage of the middle colic artery contained in the mesocolon.

The first step is the separation of the omentum from the greater curvature of the stomach and from the hepatic and splenic flexures. These flexures are now mobilized by division of each phrenicocolic ligament, though this may occasionally be unnecessary if there is a long transverse colon. The middle colic artery is now divided at its origin and the mesocolon separated from its attachment to the posterior abdominal wall. Points for resection are selected, the marginal vessels and mesocolon divided and end-to-end anastomosis performed.

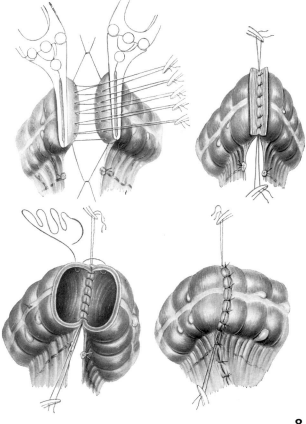

8

CARCINOMA OF SPLENIC FLEXURE AND DESCENDING COLON

Sites of ligation

9

Splenic flexure and upper descending colon

Growths of the splenic flexure and upper descending colon may spread both to glands beside the middle colic artery and to those beside the inferior mesenteric artery. A very radical removal involving ligation of both these vessels at their origin would require removal of most of the transverse and left colon and make restoration of continuity difficult. Such extensive removal is very seldom necessary or justified. It usually suffices to tie the left branch of the middle colic near its origin from the main trunk and the left colic near its origin from the inferior mesenteric artery.

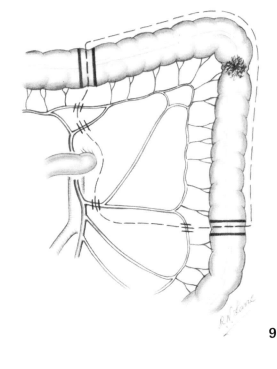

9

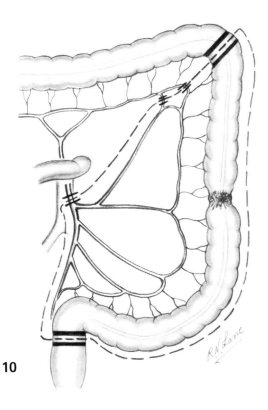

10

10

Tumours of descending colon

When dealing with tumours of the descending colon, ligation of vessels similar to that shown in *Illustration 9* may suffice. If lymph node involvement seems to indicate a more radical clearance then the inferior mesenteric artery should be ligated at its origin and the wider removal of bowel as shown here will probably be needed if good blood supply to both ends of bowel is to be ensured.

11

Mobilization of descending colon (I)

Starting at the outer side of the sigmoid colon, the line of the peritoneal attachment is divided to the splenic flexure and the colon gradually mobilized medially.

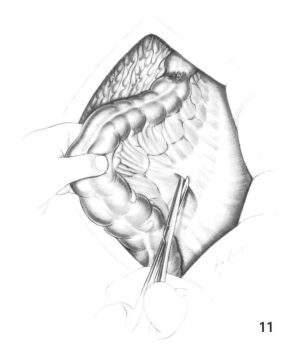

11

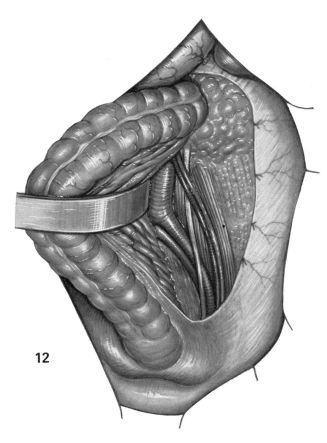

12

12

Mobilization of descending colon (II)

When fully mobilized the perinephric fat, the left ureter, the ovarian or spermatic vessels, the lowest part of the aorta and the left common iliac artery are exposed. Mesocolic vessels can now be clearly seen also.

13

Freeing of splenic flexure

The lesser sac is entered below the gastro-epiploic vessels on the greater curve of the stomach and the dissection continued towards the spleen, ligating and dividing the gastrocolic omentum. The final freeing of the splenic flexure must be done very carefully with good access, lighting and retraction, as the bowel is often in very close relation to the spleen, the capsule of which tears easily. There are often a few small vessels in the adhesions between the spleen and colon and often a 'pedicle' can be gently isolated and then clamped before division. The left colon and splenic flexure are usually then freed enough to allow their delivery outside the abdomen.

The mesocolon can be divided as required, the length of bowel containing the tumour removed and continuity restored by end-to-end anastomosis without any tension.

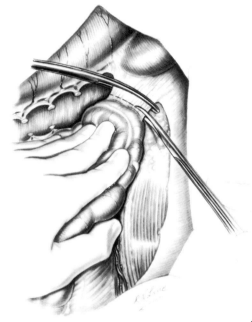

13

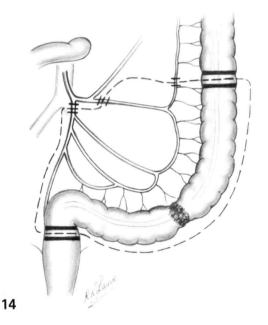

14

CARCINOMA OF SIGMOID COLON

14

Sites of ligation

For most cases of carcinoma of the sigmoid colon the superior haemorrhoidal and sigmoid arteries should be tied at their origins from the inferior mesenteric, that is just below the origin of the left colic artery. This ensures an excellent blood supply to the left colon, which is anastomosed to the upper rectum at the level of the sacral promontory.

15

Sites of ligation

If a more radical lymphatic removal is indicated, the inferior mesenteric artery is ligated at its origin from the aorta. One is then relying on the marginal artery from the middle colic to supply the descending colon and it may be necessary to remove more of the descending colon to ensure that the proximal colon is viable; in that case the splenic flexure may have to be mobilized so that the remaining colon can be brought to the rectum without tension.

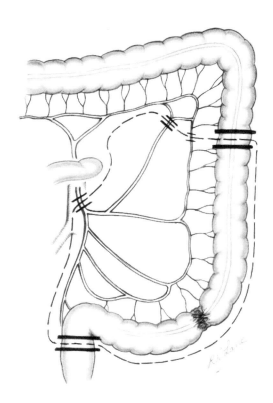

15

16

Preparation for anastomosis

Following ligation of the main vessels the mesentery is divided out to the bowel at the level decided. After gentle mobilization of the rectosigmoid from the sacral promontory, the dissection is also taken through the retrorectal tissue, again ligating and dividing the superior haemorrhoidal vessels, which are here running down behind the rectum. When the rectal wall has been bared, a right-angled clamp is applied across the upper rectum, which is then washed out with cytotoxic solution through a proctoscope *per anum.*

The upper end is divided between clamps and a soft occlusion clamp may be applied about 2·5 cm higher to prevent soiling during anastomosis or a cotton-wool ball inserted for the same purpose if clamping is difficult. This should be removed before the anastomosis is completed or gently pushed through the anastomosis. The upper end should be gently mopped out with antiseptic anticancericidal solution.

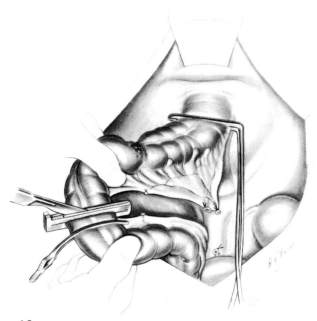

16

17a & b

The anastomosis

The author prefers a two-layer inverting anastomosis, outer seromuscular silk 3/0 interrupted stitches and an inner all-coats continuous 2/0 chromic catgut. Some surgeons prefer a single-layer inverting anastomosis with non-absorbable sutures. It is best to insert all the sutures of the outer posterior layer with the bowel ends separated and then slide the upper end down to the lower before tying them. The continuous all-coats suture is then started in the mid-line posteriorly, brought round on each side, and finished anteriorly. Further interrupted silk stitches anteriorly complete the anastomosis. The mesentery is sutured to the pelvic peritoneum on the right side with a running catgut stitch. Drainage depends upon the surgeon's preference but is not usually necessary unless there is much oozing. The abdomen is then closed. The anus may be dilated at the end of the operation. This allows an easier escape of flatus which reduces intraluminal tension.

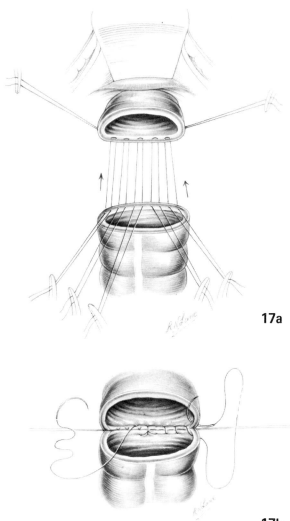

17a

17b

POSTOPERATIVE CARE

Postoperative care is essentially the same as that for any major abdominal operation. Blood loss should be made good during and immediately after the operation. Postoperative breathing exercises are commenced as soon as possible. The use of prophylactic antibiotics is a matter of personal decision. Since a period of postoperative intestinal paresis is to be expected, nothing should be given by mouth and the patient is maintained on intravenous fluids until there is positive evidence of the full return of peristalsis by the passage of flatus. Routine postoperative gastric suction is used by many surgeons; others institute this only when it appears desirable.

If a drain has been inserted at the end of the operation, it should usually be shortened by about 2 cm on the third postoperative day, and removed on the fourth or fifth day when the bowel has functioned normally.

[The illustrations for this Chapter on Colectomy for Malignant Disease were drawn by Mr. R. N. Lane.]

Colectomy for Malignant Disease of the Colon: The 'No Touch' Isolation Technique

David G. Jagelman, M.S., F.R.C.S. (Eng.)
Department of Colon and Rectal Surgery,
The Cleveland Clinic Foundation,
Cleveland, Ohio

and

Rupert B. Turnbull, Jr., M.D., C.M., F.A.C.S.
Department of Colon and Rectal Surgery,
The Cleveland Clinic Foundation,
Cleveland, Ohio

PROCEDURES

Carcinoma of the colon continues to be one of the most common malignancies in surgical practice and the vast majority of patients succumbing to this disease have evidence of massive venous spread of their tumour. It has long been suspected that cancers may be disseminated by the trauma of surgical removal (Tizzer, 1913). We feel strongly that early vascular isolation of the bowel cancer segment should be performed to limit any venous dissemination at the time of surgery (Turnbull *et al.*, 1967). A direct approach to the origin of the artery and vein concerned also allows a maximum excision of the mesenteric lymphatic drainage of the tumour and thereby a more complete cancer procedure. This method has been termed the no touch isolation technique and was first described in 1952 by Barnes.

Carcinoma of the caecum and ascending colon should be treated by right colectomy with ileotransverse anastomosis. In our opinion, carcinoma of the mid-transverse colon is best treated with total colectomy and ileorectal anastomosis. This procedure should also be considered for patients with synchronous colonic carcinoma and adenomatous polyps, particularly those in the younger age group, or in a patient with a double primary colonic cancer. Carcinoma of the splenic flexure and left colon is treated by left colectomy and colorectal anastomosis. Carcinoma of the sigmoid colon is treated by rectosigmoidectomy with anastomosis of the descending colon to the rectum.

PRE - OPERATIVE

Patients who enter the hospital for elective resection for cancer of the colon will have undergone radiological studies of the colon and sigmoidoscopic examination to 25 cm. A general physical examination is performed with particular reference to cardiovascular and respiratory status. Haemoglobin, urea and electrolyte determination, liver function tests, and urine analysis are undertaken routinely. Chest x-ray and intravenous pyelography are ordered. Anaemia is corrected by appropriate blood transfusion and blood is grouped and cross-matched for the day of surgery.

A colon without faeces and a suppressed aerobic and anaerobic colonic bacterial flora has been shown to significantly reduce the morbidity and mortality of elective colonic resections. To achieve this the patient is admitted 2 days before surgery and is placed on a low-residue diet for the first day and a fluid-only diet the second day. The day prior to surgery the patient is given 30 ml of flavoured castor oil at 7:00 a.m. This is followed by half-strength Clysodrast enemas (bisacodyl 3 mg plus tannic acid to 5 g) at 10:00 a.m. and 4:00 p.m. and finally a litre saline enema at 10:00 p.m. until the returns are clear. The oral antibiotic bowel preparation is the Nichols–Condon method (Nichols *et al.,* 1973), this being the only preparation so far described that allows for a suppression of both the aerobic and anaerobic colonic flora. Neomycin 1 g and erythromycin base 1 g is given at 1:00 p.m., 2:00 p.m. and 11:00 p.m. the day before surgery. Lactated Ringer's solution is given intravenously overnight to guard against dehydration produced by the castor oil and resulting diarrhoea. On the day of surgery the colon is lavaged on the operating table with normal saline until the returns are clear and the rectal tube is left *in situ* to allow any drainage from the colon of irrigating fluid during the operation. The patient is anaesthetized with intravenous Pentothal (thiopentone sodium) and an endotracheal tube inserted. A Foley catheter is routinely placed in the bladder to empty it of urine and allow assessment of adequate renal function during and after the procedure.

Surgical method

Skin preparation of the abdomen is performed with 10 per cent Betadine solution (povidone-iodine containing 1 per cent available iodine). The abdomen is opened via a mid-line incision and this can be extended upward to the xiphisternum or down to the pubis according to the need of access to the peritoneal cavity. The cancer-bearing segment is inspected, but not palpated. A search for spread of the tumour is then undertaken by looking for peritoneal nodules and by palpation of the liver. The remainder of the colon is inspected for synchronous pathology. The lymphovascular pedicles of the bowel cancer segment are then isolated, divided, and ligated at their origins. The bowel is then sectioned between clamps at a suitable distance from the tumour. The cancer-bearing segment of the colon is then isolated from a lymphovascular viewpoint, and is then removed. Surgical tapes are placed and tied around the bowel a few inches from the line of resection to avoid spillage of intestinal contents upon opening of the bowel for the anastomosis.

CARCINOMA OF THE RIGHT COLON. RIGHT COLON RESECTION. THE 'NO TOUCH' ISOLATION TECHNIQUE

1

Extent of resection

Carcinoma of the right colon is treated by resection of the terminal few inches of ileum, caecum, ascending colon and right side of transverse colon, together with the bowel mesentery and lymphatic pathways up to the origins of the ileocolic, right colic arteries and the right (hepatic) division of the middle colic artery.

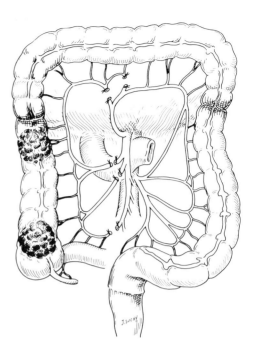

1

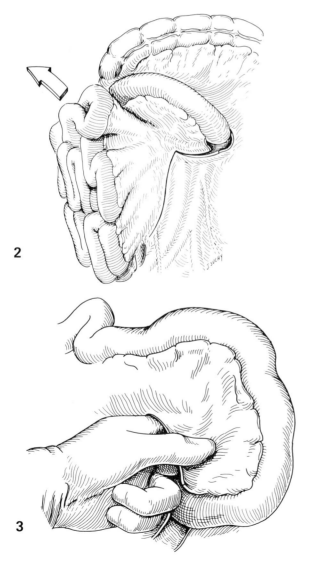

2

THE OPERATION

2

With the surgeon standing on the left side of the patient, a retroperitoneal approach to the lympho-vascular pedicles of the right colon is preferred. The small intestine is reflected to the right side of the abdomen and the duodenojejunal flexure exposed. The peritoneum is incised from this point towards the caecum.

3

The index and middle fingers are inserted along the lateral border of the third portion of the duodenum dissecting the duodenum out of the base of the small bowel mesentery. The index finger easily reaches the first part of the duodenum. This also allows for the assessment of possible duodenal invasion of a right sided colonic carcinoma.

3

4

With the fingers of the left hand lying along the lateral border of the duodenum the small bowel is now replaced in the abdomen thus lying over the palm of the left hand. The superior mesenteric, ileocolic and right colic arteries are now lying across the left index finger. The tip of the finger can be seen protruding through a window in the mesentery between the ileocolic artery and the right colic artery.

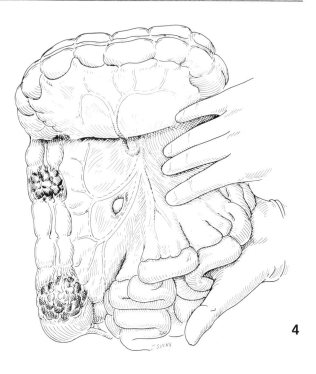

4

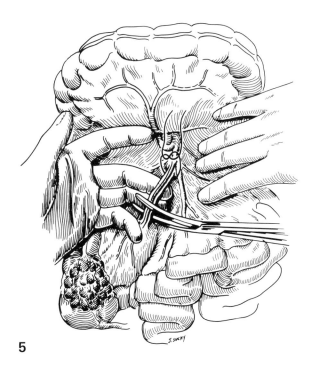

5

5

By palpation the origin of the ileocolic lympho-vascular bundle from the superior mesenteric artery where it crosses the third portion of duodenum, is defined, ligated and divided.

6

Next, the right colic artery is selected, ligated and divided at its origin.

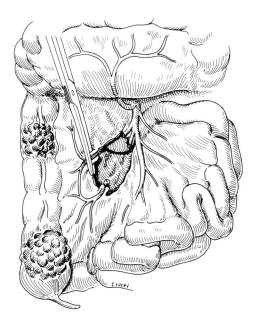

6

7

The hepatic flexure division of the middle colic artery is similarly isolated, clamped and ligated. After the main colonic vessels have been ligated and dissected the ileocolic mesentery is divided from the duodenum to the ileum approximately 12 cm proximal to the caecum. A broad linen tape is placed around the ileum just proximal to the line of division and knotted tightly to prevent intestinal spillage at the time of subsequent anastomosis.

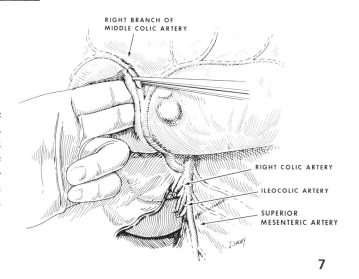

7

8

The lesser sac is entered along the greater curvature of the stomach. The gastrocolic omentum is stripped down from the greater curvature of the distal stomach. This frees the right side of the transverse colon from the stomach and duodenum. If the tumour is near the hepatic flexure, the gastrocolic omentum is taken down flush with the gastric wall, that is to say inside the gastro-epiploic arch.

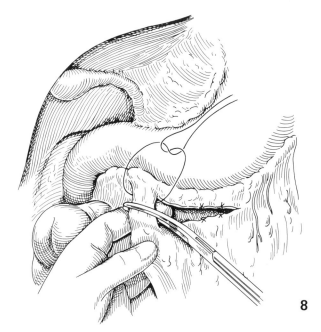

8

9

9

The remaining mesentery and mesenteric vessels of the transverse colon are then clamped and divided. The point of anastomosis of the mid-transverse colon is then selected, clamped and divided. A linen tape is placed just distal to the line of transection on the transverse colon to prevent retrograde faecal spillage at the time of anastomosis.

10

The isolated cancer-bearing segment is then reflected laterally and removed in a prograde manner. The mesentery of the ascending colon is separated from the ureter and gonadal vessels and from the surface of the right kidney. Finally all of the peritoneum of the right paracolic gutter is removed with the cancer-bearing segment.

An end-to-end ileocolic anastomosis is then performed, and the mesenteric defect is obliterated by interrupted 000 Tevdek (braided polyester impregnated with Teflon) sutures. The abdomen is closed with interrupted 0/0-gauge stainless steel wire sutures through all layers.

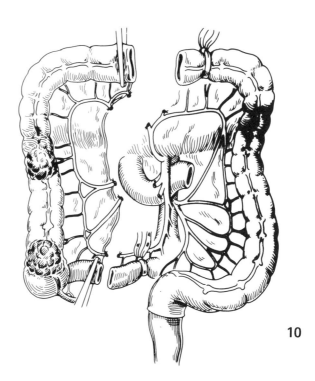

10

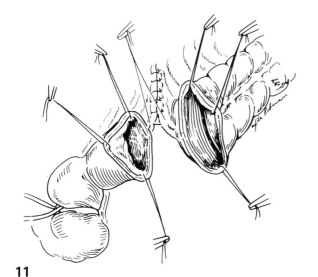

11

METHOD OF ANASTOMOSIS

An end-to-end anastomosis is preferred. If there is a disparity of size of bowel lumen an antimesenteric (Cheatle) slit is used to open up the smaller lumen. This ensures a wide open anastomosis. The bowel is checked for good pulsatile blood supply and the bowel ends are swabbed with 40 per cent alcohol as a cancericidal agent.

11

0/0 Chromic catgut stay sutures are placed around the circumference of both bowel ends to allow visualization of the diameter of the lumen and close approximation of the ends. The stay sutures allow mobility of the bowel ends and thus the use of tissue forceps may be avoided as these may traumatize the mucosa.

12

The mesenteric defect is closed with interrupted 000 Tevdek. Through-and-through vertical mattress sutures (all-layers) of 000 chromic catgut are used for the mesenteric side of the bowel.

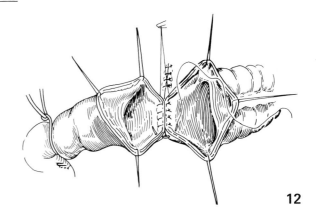

12

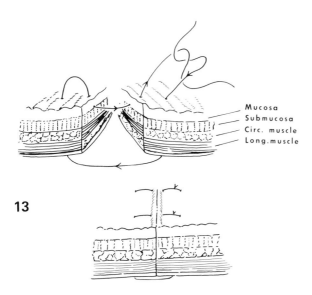

Mucosa
Submucosa
Circ. muscle
Long. muscle

13

13

The vertical mattress is formed by returning the needle through the mucosa only. This allows close anatomical approximation without any mucosal eversion.

14

The lumen of the ileum is enlarged by performing an antimesenteric (Cheatle) slit. The corners of the slit are not trimmed.

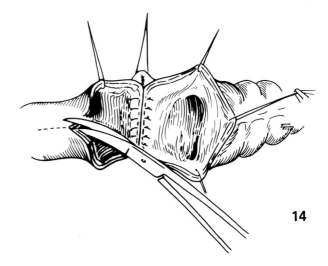

14

15

The posterior (mesenteric) half of the anastomosis has already been made. The anterior half is made with interrupted 000 chromic catgut through all layers except the mucosa. When tied the muscular walls of the bowel are approximated while the edges of the mucosa are brought into apposition. The sutures are placed from both sides towards the middle of the antimesenteric border.

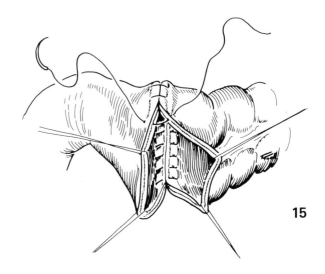

15

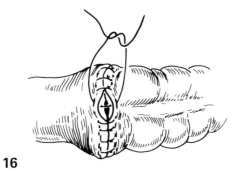

16

16

The completed first layer of the ileocolic anastomosis is shown, the ends of the ileum and colon being exactly the same circumference.

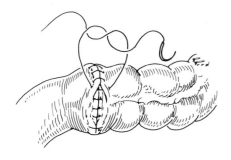

17

A second layer of superimposed interrupted seromuscular sutures of 000 Tevdek is placed around the circumference of the anastomosis to complete the procedure.

17

CARCINOMA OF THE DISTAL TRANSVERSE COLON AND LEFT COLON

18

Extent of resection

Carcinoma of the distal transverse colon and descending colon is treated by early ligation of the appropriate lymphovascular pedicles, i.e. the inferior mesenteric and splenic branch of the middle colic. Division of the transverse colon in its mid-portion and division of the rectum at the level of the sacral promontory and an end-to-end colorectal anastomosis is performed.

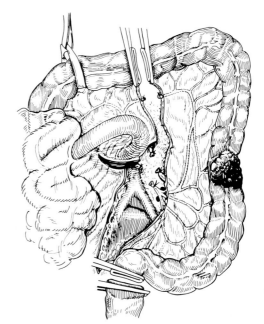

18

THE OPERATION

19

The sigmoid colon is gently lifted upwards and out of the abdomen and the peritoneum on its lateral border is incised.

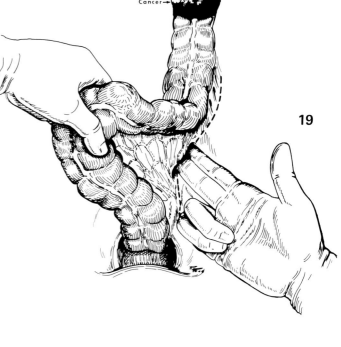

19

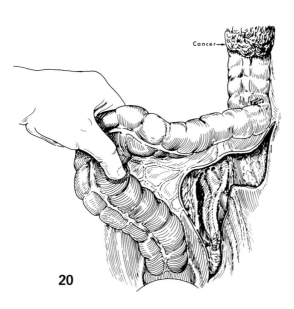

20

20

With a mixture of sharp and blunt dissection the avascular plane anterior to the gonadal vessels and ureter is defined and entered, anterior to the sympathetic chain.

21

It is then possible to pass the left hand under the sigmoid colon and define the origin of the inferior mesenteric lymphovascular pedicle on the aorta.

The inferior mesenteric artery and vein are then clamped and divided individually. If the tumour is in close proximity to the site of mobilization of the sigmoid and descending colon a direct ligation in continuity of the inferior mesenteric artery and vein is performed prior to mobilization of the sigmoid. The vessels can then be divided following full mobilization of the sigmoid and left colon, vascular dissemination having thus been prevented during mobilization.

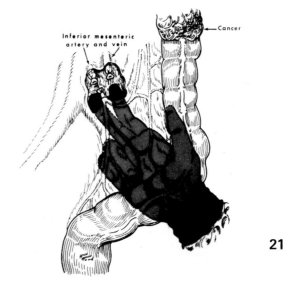

The splenic flexure branch of the middle colic artery is next ligated and divided by lifting up the transverse colon and incising into the mesentery. The left colon is then isolated from a lymphovascular viewpoint. A point of division is then selected in the mid-transverse colon and the rest of the gastrocolic omentum and transverse mesocolon is divided, individual vessels being tied as they are transected. The bowel is then divided between clamps. Dissection is continued along the greater curvature of the stomach to remove the gastrocolic omentum as far as the splenic flexure.

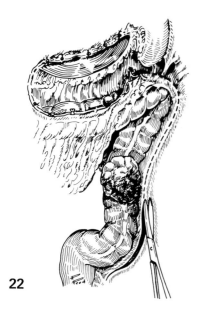

22

The incision along the left paracolic gutter is then extended upwards toward the splenic flexure and finally by gently grasping both limbs of the colon at the splenic flexure the peritoneum can be divided laterally to allow the colon to be brought down out of its splenic bed. The descending colon and its mesentery can be swept across from the anterior surface of the left kidney as far as the ligament of Treitz.

23

The lateral peritoneal incision is continued down toward the rectum on the left side and the peritoneum from the origin of the inferior mesenteric artery is divided down to the level of the sacral promontory on the right side. Before transecting the rectum it is irrigated with 40 per cent alcohol as a cancericidal agent by means of a syringe and needle introduced into the lumen of the bowel from above the level of the tumour. The rectum is transected at the level of the sacral promontory without entering the presacral space.

The specimen can then be removed. Colorectal anastomosis is then performed between the transverse colon and the rectum at the level of the sacral promontory.

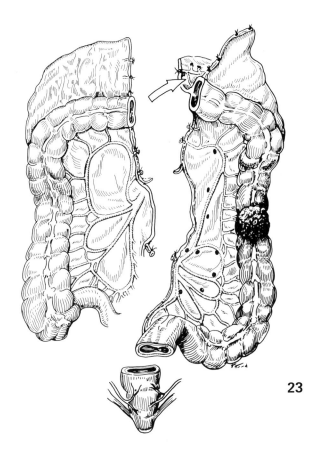

23

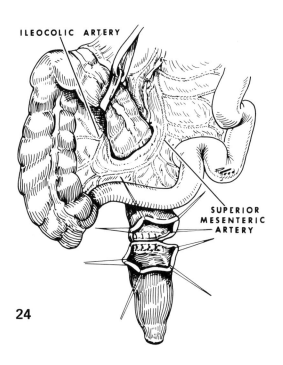

ILEOCOLIC ARTERY

SUPERIOR MESENTERIC ARTERY

24

24

If there is difficulty in approximation of the bowel ends without tension or if there appears to be undue distortion of the small intestine and its mesentery, the transverse colon should be brought through an opening in the mesenteric vascular window of the terminal ileum between the ileocolic artery and the superior mesenteric artery. The right side of the gastrocolic omentum needs to be divided as far as the duodenum to allow extra mobility of the remaining transverse colon. By the use of this technique colorectal anastomosis can be achieved without tension. The opening in the mesentery is sutured to the transverse colon to prevent the possibility of herniation of small bowel through the mesenteric window.

The colorectal anastomosis is performed as previously described including the use of the Cheatle slit if necessary to achieve equal size of the lumen of the two ends of intestine.

CARCINOMA OF THE SIGMOID COLON

25

Carcinoma of the sigmoid colon is treated by early vascular ligation of inferior mesenteric artery and vein and by division of the colon at the mid-descending level and division of the rectum just below the sacral promontory. The mobilization and resection is as for the left hemicolectomy previously described.

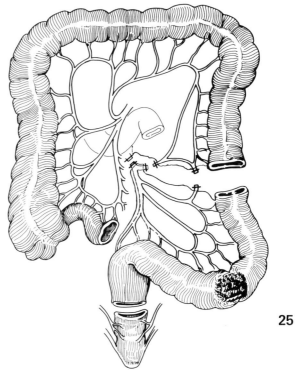

25

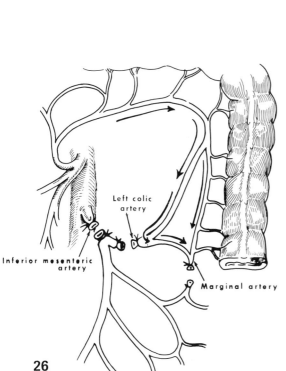

26

26

After having divided the inferior mesenteric artery at its origin, the left colic branch is identified. This is divided proximal to its bifurcation. It is hoped that retrograde blood flow will pass down the preserved left colic bifurcation and supplement the marginal artery in supplying the colon at the point of transection. The anastomosis is performed in the manner previously described.

References

Barnes, J. P. (1952). 'Physiologic resection of the right colon.' *Surgery Gynec. Obstet.* **94**, 723

Nichols, R. L., Broido, P., Condon, R. E., Gorbach, S. L. and Nyhus, L. M. (1973). 'Effects of preoperative neomycin-erythromycin intestinal preparation on the incidence of infectious complications following colon surgery.' *Ann. Surg.* **178**, 453

Turnbull, R. B., Kyle, K., Spratt, J. and Watson, J. (1967). 'Cancer of the colon: the influence of the no touch isolation technique on survival rates.' *Ann. Surg.* **166**, 420

Tizzer, E. E. (1913). 'Factors in the production and growth of tumour metastases.' *J. med. Res.* **28**, 309

[The illustrations for this Chapter on Colectomy for Malignant Disease of the Colon: The 'No Touch' Isolation Technique were drawn by Mr. R. Reed and Mr. J. Suchy.]

Abdominoperineal Excision of the Rectum

P. R. Hawley, M.S., F.R.C.S.
Consultant Surgeon, St. Mark's Hospital, London

PRE-OPERATIVE

There are three established methods of combined excision: the abdominoperineal (Miles), perineo-abdominal (Grey-Turner and Gabriel) and the synchronous (Lloyd-Davies).

In the first two methods the patient is turned between the abdominal and perineal stages. In the synchronous method the abdomen and the perineum are exposed throughout the operation by using the Lloyd-Davies leg supports and placing the patient in the lithotomy-Trendelenburg position. This latter method has superseded both the earlier methods and is either carried out by an operator doing the abdominal and then the perineal part of the operation, or, preferably, by two teams of surgeons working synchronously.

Indications

The operation is indicated where there are: (*1*) primary malignant tumours of the rectum and the anal canal (*2*) secondary extension into the rectum from malignant disease in adjacent organs, for example the vagina or uterus and (*3*) when the rectum has to be excised in Crohn's disease or as part of a procto-colectomy for ulcerative colitis when surgery is indicated. However, in patients with ulcerative colitis and some patients with Crohn's disease a more con-servative method of excising the rectum is preferable, as described in the Chapter on 'Conservative Excision of the Rectum in Inflammatory Bowel Disease', pages 26–29.

Contra-indications

The operation is contra-indicated in patients totally unfit on general grounds; cases with gross hepatic metastases; and patients with diffuse perineal metastases. However, the operability rate should approach 95 per cent.

Pre-operative preparation

The patient is admitted at least 3 days before opera-tion for assessment and bowel preparation. The chest is x-rayed and an intravenous pyelogram is carried out on patients with advanced tumours, particularly when in the upper third of the rectum. Laboratory tests include a blood count, blood grouping, urea and electrolyte examination. Urine examination is carried out and any anaemia treated by blood transfusion. It is advisable that the haemoglobin should be at least 11 g per cent before operation.

As a general rule prostatic obstruction is best dealt with in the postoperative period as all patients will need a Foley or a Gibbons catheter in place during the operation and for the first week postoperatively.

118

Bowel preparation

Mechanical bowel preparation is carried out in all cases except those presenting with intestinal obstruction. Three days before operation the patient is given 30 ml of castor oil by mouth and placed on a low-residue diet. On the second pre-operative day the patient is given fluids only by mouth. This is continued on the day before operation when the patient is given another 30 ml of castor oil by mouth. In most cases a rectal washout or enema will not be necessary after this preparation, but if felt necessary a phosphate enema can be given on the evening preceding surgery, 1·5 g in a litre of water being administered.

The operation and immediate postoperative period is covered with a broad-spectrum antibiotic which is administered intravenously during the course of the operation and for 48 hr afterwards. Suitable antibiotics include ampicillin or one of the cephalosporins.

Anaesthesia

A suitable general anaesthetic is administered. As soon as the patient is anaesthetized a self-retaining catheter is inserted into the bladder and connected to a uribag. In males the catheter and the scrotum is fixed to the right thigh with adhesive strapping so that it is clear of the surgeon carrying out the perineal dissection. An intravenous infusion is essential and is commenced before the start of the operation. The anus is closed by an encircling stitch (see Illustration 17).

THE OPERATION

SYNCHRONOUS METHOD OF EXCISION OF THE RECTUM

1

Position of patient

Note the Lloyd-Davies leg supports and the litho-tomy-Trendelenburg position with the sacrum raised on a vac-pac surgical positioning pad or a Goligher sacral rest. With the patient in this position two surgeons may work together, one in the abdomen and the other in the perineum, with no hindrance to either.

The position may be used by a surgeon working alone and an abdominoperineal or perineo-abdominal operation performed. The distinguishing features between these two methods are the timing of the various procedures and the amount of dissection carried out from either the abdominal or perineal aspect.

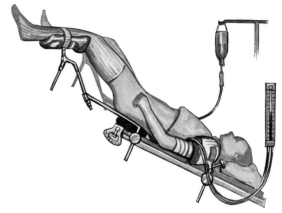

1

Abdominal exploration and dissection

2

The incision

A long lower left or right paramedian muscle sliding incision is made and extends from the pubis to about 5 cm above the umbilicus. The abdomen is then systematically examined, commencing with the liver, the whole colon and concluding in the pelvis.

The site of the colostomy is here shown at a point about 6 cm along the line from the anterior superior iliac spine to the umbilicus. In an obese patient the colostomy needs to be sited more superiorly. If the abdomen has been opened through a right paramedian incision the colostomy can be sited through the left rectus muscle.

2

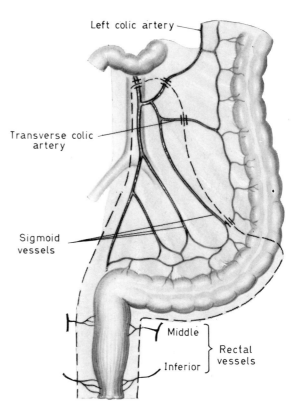

3

Extent of bowel removal

The plan of the vascular and lymphatic field which is to be removed shows an average arrangement of the vessels to be ligated: inferior mesenteric, left colic, transverse colic, middle and inferior rectal.

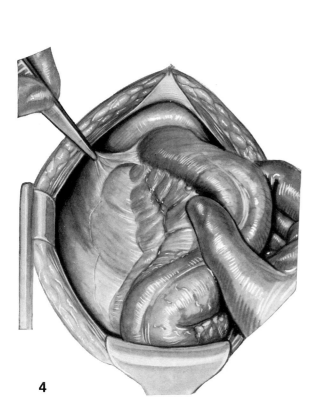

4

4

Mobilization of the colon

The wound edges are covered with moist packs and a self-retaining retractor of the Comyns—Berkeley type inserted. Small intestine can be packed away in the upper abdomen, or alternatively can be lifted out of the abdomen and placed under a warm pack or, preferably, in an Aldon bag. The iliac portion of the colon is then mobilized by incising the congenital peritoneal folds attached to the lateral aspect of its mesentery. The left ureter is identified and swept away from the vascular pedicle. The sigmoid colon is retracted to the left and the peritoneum incised to the right of the mid-line. The vascular supply of the rectum can now be approached from either side of its mesentery.

5

Ligation of the pedicle

The inferior mesenteric artery and vein are isolated by passing a finger between the mesentery and the anterior surface of the aorta. If lymph nodes are not obviously involved with tumour the presacral sympathetic plexuses should be identified and left intact. In all cases where large nodes are palpable and in tumours of the upper third of the rectum it is advisable to clear all the tissue anterior to the aorta including the sympathetic plexuses. The inferior mesenteric artery should be tied close to its origin from the aorta with thread or silk ligature. The inferior mesenteric vein lying to the left of the artery is then ligated and divided. The colostomy will be supplied by the middle colic vessels via the bifurcation of the left colic artery (which should always be preserved) and the marginal artery of the descending colon.

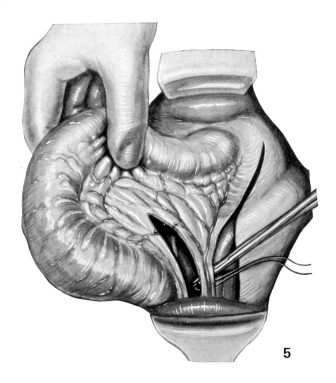

5

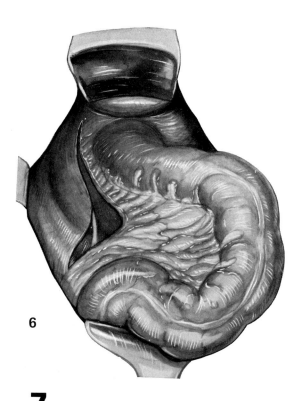

6

6

Pelvic dissection

No attempt at pelvic dissection should be made until the vessels have been ligated, except in large tumours where an initial trial dissection is carried out to assess if excision is possible. The peritoneal incisions are carried down on each side of the rectum to the level of the vesicles.

7

Production of line of cleavage

The rectosigmoid mesentery is lifted forwards from the promontory of the sacrum and a pair of blunt-ended scissors inserted in the mid-line downwards and backwards immediately in front of the first piece of the sacrum and behind the mesorectum; a presacral line of cleavage is thus defined.

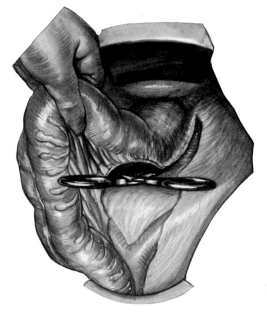

7

8

Further mobilization

The fingers and finally the hand are introduced into the presacral space and the mesorectum deliberately pushed forwards from the front of the presacral fascia and the sides of the pelvis as far downwards as the coccyx. Any tough strands of pelvic fascia are divided with scissors. At this stage the abdominal and perineal dissections meet behind the mesorectum, the rectum being completely freed posteriorly (not illustrated).

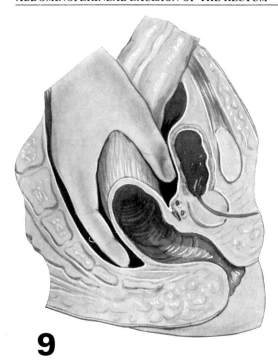

8

9

Peritoneal incisions

The peritoneal and subperitoneal tissues which have been incised on either side of the rectum are now joined anteriorly by dissecting across the peritoneal floor 1 cm in front of the lowest part of the peritoneal pouch.

The course of both ureters should be carefully noted at this stage and in bulky tumours in the mid-pelvis both ureters should be exposed throughout their course to the bladder to avoid damage.

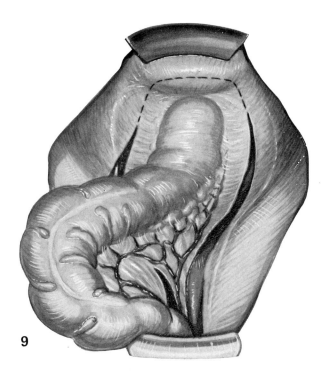

9

10

Incision of the fascia of Denonvillier

The apex of the incised peritoneum is drawn upwards and the base of the bladder and both vesicles (or vaginal wall in the female) exposed by blunt-nosed scissor dissection. A lipped St. Mark's retractor is inserted behind the vesicles which are drawn upwards exposing the fascia of Denonvillier on the anterior rectal wall. This is incised transversely and a distinct line of cleavage extending downwards as far as the apex of the prostate will be found with the fingers. While in this space the fingers are swept laterally to define the anterior border of the lateral ligaments.

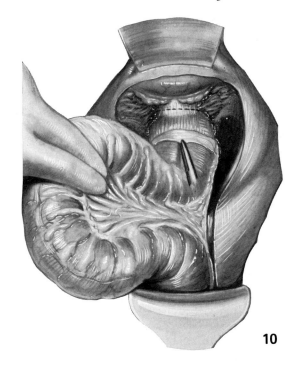

10

11

Division of the lateral ligaments

Each lateral ligament is in turn made taut by displacing the rectum to the opposite side with the left hand and then dividing with scissors well out on the pelvic wall as far downwards as possible. Any remaining portions will be divided by the perineal operator. The middle haemorrhoidal arteries should then be picked up and ligated if necessary.

The abdominal dissection is now complete, the remaining dissection being left to the perineal operator.

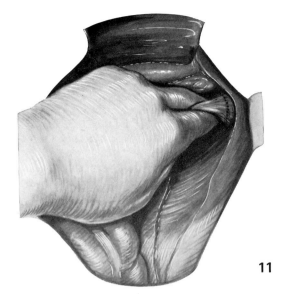

11

12

Division of colon

The colon is prepared for division by dividing the arcade between the left colic artery and the first sigmoid artery at a point which will allow 2 cm of viable colon to project through the abdominal wall at the site of the colostomy. The mesentery should be divided at right angles to the bowel. The bowel is divided between small clamps such as those of Zachary Cope. The perineal dissection having been completed, the excised colon and rectum are withdrawn through the perineum.

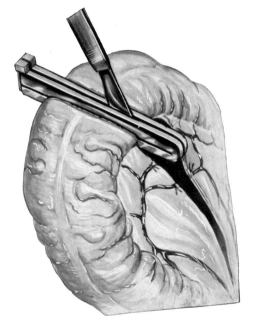

12

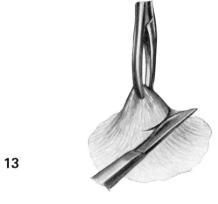

13

13

Colostomy incision

A circle of skin 1·5—2 cm in diameter is excised at a point one-third of the way along a line from the anterior superior iliac spine to the umbilicus.

A complete trephine is made through the abdominal wall to avoid constriction of the bowel. The superficial fascia is sutured to the external oblique aponeurosis in four places in order to eliminate a subcutaneous colostomy bulge. In pendulous abdomens the colostomy should be made 5—8 cm higher in order that it may be visible to the patient.

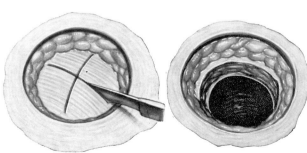

14

Passing the colon through the incision

The left border of the laparotomy wound is now elevated by passing a long forceps through the colostomy incision exposing the paracolic gutter. A non-absorbable thread purse-string suture is inserted from the lateral edge of the colostomy site, including some muscle fibres, and continued under the peritoneum of the paracolic gutter to the mesenteric border of the colon. When tied the space to the outer side of the colostomy is obliterated and this prevents small bowel obstruction through what would otherwise be a narrow foramen. The proximal clamped colon is passed through the colostomy incision.

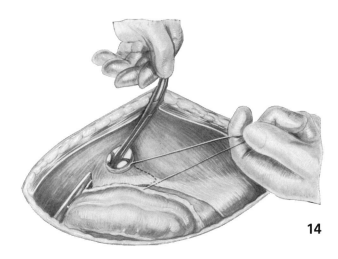

14

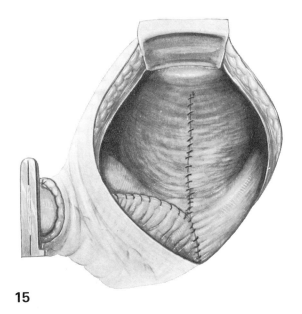

15

15

Closure of the abdomen

Before the pelvic peritoneum can be closed it is important for both the abdominal and perineal operators to obtain complete haemostasis. The pelvis is then irrigated with a suitable chemotherapeutic solution in order to minimize the risk of pelvic recurrence. Five hundred millilitres of a 1 : 500 mercuric perchloride solution is suitable for this purpose. The peritoneum from the lateral walls of the pelvis and the iliac fossae are gently mobilized with the fingers and the edges sutured together over the empty pelvis by an invaginating continuous Lembert suture to diminish the chance of adhesion formation using 2/0 chromic atraumatic catgut.

The main pedicle ligature is covered during this process and the suture continued laterally between the free edge of the mesocolon and the peritoneum of the left iliac fossa to the point of exit of the colon. The abdomen is closed without drainage and the wound sealed with Whitehead's varnish and a waterproof top dressing.

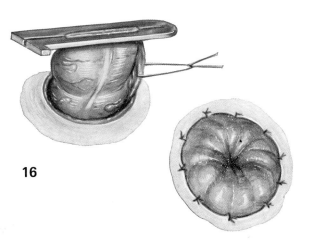

16

16

Formation of the colostomy stoma

The Zachary Cope clamp is now removed and the colon trimmed to leave 1·5–2 cm projecting above the skin surface. The edges of all coats of the colon are carefully sutured to the surrounding skin with interrupted 2/0 chromic catgut sutures. This produces a very satisfactory stoma with no tendency to skin stenosis.

PERINEAL DISSECTION IN THE MALE

17

The incision

A swab soaked in 1 : 500 mercuric perchloride solution is inserted into the anal canal and the anus is then closed with a strong subcutaneous purse-string suture to prevent soiling. No dissection is commenced until the abdominal surgeon has completed the exploration and decided that a combined excision is the correct procedure.

An elliptical incision is made round the anal canal from a point mid-way between the anus and the bulb of the urethra anteriorly and extending backwards to the sacrococcygeal articulation. This incision is deepened until the lobulated fat of the ischiorectal fossae is seen and the coccyx exposed.

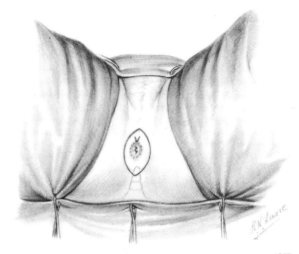

17

18

Removal of part of the coccyx

The coccyx is not routinely removed but in males with a narrow pelvis, and in patients with a large posterior tumour situated in the lower third of the rectum removal facilitates the dissection and extends the clearance of the tumour.

The coccyx is now flexed with the thumb to open up the coccygeal joint and the point of a scalpel is inserted. The distal portion of the coccyx is separated, care being taken to keep the knife close to the superior surface of the bone to avoid damaging the rectum. The middle sacral vessels may require diathermy coagulation or ligation at this stage.

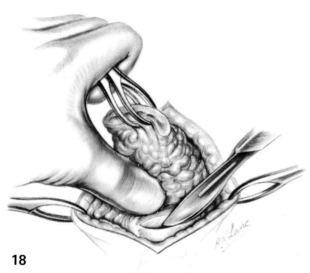

18

19

Isolation and division of the iliococcygeus muscles

Small lateral incisions are made with a scalpel on either side of the coccyx through the fibrous attachment of the coccygeus muscle and a finger is inserted on each side in a forward and outward direction to separate the levator muscles from the underlying rectal fascia of Waldeyer. The overlying ischiorectal fossa fat and the iliococcygeus muscles are now divided well out on the lateral walls of the pelvis. The inferior haemorrhoidal vessels require diathermy coagulation or ligation.

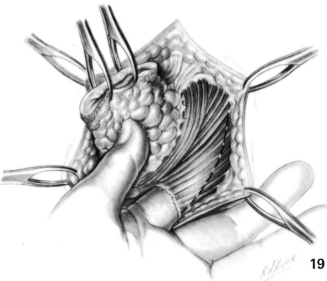

19

20

Exposure of the mesorectum

A St. Mark's pattern self-retaining perineal retractor is then placed in position and the fascia of Waldeyer which can be clearly seen incised just in front of the divided coccyx. If this fascia is not divided the presacral fascia will be stripped from the sacrum producing nerve damage and severe haemorrhage from the presacral venous plexus. This incision is continued laterally at the outlet of the bony pelvis to expose the mesorectum.

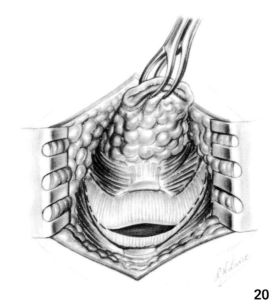

20

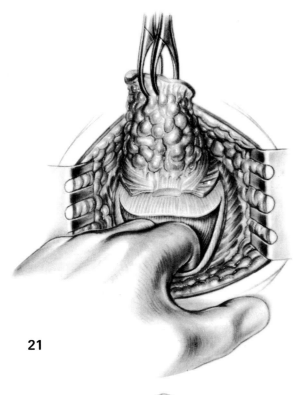

21

21

Separation of mesorectum

The fingers are inserted in front of the cut edge of the fascia and the mesorectum can be separated from the front of the presacral fascia and the lateral pelvic walls to the level of the sacral promontory.

Perineal and abdominal operators meet in this plane at this stage in the operation (*see Illustration 8*), the rectum being completely freed posteriorly.

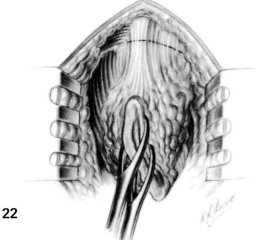

22

22

Anterior dissection

The rectum is then retracted posteriorly and transverse incisions are made on either side of the wound to expose the superficial and then the deep transverse perineal muscles. The plane of the dissection must be behind these muscles to avoid injury to the urethra and when the deep transverse perineal muscles are completely exposed by dividing the decussating fibres of the external sphincter muscle whitish longitudinal fibres of the anterior rectal wall will be seen.

23

Separation and division of the pubococcygeus muscles

The broad strap-like pubococcygeus muscles now become evident on either side of the rectum and prostate or vagina. A finger is inserted between the superior borders of these muscles, separating them from the underlying pelvic fascia while they are being divided almost completely from their origins on each side.

The underlying fascia, which is the lateral continuation of the fascia of Denonvillier and Waldeyer, is then divided to expose the rectal wall. The prostate will then be clearly felt anteriorly and the plane between the rectum and prostate defined. If the surgeon does not cut this fascial layer he will not enter the plane between the rectum and prostate and his dissection will be carried forward lateral to the prostate, producing a deep fossa anterior and lateral to the prostate and causing an unnecessary large wound and significantly increasing haemorrhage from the wound.

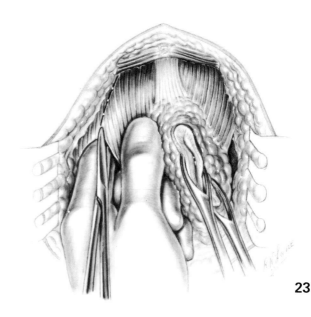

23

24

Separation and division of fibromuscular bundle

The thick inferior borders of the puborectalis muscles, together with longitudinal muscle fibres passing from the anterior rectal wall to the apex of the prostate and membranous urethra (recto-urethralis muscle) still hold the anorectal junction forwards in the middle line.

This barrier is separated into two bundles by blunt dissection with an artery forceps. The forceps are directed towards the apex of the prostate which is located with the index finger of the left hand and must lie parallel with the posterior aspect of the gland to avoid injury to the urethra. The separated fibromuscular bundles are divided in turn and the capsule of the prostate exposed.

Occasionally a few readily-recognized longitudinal fibres obscure the capsule and require separate division to avoid injury to the rectum and expose the true plane of cleavage which will already have been found by the abdominal operator.

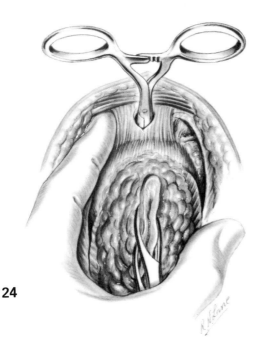

24

25

Division of the pelvic fascia

The visceral pelvic fascia, which is condensed anteriorly and passes forward to the lateral aspects of the prostate, is divided, exposing the whole of the posterior aspect of the prostate and then the seminal vesicles above. At this stage the abdominal and perineal operators meet anteriorly.

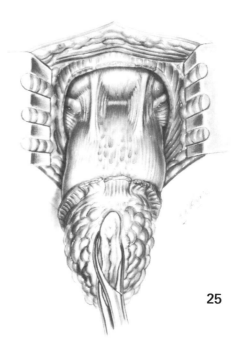

25

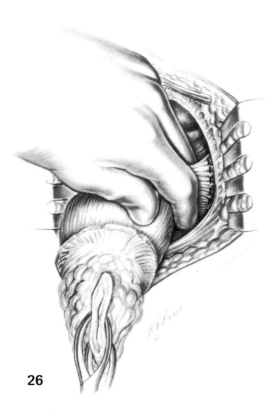

26

26

Removal of the rectum

The anterior and posterior aspects of the rectum are now completely isolated and only the remaining lower portions of the lateral ligaments require division. The bowel is alternatively displaced to the opposite side and the stretched ligament divided close to the pelvic wall. The excised rectum and sigmoid colon is then passed down from the abdomen and removed through the perineum. Haemostasis is secured and to avoid the risk of reactionary haemorrhage the blood pressure at this stage of the operation should not be much lower than the patient's normal. Open veins may be located by levelling the table.

27a & b

Closure of the perineal wound

It is necessary to pack the perineal cavity firmly with dry gauze in the rare case where severe haemorrhage persists. This is removed 3 days later. When the peritoneal pelvic floor cannot be closed a thin plastic bag lightly packed with gauze is inserted into the pelvic cavity to prevent downward prolapse of the small intestine. This is left in place for 3–5 days.

In the majority of cases the perineal wound in males can be completely or partially closed. No attempt is made to suture the levator muscles or the pelvic fat. In cases where really good haemostasis is not attained, or where there is pre-existing infection or the wound has been soiled by perforating the rectum, the wound is closed as shown in *Illustration 27a*. The skin anteriorly and posteriorly are closed with vertical mattress sutures leaving a space in the middle of the wound through which three fingers can be inserted. The corrugated drain is placed into the pelvic cavity through this open aspect of the wound and sutured to the skin. When good haemostasis is attained and

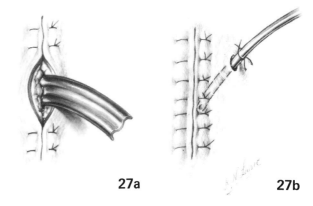

27a   **27b**

there is no pre-existing sepsis or soiling, one or two suction-drainage tubes, preferably of the sump type such as the Shirley drain, are inserted into the pelvis through lateral stab incisions and the wound closed completely with vertical mattress sutures. Continuous suction is started immediately and maintained for between 5 and 7 days. The wound is sealed with gauze dressings using Whitehead's varnish and adhesive tape which is left undisturbed until the sutures are removed on the tenth postoperative day.

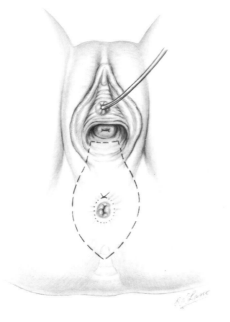

28

PERINEAL WOUND DISSECTION IN THE FEMALE

28

The incision

In excising the rectum for malignant disease, unless the tumour is small and situated in the mid-line posteriorly, the posterior vaginal wall should always be excised in continuity with the rectum. The incision therefore extends from the posterior lateral aspects of the labia around the anus to the coccyx.

29

The extent of the anterior dissection

Excision of the rectum procedes as in the male until the anterior part of the dissection is reached. The anterior incisions are then carried upwards through the lateral aspects of the vagina as far as the posterior fornix. A transverse incision is then made through the posterior fornix to join the two lateral incisions. This is deepened to expose the rectal wall, at which point the abdominal and perineal operators meet anteriorly. The lateral ligaments are then divided and the specimen removed.

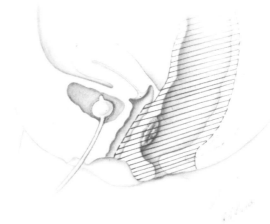

29

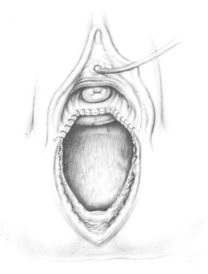

30

30

Haemostasis

No attempt at reconstructing the vagina is necessary. Haemostasis is attained by oversewing each half of the cut edge of the vagina with a continuous 2/0 chromic catgut suture.

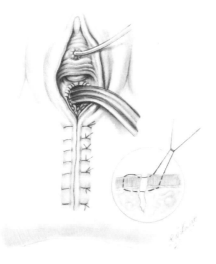

31

31

Perineal closure

As in the male no attempt is made to suture the cut edges of the levator muscle or the pelvic fat. The incision is closed with interrupted mattress sutures as far forward as the cut edges of the labia which are approximated. A corrugated drain is placed into the pelvic cavity through the re-formed vaginal orifice.

POSTOPERATIVE CARE AND COMPLICATIONS

These are of particular importance after operations which have included removal of the rectum because not only may the patient suffer from any of the complications of a major abdominal operation but, in addition, the colostomy, urinary tract and perineal wound require special attention.

Intravenous infusion

The infusion of whole blood given during the operation may be continued afterwards. It is followed by intravenous dextrose and electrolyte solutions until normal peristalsis returns and flatus is passed through the colostomy. This usually occurs between the third and fifth postoperative days.

Gastric complications

Gastric aspiration through a nasogastric tube is unnecessary in the majority of patients. Small quantities of water by mouth are commenced as the postoperative ileus is relieved.

The perineal wound

The perineal wound is closed with suction-drainage in most male patients. The dead space between the skin and the pelvic peritoneum will be obliterated more rapidly if the patient is encouraged to sit up or if the head of the bed is raised as soon as the general condition of the patient permits, usually after a period of 24 hr. If a corrugated drain is present, it is removed on the third postoperative day but the skin sutures are retained for 10 days, the scar then being supported by suitable adhesive tape. In the male patient in whom the perineal wound has been closed by primary suture, continuous suction is maintained until drainage is minimal usually for a period of between 5 and 7 days. The suction catheter is then withdrawn and the skin sutures removed on the tenth postoperative day. If it has been necessary to pack the wound the gauze is gradually removed from the plastic bag during the first 3–5 days, after which the bag itself is removed. The perineal cavity is dressed twice daily with an antiseptic solution until it is nearly flat, when skin healing takes place by secondary intention. It is important to remove all retained blood clots.

Retention of urine

In any radical operation some temporary or permanent damage to the nerves of the bladder is inevitable. All patients have an indwelling catheter of the Gibbon or Foley type connected to a sterile plastic bag on open drainage. On the fifth day the catheter is removed and a trial made to establish normal micturition. This may be helped by carbachol or a similar drug by mouth or by injection. Those who fail are given open drainage as before for another 24–48 hr when a further trial is made. The process may be repeated several times and even when micturition appears to be established it is important to ensure that there is little or no residual urine. Patients with prostatic enlargement may require either a transurethral resection or an open prostatectomy. Those with complete bladder paresis may be assisted by a small transurethral resection; bladder emptying is then accomplished at regular intervals by suprapubic pressure. This is however very rare.

The colostomy

The action of the colostomy is usually spontaneous and it will be found that on the fourth or fifth day after the operation flatus will be passed. Should delay occur a glycerin suppository may be inserted into the colon, but in the absence of distension it is usually wise to leave the bowel alone until it begins to function normally. Only occasionally will an enema be required. A transparent adhesive colostomy appliance will have been placed over the colostomy at the end of the operative procedure. No other dressings are required, though the colostomy stitches should be removed in 10 days if they have not resorbed.

[*The illustrations for this Chapter on Abdominoperineal Excision of the Rectum were drawn by Mr. R. N. Lane.*]

Abdominoperineal Excision of the Rectum

Malcolm C. Veidenheimer, M.D.
Section of Colon and Rectal Surgery,
Lahey Clinic Foundation, Boston, Massachusetts

Low-lying rectal cancers are usually treated by an abdominoperineal excision of the rectum. This may be accomplished in the traditional way of Miles or by the synchronous combined method. The Miles approach involves an abdominal dissection and mobilization of the rectum, which is then buried beneath the reconstituted pelvic floor. The rectum is subsequently excised through the perineal route. Traditionally, this manoeuvre was accomplished by turning the patient into the left lateral position, although it may also be carried out with the patient in the lithotomy position.

The synchronous combined operation is the approach we favour. This operative technique involves two teams operating synchronously once the operability of the lesion has been determined by the abdominal operator. We believe such an approach allows readier access to the anatomical structures, especially in the presence of large bulky tumours and a narrow pelvis in men.

Indications

Abdominoperineal excision is the customary treatment for rectal cancers low enough to be palpated by the examining finger. Higher lesions may permit an anterior resection with reconstitution of intestinal continuity. Controversy exists regarding the management of small low-lying cancers of the rectum, and alternate forms of therapy to the abdominoperineal operation described here are to be found elsewhere in this book. The abdominoperineal excision of the rectum may also be performed because of rectal involvement by primary tumours of other pelvic organs. Even in the presence of extensive metastatic disease, if the patient's life expectancy is more than a few months, we believe that greater patient comfort can be achieved if the primary lesion is removed. Abdominoperineal excision of the rectum is also performed for inflammatory bowel disease; in this instance, however, the dissection is carried closer to the bowel than is described in this chapter in an effort to preserve as much of the nerve supply to the bladder and organs of sexual function as possible (*see* Chapter on 'Conservative Excision of the Rectum in Inflammatory Bowel Disease', pages 26–29).

Pre-operative preparation

All patients undergoing abdominoperineal excision are instructed to take a liquid diet for 2 days before operation. The bowel is cleansed by the use of laxatives taken orally unless the rectal tumour has produced obstruction. We do not routinely utilize an antibacterial preparation in the absence of a colonic anastomosis.

Pre-operative intravenous pyelography is carried out in all of our patients having bowel surgery to assess renal function and ureteral anatomy. Chest radiography and liver profile studies are also carried out in the pre-operative period. Two units of whole blood are cross-matched and are available if needed during the surgical procedure.

Anaesthesia

The two methods of administration of anaesthesia for this procedure are by the general route, using an endotracheal tube, or by the spinal form, which is supplemented by Pentothal (thiopentone sodium), nitrous oxide and oxygen. A cardiac monitor is utilized throughout the procedure. A size 16 Foley catheter with a 5 ml bag is inserted into the bladder in the operating room under sterile conditions.

THE OPERATION

1

The patient is positioned with legs in stirrups. Partial flexion of the thighs permits ready access to the abdomen by the abdominal team of operators, but the use of the stirrups allows access to the perineum by the perineal operators. A moderate degree of Trendelenburg tilt aids in the dissection.

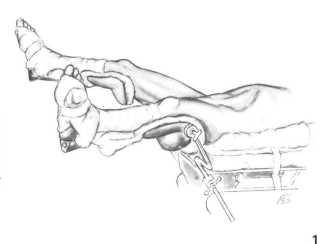

1

2

The location of the incision is important not only in consideration of access to the abdominal contents but also in consideration of deformity of the abdominal wall and the relationship of such deformity to the placement of an abdominal stoma. Because of the importance of such a consideration, all of our incisions are made in the mid-line so that neither the right nor left half of the abdomen has scarring that might interfere with the selection of a site for a stoma.

The colostomy, ideally, should be situated over the rectus muscle and beneath the belt-line at a distance from the iliac crest, umbilicus, and rib margin that will permit easy application of an appliance. Paracolostomy herniation is less likely to occur if the stoma is placed through the rectus muscle rather than in a pararectal situation or more laterally in the oblique musculature of the abdominal wall.

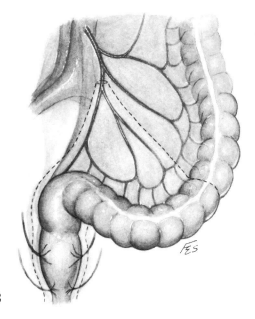

2

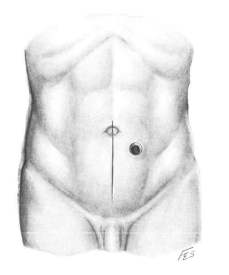

3

3

The operation of abdominoperineal excision evolves around the control of the three major areas of blood supply to the rectosigmoid and rectum. These are the sigmoidal and superior haemorrhoidal branches of the inferior mesenteric artery, the middle haemorrhoidal arteries, which pass through the lateral ligaments of the rectum, and the inferior haemorrhoidal vessels, which are to be found in the ischiorectal fossa. We do not believe in ligation of the inferior mesenteric artery at its origin because nodal involvement at that level is found only in patients with incurable rectal cancer. We, therefore, ligate distal to the main inferior mesenteric trunk and thus ensure a more viable blood supply to the colostomy.

4

After the insertion of a self-retaining Balfour retractor and a plastic wound protector, the abdomen is explored for evidence of spread of the primary disease. Mobilization of the sigmoid and rectosigmoid colon begins in the left paracolic gutter to obtain sufficient mobility to bring the bowel to the abdominal wall at the level of the proposed colostomy.

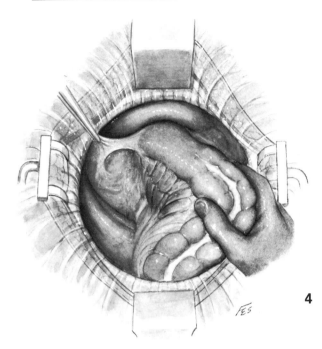

4

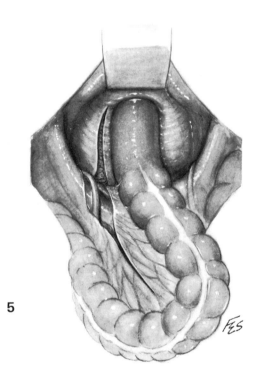

5

5

The peritoneum on the left aspect of the sigmoid and rectosigmoid is incised with scissors. The site of this incision is guided by the location of the branches of the inferior mesenteric artery mentioned in *Illustration 2*. The left ureter must be observed and protected during the course of this dissection. All patients should have pre-operative intravenous pyelography to determine the course and number of ureters present from each kidney. Dissection of the peritoneum is continued anteriorly to the base of the bladder.

6

The peritoneal incision on the right side of the sigmoid and rectosigmoid is performed in a similar fashion. Again, the ureter is preserved. A gauze pad protects the small bowel from the operative field. The vasculature is ligated between clamps.

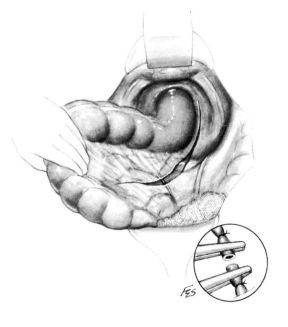

6

7

The peritoneal incisions have been joined across the base of the bladder anteriorly just anterior to the bottom of the rectovesical pouch, and the retrorectal presacral space is entered in front of the sacral promontory by inserting dissecting scissors into this region while maintaining gentle anterior traction upon the rectosigmoid. The loose areolar tissue in the presacral space is relatively avascular and usually readily entered.

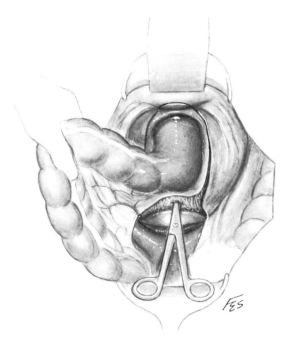

7

8

Once the presacral space has been demonstrated with sharp dissection, the right hand is inserted into this region, and the presacral dissection is carried out by means of blunt finger dissection and gentle anterior displacement of the rectum.

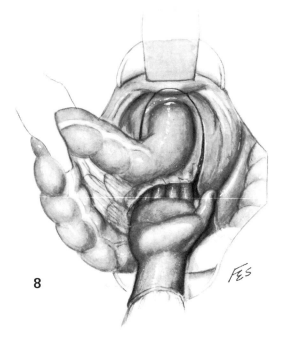

8

9

The rectum is freed from the presacral fascia distally to the level of the tip of the coccyx. The dissection is performed in a plane anterior to the presacral fascia and thus damage to the presacral veins is avoided. Occasionally, branches of the middle sacral artery will require ligation.

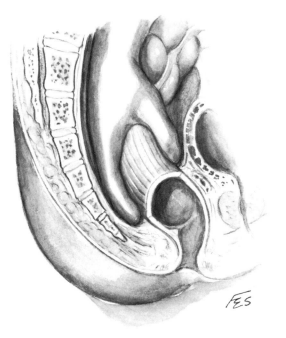

9

10

The anterior dissection, aided by retraction on the bowel, is now carried to a deeper plane. The posterior wall of the bladder and the seminal vesicles are demonstrated by a combination of sharp and blunt dissection. Denonvillier's fascia must be incised by sharp dissection, as depicted here, to mobilize the rectum farther from the prostate and seminal vesicles.

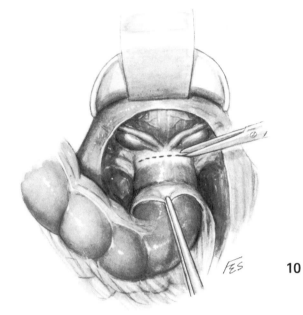

11

Once this layer has been incised, the bladder, prostate and seminal vesicles may be swept away from the rectum by finger and scissor dissection displaying the now bared longitudinal muscle wall of the anterior rectal surface. By means of retraction of the bladder and prostatic area and counter-traction on the rectum, the dissection is carried distally until the apex of the prostate and the urethra with its contained catheter can be palpated.

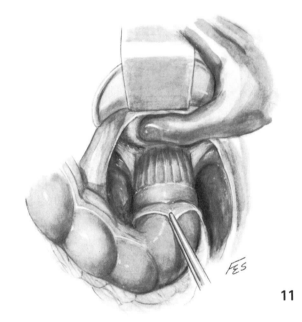

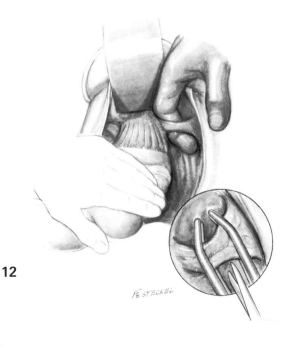

12

Attention is now turned to the middle haemorrhoidal vasculature. By means of a corkscrew motion with the index finger passed along the right and then left lateral borders of the rectum, the lateral ligament with its contained middle haemorrhoidal vessels is isolated from the surrounding fascial structures, clamped, cut and ligated. Upon conclusion of this step of the procedure, the rectum is completely isolated anteriorly, laterally and posteriorly. A few strands of remaining fascia may require division with scissors, but no important vascular control will be required to complete the abdominal dissection.

13

The site of the colostomy is now prepared by grasping the skin in a Kocher clamp and excising a circular segment of skin, the diameter of which should approximate the diameter of the sigmoid colon to be used for the sigmoid colostomy. The subcutaneous fatty tissue is retracted, and the anterior sheath of the rectus muscle is incised in a cruciate fashion. The rectus muscle fibres are split in a longitudinal direction, and the peritoneal cavity is entered with scissors. The colostomy aperture in the peritoneum, muscle and skin must be of a size to admit two fingers.

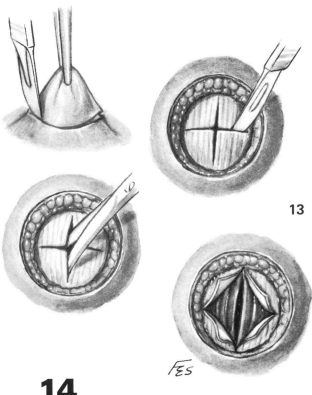

13

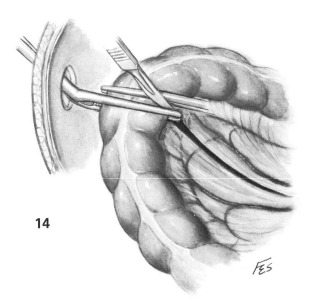

14

14

An angled Kocher clamp is passed through the colostomy incision into the abdominal cavity to grasp the sigmoid colon at the site of the proposed colostomy. The distal rectosigmoid is also clamped, and the bowel is divided between these two clamps. The proximal bowel is withdrawn through the abdominal wall to lie without tension on the anterior abdominal surface.

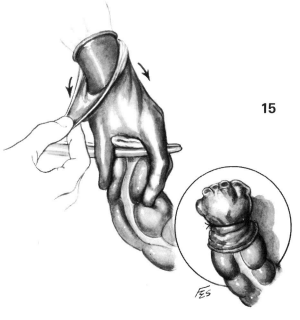

15

15

The distal divided bowel is sealed from contamination by grasping it in a doubly gloved hand and tying the removed outer glove over the stump of rectosigmoid as the clamp is removed from the bowel.

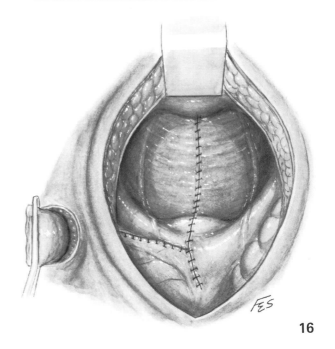

16

16

The rectum is then buried in the pelvic cavity, and by finger dissection the peritoneum on either lateral wall is mobilized to a degree that will permit closure with a continuous chromic catgut suture. We do not close the lateral gutter in relation to the afferent limb of the colostomy.

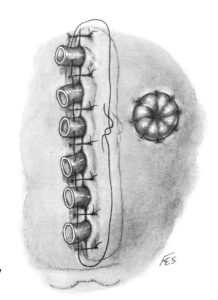

17

17

The colostomy is completed by immediate mucocutaneous suture using about eight sutures of 4/0 chromic catgut. A disposable colostomy bag is applied to the colostomy in the operating room. Note the clothesline drain: a series of 0·5 cm Penrose drains suspended from a silk suture. These drains, measuring 3–5 cm in length, are inserted between each skin stitch and removed on the fourth postoperative day. We believe copious irrigation of the wound before skin closure and the use of the clothesline drain diminish the incidence of wound infection.

The perineal dissection is commenced once the operability of the lesion has been ascertained by the abdominal surgeon. Thus, the dissection can be performed synchronously from both the abdominal and perineal routes. If two teams are not available to perform the abdominoperineal excision, the abdominal dissection, as depicted in *Illustrations 1–17*, may be performed first and the perineal dissection performed as a separate operative approach after the colostomy has been fashioned and the abdominal incision has been closed. However, both the abdominal and the perineal dissections are facilitated by use of the synchronous technique.

The perineal dissection

18

A purse-string suture of heavy catgut is placed around the anal verge to close the anus. A rectangular incision is made surrounding the area of the anus, including a generous margin of peri-anal skin, and extending from the tip of the coccyx posteriorly to the bulb of the urethra anteriorly. The edges of the skin are grasped by Lahey double-hook clamps, and the peri-anal skin is grasped anteriorly and posteriorly with Kocher forceps.

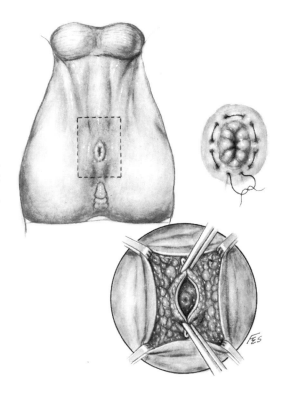

18

19

The dissection begins laterally. Blunt scissors are used to divide the peri-anal fat and to enter the ischiorectal fossa. Usually there are two distinct vascular bundles lying anteriorly and posteriorly deep in the ischiorectal fat. These are the inferior haemorrhoidal vessels, and they will require ligation.

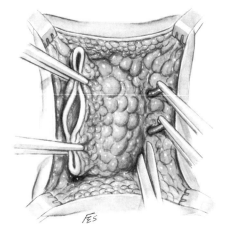

19

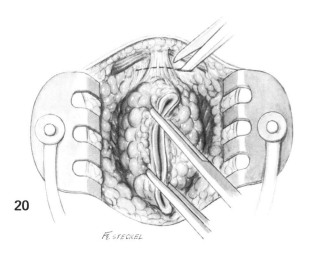

20

20

Once the ischiorectal fossa has been entered bilaterally and posteriorly to the level of the tip of the coccyx, the anterior dissection is deepened in a plane at the posterior border of the deep transverse perineal muscle.

21

A self-retaining retractor facilitates this dissection. The presacral space is now entered by inserting scissors into this plane at the level of the coccygeal tip. It is important that these scissors be inserted in a truly anterior direction so that they penetrate the presacral fascia and do not strip this fascia from the front of the sacrum. Thus, haemorrhage from the presacral veins will be avoided. At this juncture, the abdominal and the perineal dissections meet, and the rectum and anus will be free in the mid-line posteriorly.

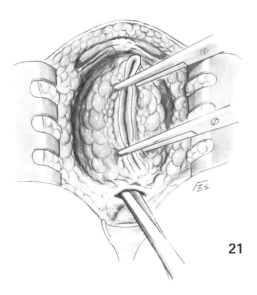

21

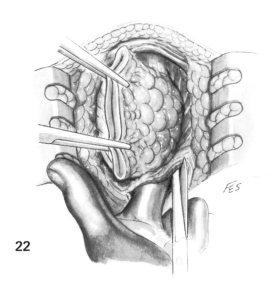

22

22

A finger inserted through the precoccygeal incision will enter the already dissected pelvic space. This finger is swept across the superior aspect of the levator muscles on the left and right sides of the pelvis, and the levator muscles are divided along their pelvic wall attachment with scissors. This plane is usually avascular.

23

The rectum is delivered from the pelvis and by traction in an anterior direction, the remaining attachments of the recto-urethralis muscle and fascia in the region of the urethra may be divided with safety. The palpating finger should readily ascertain and protect the urethra with its contained catheter.

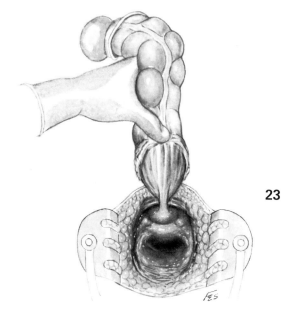

23

24

The perineal wound is copiously irrigated and then closed using interrupted chromic catgut sutures in the ischiorectal fat. A suction sump drain is placed into the pelvic cavity and brought out through the posterior aspect of the perineal wound. The perineal wound is closed using interrupted silk sutures.

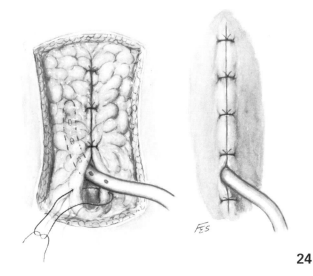

24

POSTOPERATIVE CARE

The patient is not given anything orally until gas is passing freely through the colostomy. This usually takes 24–48 hr. After this time, a liquid diet is prescribed.

Our patients sit on the edge of the bed the evening of operation and are asked to sit in a chair the day after operation. Ambulation continues in an increasing way throughout the hospital stay.

The clothesline drain is removed on the fourth postoperative day as is the perineal suction catheter. At this time, the perineal sinus is irrigated with normal saline solution three times a day, and the patient commences sitz baths three times each day. The perineal sutures are removed on the sixth or seventh day, and the sutures of the abdominal incision are removed on the seventh postoperative day.

The Foley urethral catheter is left indwelling for 1 week after abdominoperineal excision. In patients whose prostatic enlargement has interfered with urinary tract function, transurethral resection of the prostate may be necessary after abdominoperineal excision because of interference with bladder function consequent upon the excision of the rectum. We prefer to defer such a procedure for some weeks even if it is necessary for the patient to leave the hospital with an indwelling catheter.

The colostomy may be cared for by irrigation every second day or by permitting spontaneous activity. The patient is instructed in both forms of care and makes a decision regarding choice of care after becoming accustomed to the colostomy. Instructions regarding colostomy irrigations are commenced 1 week after operation at a time when the colostomy has become firmly adherent to the abdominal wall. During the hospital stay the colostomy is cared for by means of disposable plastic colostomy bags.

[*The illustrations for this Chapter on Abdominoperineal Excision of the Rectum were drawn by Mr. F. E. Steckel.*]

Anterior Resection

J. C. Goligher, Ch.M., F.R.C.S., Hon. F.A.C.S.
Professor of Surgery, University of Leeds;
Surgeon, General Infirmary at Leeds

PRE - OPERATIVE

Indications

When anterior resection was first introduced for the treatment of carcinoma of the rectosigmoid and upper rectum in the early 1940's, there was considerable controversy as to its safety and efficacy for this purpose. But its use has been in large measure vindicated in more recent years by many large-scale studies of the early and late results in comparison with those of abdominoperineal excision (Waugh et al., 1955; Mayo and Fly, 1956; Mayo et al., 1958; Deddish and Stearns, 1961; Cullen and Mayo, 1963; Morgan, 1965; Vandertoll and Beahrs, 1965). Although nearly all these enquiries are open to some criticism on the validity of their comparative data (Goligher, 1962), their findings have convinced most surgeons that anterior resection can offer as good a chance of cure as does abdominoperineal excision for many patients with growths in the rectosigmoid or upper third or half of the rectum. It may thus now be regarded as an established surgical procedure for the treatment of suitable carcinomas in these situations; but, if disappointments are to be avoided, great care must be exercised in the choice of patients for this operation. The main criteria of selection are the following.

Height of growth and physical characteristics of patient

These are by far the most important considerations in deciding on the suitability of a case for anterior resection – or other form of sphincter-saving resection. It is only for growths of the upper two-thirds of the rectum and the rectosigmoid (that is, with their lower margins lying anywhere between 7·5 and 15 cm from the anal verge on sigmoidoscopy) that sphincter-saving resection need be considered at all. At first sight it might seem that, if the growth is situated as low as 7·5 or 8 cm and the upper end of the anal canal is at 3·5 cm, it would be impossible to achieve a 5 cm (2 inch) margin of clearance below the lesion, as is usually considered essential in a radical sphincter-saving resection for cancer (Quer et al., 1953; Grinnell, 1954; Goligher, 1975), without removing the upper part of the anal sphincters. It must be remembered, however, that once the lateral ligaments have been divided and the rectum has been fully mobilized and straightened out, a point on the rectal wall 7·5 cm from the anal verge may rise to 11 or 12 cm (see Illustration 5), making a radical resection with conservation of the sphincters at least theoretically possible. Whether an anterior resection will be technically possible or not at these lower levels will depend to a large extent on the sex and build of the patients, as well as on the surgeon's familiarity with this type of operation. The greater width of the female pelvis considerably facilitates the performance of anterior resection, and in a thin woman it is easily possible to carry out an adequate resection of this kind for a carcinoma lying as low as 8 cm from the anal verge. But in an obese woman or in a male patient, even if emaciated, this operation is seldom practicable for growths lower than 10 to 11 cm, whilst in obese males lesions as high as 12 to 13 cm may be found technically extremely difficult for anterior resection. Clearly, if anterior resection is the only form of resection with conservation of the sphincters being practised by a surgeon however skilled he may be in its use, a few of the female patients and a larger proportion of the male patients with carcinomas in the middle third of the rectum, which on pathological grounds would be deemed suitable for sphincter-saving resection, will be denied the opportunity of having this type of operation and condemned to an abdominoperineal excision and a permanent colostomy. There is thus a need for the complementary practice of other forms of sphincter-saving resection, such as the abdomino-anal or abdominosacral resection (*see* pages 157–198), if the maximum use of sphincter conservation is to be made in the radical treatment of rectal cancer.

From the foregoing it will also be appreciated that a firm decision as to whether a sphincter-saving resection is going to be feasible or not, and which type of operation will be most suitable, cannot be reached until the abdomen has been opened, and often not until the rectum and the carcinoma have been fully mobilized.

The grade of malignancy of the growth

It is known that unusually extensive spread in the rectal wall – sometimes up to 7–10 cm distant from the macroscopic edge of the primary lesion – may occur in connection with anaplastic rectal carcinomas. Clearly, in such cases a conventional resection with anastomosis might result in a troublesome local recurrence, and a sphincter-saving resection is probably better avoided in any patient whose pre-operative sigmoidoscopic biopsy shows a highly active growth.

In this case it may be pointed out that a villous papilloma, the lower edge of which seems to be benign as shown by the complete absence of induration on palpation with the finger, may be safely removed by a resection excising as little as 0·5–1 cm of normal bowel wall distal to the growth.

The presence of hepatic metastases

When secondary deposits are present in the liver and the condition is incurable, considerable palliation may nonetheless accrue from removal of the primary growth, which is responsible for most of the patient's symptoms. Obviously the palliative value of such an excision will be greatly enhanced if it can be carried out as a sphincter-saving resection instead of as an operation involving the establishment of a permanent colostomy. Bearing this in mind the surgeon may feel tempted to stretch the indications for resection with conservation of the sphincter in such patients. If he is not careful, however, he may incur for his patient a high incidence of complications which may greatly prolong the period of convalescence and thereby diminish the amount of palliation afforded. It is generally wiser, therefore, not to accept any relaxation in the usual criteria of selection for sphincter-saving resection when considering palliative cases.

Special pre-operative measures
Preliminary or simultaneous transverse colostomy

If the patient is acutely or subacutely obstructed a proximal colostomy alone should be performed in the first instance. This is best sited in the extreme right of the transverse colon, at a small transverse wound in the right subcostal region, which leaves the left half of the abdomen unencumbered by a stoma at the subsequent resection 2 or 3 weeks later. In the interval between the establishment of the colostomy and resection, the colon is prepared by daily washes-through from the colostomy to the anus or vice-versa, and by insertion of suppositories containing phthalyl-sulphathiazole or neomycin. In the usual unobstructed case, however, a preliminary colostomy is unnecessary, but if at operation the bowel is found to be more heavily loaded than was anticipated, or if the anastomosis was effected only with difficulty, it may be advisable to establish a temporary defunctioning transverse colostomy at the end of the resection. In fact many surgeons, impressed by the frequency of dehiscence of the anastomosis after *low* anterior resection, make it virtually their routine to perform a simultaneous transverse colostomy at the conclusion of any really low resection.

For the average patient the local and general preparation differs in no essential respect from that employed for abdominoperineal excision (*see* pages 118–119), but mechanical preparation of the bowel is especially important since an empty colon facilitates the conduct of these operations and probably results in a smoother recovery. In the anaesthetic room an indwelling urethral catheter is inserted, the bladder completely emptied by compression, and an intravenous infusion started in the right arm.

Anaesthesia

General anaesthesia supplemented by relaxant drugs is the most satisfactory routine for these operations, although spinal and epidural anaesthesia have their advocates.

Position of patient

The general set-up for sphincter-saving resections is identical with that for abdominoperineal excision, for, as has already been emphasized, the feasibility of carrying out a sphincter-conserving type of operation usually emerges clearly only at laparotomy, and indeed often only after a certain amount of dissection. It may well be, therefore, that the intervention will finish up as an ordinary combined excision. If the synchronous combined technique is preferred for abdominoperineal excision, the patient is placed in the modified lithotomy-Trendelenburg position (*see* page 120), which also allows a change in plan of operation should resection with restoration of continuity be contra-indicated. This particular position has in addition certain technical advantages for the conduct of sphincter-saving resections, for it affords ready access to the anal region whilst the abdomen is still open.

THE OPERATION

LOW ANTERIOR RESECTION

1

Incision, abdominal exploration, mobilization of sigmoid colon and exposure and ligature of inferior mesenteric vessels

The initial steps of this operation are identical with those of the abdominal phase of abdominoperineal excision (*see* pages 120–125, *Illustrations 2–16*), and consist of: opening and exploration of abdomen through a long left paramedian rectus-displacing incision extending from the pubis to at least 8–10 cm above the level of the umbilicus; ligation of the bowel with a strong silk tie 8–10 cm above the growth to control upward displacement of free cancer cells in the lumen; mobilization of the sigmoid loop by division of the developmental adhesions on the lateral side of the sigmoid mesocolon; identification of the left ureter and exposure of the inferior mesenteric vessels through incisions in the peritoneum on either side of the base of the mesocolon, extended upwards on the right side in front of the abdominal aorta to the lower border of the third part of the duodenum. The inferior mesenteric artery is then ligated and divided at its origin flush with the front

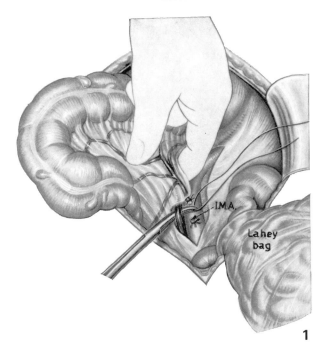

1

of the aorta, and the vein is tied separately at about the same level. (It greatly facilitates the display of these structures if, at the beginning of the operation, the loops of small gut are turned out of the abdomen into a plastic Lahey bag which retains them on the front of the upper right abdomen and lower chest out of the way of the abdominal dissection.)

2

Preparation of colon stump

The sigmoid loop is now spread out to display its vessels (aided by transillumination if necessary), preparatory to making an oblique incision with scissors in the mesosigmoid from the site of ligation of the main vessels to a point on the sigmoid colon adjudged capable of extending without tension to the top of the future rectal stump. Generally the length of colon stump required for this purpose does not need to be much longer than that used for establishing the terminal iliac colostomy in an abdominoperineal excision. Commonly, the cut traverses the ascending and transverse left colic vessels and the marginal arcade between the first and sigmoid arteries, which have to be ligated and divided. Finally the bowel itself is sectioned between two Parker-Kerr clamps applied obliquely from the antimesenteric to the mesenteric border.

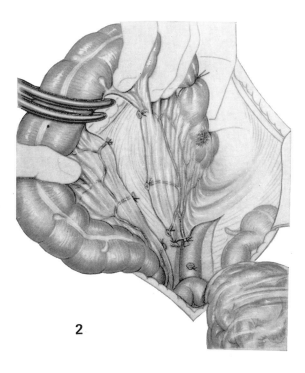

2

3

Alternative plans of ligation and preparation of colon stump

The scheme of ligations just outlined leaves the descending colon and sigmoid stump nourished solely by the middle colic artery through its bifurcation and continuation distally as the marginal artery (*A*). Almost invariably this supply is found to be adequate as shown by the colour of the bowel and the pulsation of the vessels in its wall, or, if there is any dubiety, by free arterial bleeding on snipping one of the small mural arteries. If a longer colon stump is required, it can often be prepared by retaining more of the sigmoid, supplied by the intersigmoidal marginal arcades (*B*). An alternative plan for securing a longer colon stump is to mobilize the splenic flexure, and this procedure, together with resection to the upper descending or distal transverse colon (*C*), is also forced upon the surgeon if the blood supply to a sigmoid stump, fashioned as described above, has been found inadequate. Naturally if a purely palliative resection is being undertaken a low ligation of the inferior mesenteric vessels suffices (*D*).

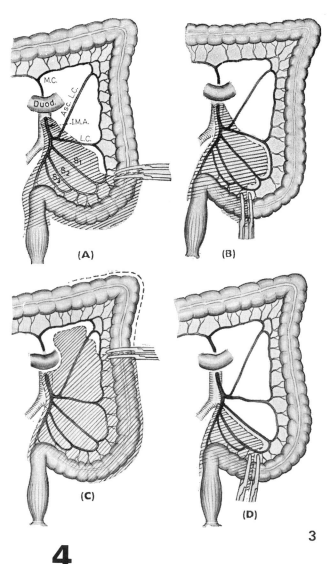

(A) (B)

(C) (D)

3

4

Separation of rectum and growth from pelvis

The rectum has now to be dissected free from its surroundings in exactly the same way as in an abdominoperineal excision. The lower ends of the incisions in the peritoneum on either side of the sigmoid mesocolon are extended downwards round the brim of the pelvis to meet anteriorly on the back of the bladder. The tongue of tissue including the upper ends of the inferior mesenteric vessels is dissected down off the common iliac vessels and front of sacrum, the separation being completed to beyond the tip of the coccyx by inserting the hand into the presacral space and lifting the rectum forwards. Next, by both scissor and blunt dissection the bladder, vasa deferentia, seminal vesicles and prostate are separated from the front of the rectum and its lateral ligaments. Finally, the lateral ligaments are divided with long heavy scissors either *in toto* or in their upper two-thirds, depending on the height of the growth.

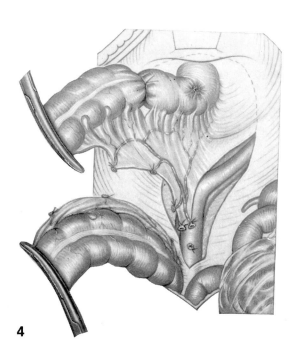

4

5

Final assessment of suitability of growth for anterior resection

The effect of mobilizing the rectum as just described – and particularly of dividing the lateral rectal ligaments – is to allow the bowel to run straight upwards from the anorectal ring without its normal anteroposterior and lateral curves. As a consequence it 'lengthens', and a growth at say 8 cm from the anal verge on sigmoidoscopy before operation may now lie at 12 cm or more from the anus. It is at this stage that the surgeon should make his final decision as to the suitability of the lesion for low anterior resection or not. With the rectum held gently taut he should estimate the top of the anorectal stump, if an anterior resection is performed, as lying 5 cm below the lower edge of the growth. If it seems that division at this level will leave a sufficient anorectal remnant to permit of a satisfactory sutured anastomosis he will proceed to anterior resection. Otherwise he will complete the operation as an abdominoperineal excision or a 'pull-through' resection.

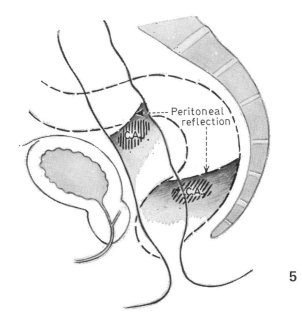

5

6

Division of mesorectum

The next step is to separate the mesorectum from the back of the rectum at the level selected for division of the bowel below the growth. This is done by scissor dissection aided by gauze dissection. The mesorectum is then clamped with two large curved artery forceps or crushing intestinal clamps and divided between them. These ends are tied off, leaving the rectum bared all round over a segment of about 3 cm long, near the lower edge of which the division of the bowel and anastomosis will take place.

The higher up on the rectum the distal line of the resection is to be taken, the easier it is to define and divide the mesorectum in this manner. Lower down, the mesorectum fans out on the back of the rectum and becomes less substantial, so that in very low resections its preparatory isolation and division may not be feasible or necessary.

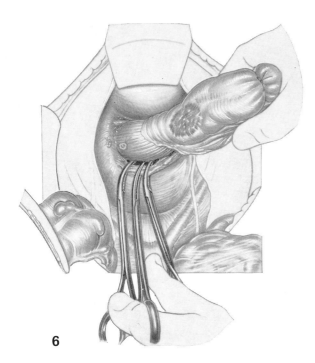

6

Irrigation of rectal stump

Before dividing the rectum and proceeding to the anastomosis of the colon and the rectal stump it is a good plan, if the patient is in the modified lithotomy-Trendelenburg position, to cleanse the distal bowel by irrigation from below. This is useful in reducing the amount of faecal contamination when the rectum is eventually divided, for, however quick the surgeon may be with his sucker, there is liable to be some leakage of faeces at this stage. It also has the advantage that it washes away — and, if suitable agents are used, may destroy — loose malignant cells mixed with the faeces, and this diminishes the risk of their becoming implanted in the suture line when the anastomosis is done.

7

Clamping of rectum

As a preliminary to irrigation of the rectal stump a curved Parker-Kerr clamp — or better, a slightly angled clamp — is applied across the rectum exactly in the sagittal or anteroposterior plane to prevent further faeces descending into the lower segment of bowel. It is placed at least 5 cm below the distal edge of the growth and with its handles just above the pubis.

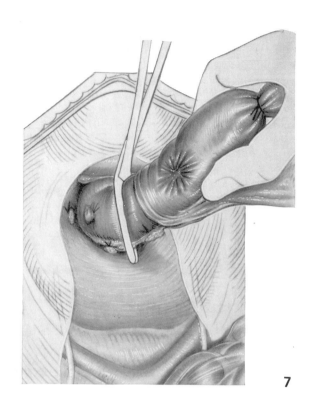

7

8

8

The irrigation

An assistant now passes a proctoscope *per anum* and, through a rubber catheter, irrigates the rectum below the clamp, first of all with 500 ml of a 1 per cent solution of cetrimide as a cleansing agent, and then with 500 ml of a 2 per cent solution of nitrogen mustard, which seems to be one of the most suitable cytotoxic agents for this purpose (Goligher, 1967).

9

Injection of cytotoxic agent into colon stump

If desired a cancericidal agent may be introduced into the colon stump also. One way of doing so is to clamp the stump 10 cm or so from its end with a spring clamp and then to inject 20 ml of 2 per cent solution of nitrogen mustard through a fine needle. This solution is left there as the anastomosis proceeds, being evacuated by suction when the terminal crushing clamp is eventually removed. An alternative plan for applying a cytotoxic agent to the colon is simply to swab out the open end of the bowel during the anastomosis, using pledgets soaked in cetrimide and then nitrogen mustard.

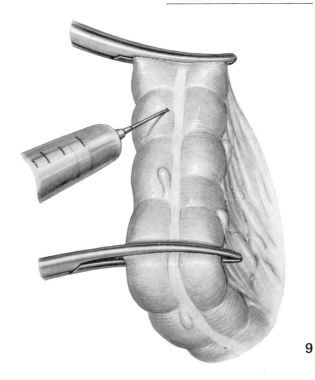

9

The anastomosis: two-layer suture technique

10

Insertion of left lateral row of Lembert sutures

In preparation for the anastomosis, the sigmoid and rectum above the angled crushing clamp are drawn vertically upwards to lift the lower rectum as far as possible out of the pelvis and facilitate the insertion of sutures into it, in the same way as traction exerted on the body of the mobilized stomach is useful during gastrectomy. The Parker-Kerr clamp controlling the end of the colon stump is rested on the left edge of the abdominal wound, with its mesenteric border directed posteriorly and separated by a distance of 10–12 cm from the rectum. A series of mattress Lembert sutures of fine serum-proof silk is now inserted between the left lateral wall of the rectum and the adjacent surface of the colon, 0·5 mm distant from the controlling clamps in each case, and left untied until all have been placed.

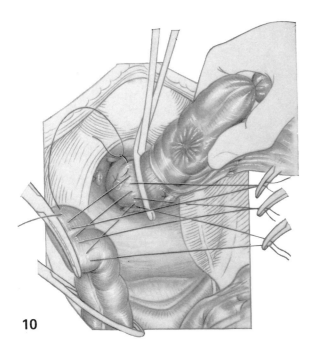

10

11

Apposition of colon and rectal stumps and tying of left lateral Lembert sutures

The colon is then slid down on these sutures to come into apposition with the rectum, and the stitches are tied, the tails of the first and last being retained for traction, all the others being cut.

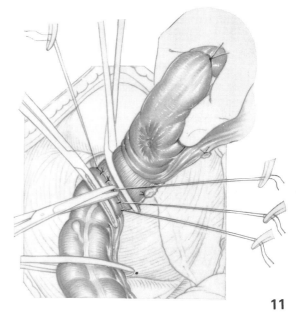

11

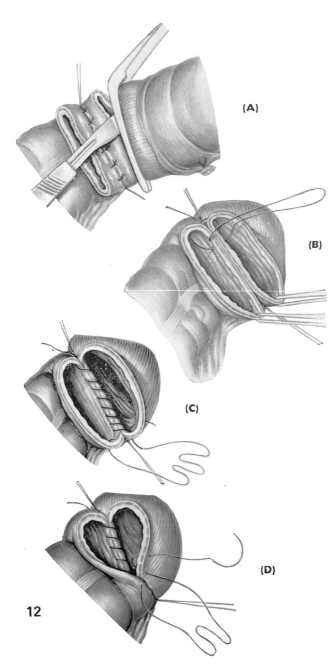

(A)

(B)

(C)

(D)

12

12

Excision of clamps and insertion of continuous through-and-through suture

The crushing clamps, together with the crushed tissue gripped by their blades, are next excised with a scalpel, and in the case of the rectum this means also removal of the entire operative specimen (*A*). If the colon stump was not previously irrigated with a cytotoxic agent, the cut edges and terminal part of the interior of the colon stump are now swabbed with a 1 per cent solution of cetrimide and then a 2 per cent solution of nitrogen mustard.

A continuous 2/0 or 3/0 chromic catgut suture on a fine half-circle atraumatic needle is used to unite the cut edges of the colon and rectum. It is started at the anterior or antimesenteric poles, being inserted from the outer aspect of the rectum to the peritoneal aspect of the colon through the full thickness of bowel lumens. When tied, the knot therefore lies outside the lumen (*B*). The needle is re-introduced through the rectal wall into the lumen for suture of the adjacent halves of the bowel edges, which is done with an ordinary over-and-over stitch. At the mesenteric poles of the lumens, however, the type of suture changes to a Connell or 'loop on the mucosa' stitch (*C*), which is continued along the remote halves of the bowel circumferences (*D*), eventually to reach the antimesenteric angles again. The Connell suture gives good inversion of the cut edges and avoids all mucosal pouting.

13

Insertion of right lateral Lembert sutures

The anastomosis is completed with a covering row of Lembert stitches of fine silk on the right lateral walls of the colon and rectum. These are inserted in mattress fashion to secure a better grip of the longitudinally running muscle fibres in the rectal wall. The tails of the sutures are left long and held by the assistant, facilitating insertion of the next stitch.

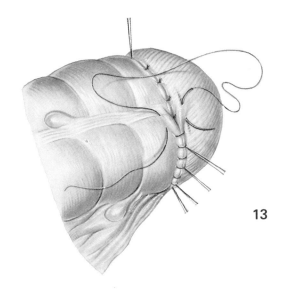

13

The anastomosis: one-layer suture technique

14

Placement of open colonic and rectal stumps for commencement of suture

Both rectal and colonic stumps having been prepared as shown in *Illustrations 2–8* of this section, the crushing clamps controlling the ends of each stump are excised leaving two open stumps about 15–20 cm apart. The plan is to insert the single layer of interrupted sutures corresponding to the posterior half or preferably two-thirds of the bowel circumference whilst the colonic and rectal stumps are thus separated, and then to slide the colon stump down into the pelvis on these sutures. As for choice of suture material, 3/0 silk or corresponding grades of plastic materials, such as Ethiflex or Tevdek, or of stainless steel wire, mounted on atraumatic needles are satisfactory but possibly chromic catgut might do as well.

It is a convenience to start with a stitch in the mid-line posteriorly corresponding to the anti-mesenteric border of both stumps. The needle is entered on the mucosal aspect of the colon 6 mm or so from the cut edge, and traverses the colonic wall to emerge from the outer surface. It is then inserted through the rectal wall from the outside, again 6 mm from the cut edge, to emerge on the mucosal surface. Next the suture returns from rectum to colon catching the edges of the rectal and colonic mucosae in the process. (The precise relationship of the suture to the layers of the rectal and colonic walls is depicted in the inset drawing.) Finally the needle is cut off the suture material and the two tails of the untied stitch are clipped together with artery forceps.

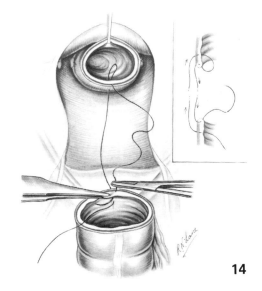

14

15

Insertion of remaining sutures in posterior two-thirds of bowel circumference

It is helpful to mark the anterior limits of the two posterior thirds of the bowel circumference by inserting a vertical mattress stitch on either side in exactly the same way as was used for the median posterior stitch, the ends being left long and clipped untied with artery forceps. Further sutures are then inserted at intervals of 4 or 5 mm between these three main marking stitches, first of all in the right posterior third and then in the left posterior third.

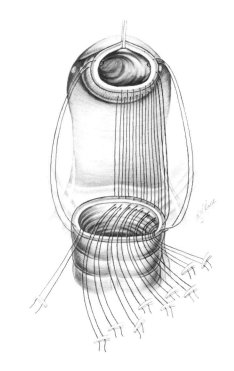

15

16

Sliding colon stump down on to rectal stump and tying sutures with knots on colonic mucosa

The next step is to gently slide the colon stump into the pelvis on the tautened strands until the posterior cut edges of the colonic and rectal stumps are in apposition. The sutures are then tied seriatim, commencing near the posterior mid-line and extending to either side in turn. The knots of these sutures lie on the mucosal aspect of the edge of the colon.

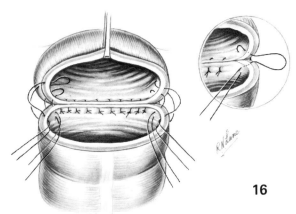

16

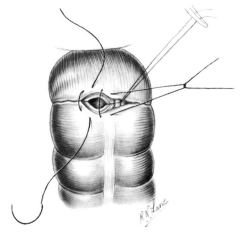

17

Closing the gap in the anastomosis corresponding to the anterior third of the bowel circumference

All that remains to be done now in regard to the anastomosis is to complete the suture of the anterior third of the bowel circumference. Vertical mattress sutures of the Gambee type with the knots on the serosal aspect may be used but are difficult to insert in a bowel situated low in the pelvis. It is easier to use transversely placed mattress sutures, as illustrated, when working at this depth.

17

18

Drainage of pelvic cavity

Opinions differ as to the best way of draining the pelvic cavity. A good method is by a suprapubic suction drain inserted extraperitoneally from the lower end of the abdominal wound beneath the pelvic peritoneum at the side of the bladder to the region of the anastomosis. Previously it was the custom to suture the pelvic peritoneum over the anastomosis, but at the present time most surgeons prefer to leave the peritoneum unsutured so that the loops of small bowel and tail of the greater omentum may drop down into the pelvis and surround the anastomosis.

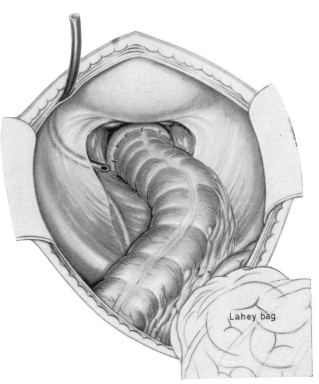

18

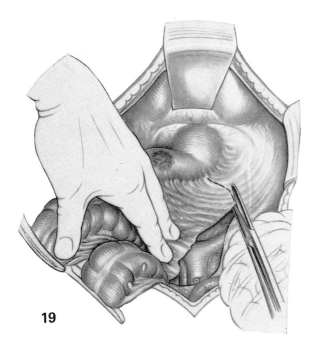

19

HIGH ANTERIOR RESECTION

In resecting carcinomas of the rectosigmoid region the same technique is employed, but the rectum is not completely lifted out of its sacral bed, the anastomosis being between the colon and the intraperitoneal part of the rectum. The preparation of the colon stump is exactly the same as that described for *low* anterior resection.

Preparation of rectal stump

19

Incision of right leaf of mesosigmoid and mesorectum

The upper rectum and lower sigmoid are drawn upwards and to the left to render the mesorectum and mesosigmoid taut. Then, starting at the lower end of the incision made in the right leaf of the mesosigmoid for exposure and ligation of the inferior mesenteric vessels, an oblique scissor cut is carried in the peritoneum to reach the back of the bowel 5 cm below the lower margin of the growth. Subsequently the peritoneal cut is deepened through the subjacent fat, especially in its posterior part.

20

Incision of left leaf of mesosigmoid and mesorectum, and clamping and division of superior haemorrhoidal vessels

Whilst the rectum is now retracted upwards and to the right, a similar incision is made in the left leaf of the mesosigmoid and mesorectum, care being taken to ensure that its termination at the back of the bowel corresponds accurately with the end of the incision in the right leaf. The underlying fat is also divided with scissors or broken through by blunt dissection in the posterior part of the cut, but anteriorly a search is made for the superior haemorrhoidal vessels as they run downwards and forwards close to the back of the bowel. These vessels are isolated, clamped with two large crushing clamps, divided and tied, thus baring the posterior wall of the rectum at this point.

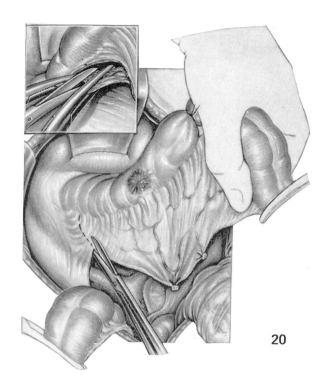

20

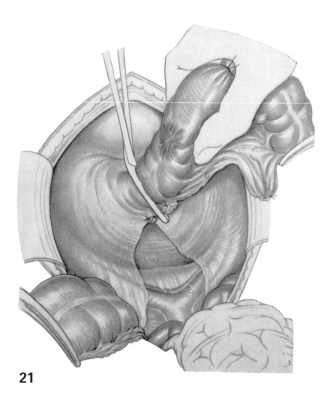

21

21

Clamping of bowel and commencement of colorectal anastomosis

A curved Parker-Kerr or slightly angled clamp is applied across the rectum in the sagittal plane immediately above the level chosen for the lower limit of the resection, and at least 4 cm distal to the inferior edge of the growth. Thereafter the anorectum below the clamp is irrigated by an assistant through a proctoscope as in low anterior resection. When this has been completed the end of the colon stump controlled by a Parker-Kerr clamp is drawn down to the left edge of the abdominal wound, and the anastomosis is commenced with the insertion of mattress Lembert sutures of fine serum-proof silk between the left lateral wall of the rectum below the angled clamp and the adjacent colon wall close to the Parker-Kerr clamp.

22

Completion of anastomosis and drainage

The subsequent steps of the anastomosis proceed exactly as in a low anterior resection. The left lateral Lembert stitches are tied, the clamps are excised and a through-and-through suture of fine 2/0 or 3/0 chromic catgut is inserted to bring the divided edges together. Lastly, a row of Lembert sutures is placed on the right side of the bowel. The final result is an entirely intraperitoneal anastomosis between the colon and a very short cuff of intraperitoneal rectum. A suction tube drain or corrugated rubber drain is laid down to the suture line through the lower end of the main wound or through a separate stab wound in the left lower abdomen.

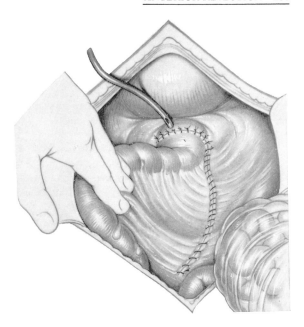

22

SPECIAL POSTOPERATIVE CARE AND COMPLICATIONS

If there has been unusual faecal contamination during the operation it is probably wise to administer systemic antibiotic therapy such as gentamicin 80 mg and lincomycin 600 mg twice daily for 4 or 5 days. Some surgeons favour a short prophylactic course of these drugs, consisting of one dose immediately pre-operatively and another one 6 hr after operation, in all cases.

Oral fluids should be restricted and the intravenous infusion continued with appropriate solutions, as indicated by daily plasma electrolyte estimations and other considerations, until vigorous peristalsis returns and flatus or faeces is passed per anum or per colostomy; glycerine suppositories may assist to that end. The suprapubic drain is retained as long as significant quantities of fluid are withdrawn, which is usually for 3 or 4 days at least. The urethral catheter is removed on the fourth or fifth day.

If a transverse colostomy was established at the time of doing a low anterior resection, it can be closed after 2·5–3 weeks if the anastomosis heals *per primam*, but in any event it is probably better to retain it for 6–8 weeks, because of the difficulties of colostomy closure sooner due to residual oedema in the everted bowel.

Anastomotic dehiscence

Separation of the anastomosis at some part of the bowel circumference, usually the posterior third, is not uncommon after *low* anterior resection. Everett (1975) has provided evidence that it is less frequent after a one-layer suture technique than after a two-layer technique, though surgical opinion on this point is divided However, it is a surprisingly innocuous complication as a rule, especially if a transverse colostomy was made at the conclusion of the resection. All that need be done under these circumstances is that the colostomy should be retained until the dehiscence has largely healed, which may require anything from a fortnight to several weeks, depending on the extent of the breakdown. Meanwhile irrigations of the rectum through a proctoscope or washes-through from the colostomy to the anus may help to clear up resulting pelvic infection. If a transverse colostomy was not established at the time of the resection, the treatment of a major dehiscence of the anastomosis with suprapubic leakage of faeces consists of making such a colostomy without delay, but lesser degrees of breakdown of the suture line may be left.

Stricture

Some degree of narrowing at the anastomosis due to reactionary oedema is a fairly frequent finding in the early weeks after an anterior resection, but this usually corrects itself spontaneously possibly assisted by the dilating effect of passing normal faeces. Only if there has been a major breakdown of the anastomosis involving, say, half the bowel circumference, is a persistent stricture likely to develop, but it is surprising how over a period of 6 or 12 months these strictures may also undergo considerable spontaneous dilatation. Rarely is it necessary to carry out dilatation with Hegar's dilators, at first under a short general anaesthetic and then daily by the patient himself for a time.

Local recurrence

Local recurrence of rectal carcinomas are easier detected after a sphincter-saving resection than after an abdominoperineal excision. Sometimes they may seem to be confined to the region of the anastomosis, but on other occasions they are more widespread in the pelvis and may also be associated with recurrence elsewhere in the abdomen. Rarely in the former group it may be possible to remove the recurrence by an abdominoperineal excision, but this may be technically a very difficult operation. Otherwise supervoltage radiotherapy may be considered.

Anal incontinence

After anterior resection, even of the low variety, the functional result is almost invariably excellent, although, due to the loss of the greater part of the sigmoid colon and much of the rectum, motions are passed at first more frequently. This gradually rectifies itself in a few months. Exceptionally rarely in very elderly patients after extremely low anterior resection there may be some incontinence of flatus and even faeces for a few weeks or months after operation or even indefinitely.

References

Cullen, P. K. and Mayo, C. W. (1963). *Dis. Colon Rect.* **6**, 415
Deddish, M. R. and Stearns, M. W. Jr. (1961). *Ann. Surg.* **154**, 91
Everett, W. (1975). *Br. J. Surg.* **62**, 135
Goligher, J. C. (1962). *Proc. R. Soc. Med.* **55**, 341
Goligher, J. C. (1975). *Surgery of the Anus, Rectum and Colon,* 3rd Edition. London: Bailliere Tindall
Goligher, J. C., Duthie, H. L., Watts, J. M. and de Dombal, F. T. (1965). *Br. J. Surg.* **52**, 323
Grinnell, R. S. (1954). *Surgery Gynec. Obstet.* **99**, 421
Mayo, C. W. and Fly, D. A. (1956). *Surgery Gynec. Obstet.* **103**, 94
Mayo, C. W., Laberge, M. Y. and Hardy, W. M. (1958). *Surgery Gynec. Obstet.* **106**, 695
Morgan, C. Naunton (1965). *Ann. R. Coll. Surg. Eng.* **36**, 73
Quer, E. A., Dahlin, D. C. and Mayo, C. W. (1953). *Surgery Gynec. Obstet.* **96**, 24
Vandertoll, D. J. and Beahrs, O. H. C. (1965). *Archs Surg.* **90**, 793
Waugh, J. M., Block, M. A. and Gage, R. P. (1955). *Ann. Surg.* **142**, 752

[*The illustrations for this Chapter on Anterior Resection were drawn by Mr. R. N. Lane.*]

Per-anal Endorectal Operative Techniques

A. G. Parks, M.Ch., F.R.C.S., F.R.C.P.
Consultant Surgeon, St. Mark's Hospital, London and
The London Hospital

and

James P. S. Thomson, M.S., F.R.C.S.
Consultant Surgeon, St. Mark's Hospital, London

INTRODUCTION

Endocavity techniques are being developed in many spheres of surgery and the rectum is particularly suitable for exploitation of these methods. It is not generally recognized that excellent exposure of the lower rectum may be obtained by holding the anal canal open by the use of suitable retractors. The latter maintain an anal aperture sufficiently large to enable the surgeon to work with special instruments and also hold the walls of the rectal ampulla apart by means of suitably shaped blades. Not only is it possible to deal with a lesion which is situated in the rectum itself and thereby immediately exposed by the open blades of the retractor, but conditions at a higher level can usually be drawn down by intussusception of the rectosigmoid region so that a sessile adenoma at 15—20 cm could be dissected off the wall of the colon under direct vision. An operating sigmoidoscope is not suitable for this work, as it gives inadequate exposure.

A lightweight retractor is illustrated, which is easily inserted and which is held in position by a groove in each blade to accommodate the anal sphincters. The blades are so shaped that, when the instrument is opened, they hold the walls of the rectum apart so that the cavity can be readily seen; in addition a third blade may be used which gives even better exposure.

Submucosal excision of sessile adenomas of the lower rectum using the endorectal route was described in 1966 (Parks) and is now an established procedure. The same technique has been used for excising certain selected malignant tumours. It is also a route through which very low anastomoses can be performed between the colon and upper anal canal with greater ease and safety than could ever be done via the abdomen. These last two uses of the method are at present being evaluated with promising initial results.

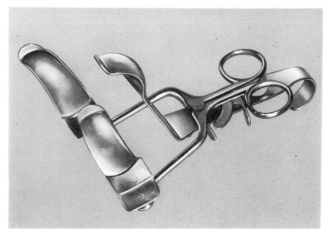

EXCISION OF SESSILE ADENOMA OF THE RECTUM

Assessment

It is usually possible to diagnose a sessile adenoma of the rectum by palpation. If the lesion is universally soft, then in all probability it is benign. If, however, there is ulceration or the presence of indurated areas, then malignant change may already have occurred. The diagnosis may be confirmed by sigmoidoscopic biopsy and this is especially helpful if malignant invasion is present. However, if the pathologist reports only a benign lesion to be present, this does not rule out the possibility of malignancy elsewhere in the tumour and for this reason a biopsy with such a report may be unhelpful. Furthermore, removal of large pieces of tumour for biopsy purposes may interfere with the technique of submucosal excision by obliterating the submucosal space; this is particularly prone to occur if diathermy is used to stop bleeding. It is far better, therefore, to perform a total excision of the whole tumour and to subject this to pathological examination.

A patient with a sessile adenoma of the rectum may be considered to have an unstable state of the entire colonic mucosa. In approximately 10 per cent of such patients there is a synchronous tumour at some other site in the large intestine. It is therefore essential to have a barium enema carried out prior to any treatment of the obvious lesion in order to detect the presence of other neoplastic lesions, benign or malignant.

It is possible to make some estimate as to whether a tumour of this sort is suitable for treatment by this method by pre-operative examination. This will certainly be the case if it is palpable digitally. It is not generally realized that impalpable benign tumours can be delivered into the rectal ampulla and excised in precisely the same manner. A sessile adenoma at 15—20 cm can usually be exposed by passing a sigmoidoscope through the open blades of the retractor; once the tumour has been reached, forceps placed upon the tumour itself, or the nearby mucosa will allow it to be coaxed downwards into view by intussusception.

Preparation

It is essential that the rectum be empty of faeces for the easy conduct of this operation and therefore the patient should receive an enema containing a contact laxative the night before and on the morning of the operation.

Anaesthesia and position of patient

The operation is most conveniently performed under general anaesthesia, muscle relaxant drugs being given to allow the anal canal to be readily dilated. Not only does this make it easier to use the instrument but it must be remembered that anal dilatation under light anaesthesia is a potent afferent stimulus and may cause cardiac irregularities. The operation may be done with equal facility whether the patient be in the lithotomy or the jack-knife position, although the latter position may be more satisfactory for anterior tumours.

Illumination may be obtained by placing a light source at the anus, using a head lamp or by using the main theatre light behind the operator. The first method, however, will provide the most satisfactory illumination.

Principle of technique

A sessile adenoma is a benign mucosal lesion and thus only the mucosa needs to be excised for its removal. This is made possible by the laxity of the submucosa, a layer which only contains blood and lymphatic vessels, together with loose areolar tissue. In its natural state it is approximately 1 mm thick but by the infiltration of a solution, such as physiological saline with adrenaline, it may be distended to some 2 cm in thickness. Thus, a sessile adenoma will be lifted-up with the mucosa from the underlying circular muscle. It is then possible to excise the adenoma by dissecting with scissors in the oedematous submucosa; this should be carried out as close to the mucosa as possible to avoid the submucosal anastomoses which will bleed if damaged. However, the addition of adrenaline to the solution (1:300,000) largely prevents bleeding. Furthermore, the tumour can be removed without any damage to the underlying circular muscle.

THE OPERATION

1

Insertion of the retractor

The retractor is gently inserted into the anus and when fully in position the blades are slowly opened. The area of interest is 'milked' between the blades by digital manipulation. A third blade can be inserted and is particularly valuable if the tumour is proliferative and bulky.

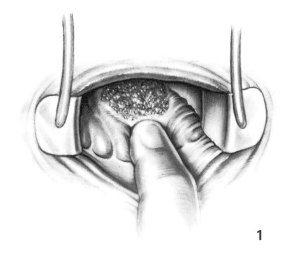

1

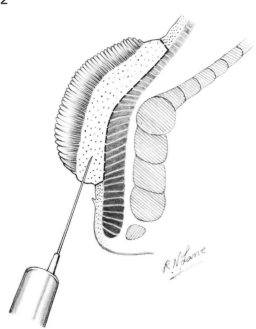

2

2 & 3

Injection of the submucosal plane

A solution of adrenaline in isotonic saline (1:300,000) is injected into the submucosa by placing a needle into this layer 1–2 cm away from the tumour itself. The solution rapidly spreads in all directions and the adenoma is seen to be lifted off the underlying muscle.

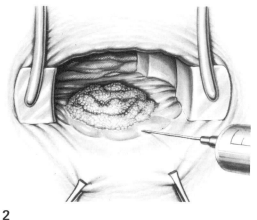

3

4 & 5

Excision of the adenoma

It is desirable that a margin of normal mucosa is excised with the tumour. Injection of the submucosal plane renders the mucosa tense and small extensions of the tumour which would otherwise be overlooked and left behind are rendered obvious and can be removed. With sharp pointed scissors an incision is made about 1 cm from the edge of the tumour. With the same scissors the oedematous submucosa is incised just deep to the mucosa and the tumour. Both of the latter are fragile and should be handled with care, using fine forceps, such as Babcock's design. It may be necessary to inject further quantities of the adrenaline solution as it tends to leak out of the submucosal plane once this has been incised. Bleeding points are controlled using diathermy coagulation, as even a small amount of blood may conceal the correct plane of dissection. Furthermore, there is a tendency for even the smallest bleeding point to continue to ooze for a long period after the operation if careful haemostasis has not been established.

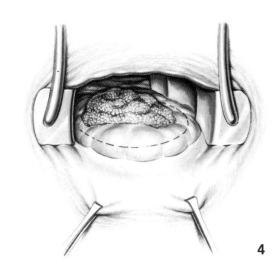

4

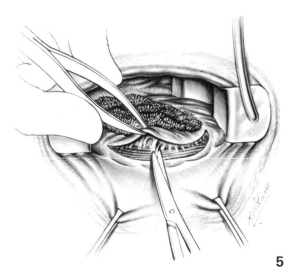

5

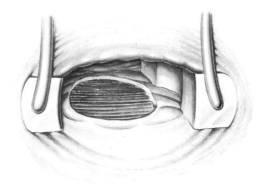

6

6

If the lesion is non-circumferential, as most are, then the wound may be left open. It will rapidly heal without infection or stenosis.

Extensive circumferential lesions

The technique is almost identical with that described above with the obvious exception that the whole tumour cannot be exposed at one time. It will therefore be necessary to withdraw the retractor and re-insert it at a different angle in order to excise tumour from an area of rectum not originally seen. Sometimes the tumour can still be removed *in toto* but often, especially if it is proliferative, it may need to be removed in segments. It is usually possible to excise a circumferential tumour in three segments. Should the lesion extend up to 12 or 15 cm it is still possible to excise it by drawing the rectal wall down into the area exposed by the retractors, using gentle retraction on the exposed muscle. Repeated injections of the adrenaline in saline solution will be required before the top of the tumour is dissected free.

7 & 8

If the tumour is circumferential for more than a few centimetres of the rectum, then stricturing is possible if the denuded area of muscle is not covered with mucosa. Circumferential wounds 10–12 cm in length can be closed satisfactorily by the process of imbricating the muscle of the rectal wall with non-absorbable sutures. Commencing at the lower edge of the wound, multiple 'bites' of the circular muscle of the rectum are taken until the upper edge is reached. About ten such sutures are placed around the rectum and these, when tied, will exert a 'concertina-ing' effect, drawing the mucosal edges together. These may then be sutured with another layer of catgut stitches. Secondary separation does not occur and healing is rapid.

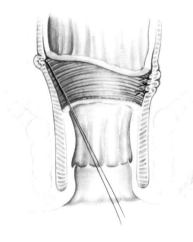

7

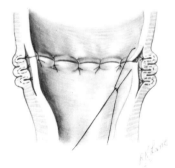

8

9

In a few cases the adenomatous process extends from the upper anal canal into the lower sigmoid colon. As much of the tumour as possible should be excised using the technique described above but the higher part of the tumour, in the upper rectum and sigmoid colon, will require an abdominal approach. An abdominal incision is made and after mobilization the rectum is divided across at a point just distal to that reached by the submucosal excision carried out through the anus. The remainder of the adenoma is removed by resecting the upper rectum and sigmoid colon. The continuity of the bowel is restored by relining the resulting rectal stump with the descending colon which is brought through the muscle tube of the rectum and anastomosed to the anal canal. This anastomosis is performed using the technique described on page 166.

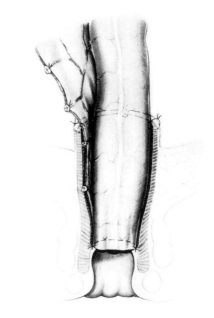

9

10

Preparation of the specimen for the pathologist

So that the histopathologist may have the maximum opportunity for examining the specimen, it should be pinned out on to a cork board and spread as widely as possible. It is then fixed by floating the cork upside down in a bath of formal saline solution.

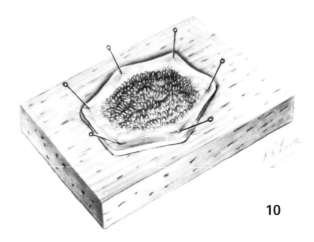

10

POSTOPERATIVE CARE AND COMPLICATIONS

Those patients who have had a purely endorectal excision need virtually no postoperative care (of any kind). A normal diet is given straight away and it is perhaps wise to administer a hydrophilic laxative to ensure that the initial bowel action is soft.

The most important and commonest complication is haemorrhage from the site of the lesion, though this is uncommon if haemostasis has been carefully established. If despite all such measures it occurs, it will be necessary to examine the wound under anaesthesia when the bleeding point can be either under-run with a suture or coagulated with diathermy.

Recurrence

It is well known that these tumours have a tendency to recur whatever method of excision is used. This may be due either to incomplete initial removal or to the independent growth of another lesion. For this reason the patient should be examined with the sigmoidoscope at least every 3 months for the first year and then at 6-monthly intervals thereafter indefinitely. Metachronous lesions elsewhere in the colon may occur after some years and these may be detected by performing a barium enema at approximately 5-yearly intervals.

LOCAL EXCISION OF RECTAL CARCINOMA

Indications

The place of local excision in the management of certain patients with rectal carcinoma is at present ill-defined. An elderly patient finds a colostomy such an indignity and degradation, both in the eyes of himself and his family, that almost any attempt is justified to avoid it. Manifestly only a relatively small tumour or a pedunculated one is suitable for this approach and it may be that with increasing experience the procedure need not be limited to the elderly. The size and height of the tumour above the anal canal, together with its grade of malignancy on histological examination, must be assessed. It should be confined to the rectal wall and mobile on palpation. Careful digital palpation of the retrorectal tissues is carried out in an endeavour to detect enlarged mesorectal lymph nodes. If present, this is a contra-indication to local excision.

Once a tumour has been excised in this limited way, the pathologist may report that the excision is inadequate or that the tumour is of higher grade malignancy than had been suspected. In this case the procedure must be regarded as an excisional biopsy and further, more radical, treatment planned. A similar argument, of course, applies to a sessile adenoma which on histopathological examination is revealed to contain infiltrating malignancy.

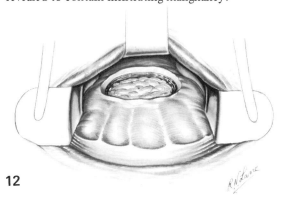

12

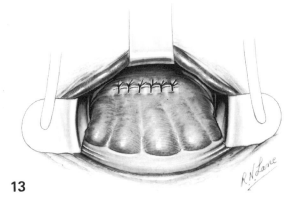

13

THE OPERATION

11

Insertion of the retractor

This is done in a similar way to that previously described.

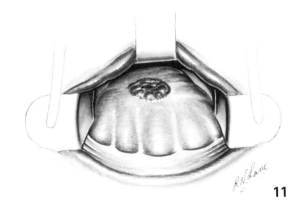

11

12

Excision of the tumour

An incision is made in the normal mucosa about 2 cm away from the edge of the neoplasm. It is necessary to incise full thickness of the rectal wall and expose the extrarectal fat. Dissection is carried out in the extrarectal fat so that the lesion, together with 2 cm of surrounding mucosa and rectal muscle, is excised as a disc. Removal is facilitated by infiltrating the extrarectal fat with isotonic saline containing adrenaline 1:300,000.

13

Closure of the wound

Haemostasis must be perfect otherwise a haematoma will collect in the loose extrarectal tissues, causing infection and breakdown. The wound is then closed transversely with one layer of non-absorbable sutures which should be tied in such a way that the bowel edge is approximated but not strangulated. Occasionally part of the suture line separates, leaving a defect which heals by secondary intention. So far spreading infection has not been encountered postoperatively and the patient is unaware of any symptoms. There is no special postoperative management other than the avoidance of constipation.

A TECHNIQUE OF COLO-ANAL ANASTOMOSIS

Introduction

The operative techniques for treating malignant disease of the rectum have largely fallen into two groups: excision of the rectum with a terminal colostomy or alternatively anterior resection with an anastomosis. Generally speaking, tumours of the lower third usually require excision of the rectum (unless local excision is possible), whereas those of the upper third may be treated by anterior resection with anastomosis. A neoplasm situated in the middle third may be managed in either way depending on the histological grading of the tumour and its extent, together with the technical problems involved in performing the more difficult operation of anterior resection. It is usually easier to perform a low anastomosis in a woman from the abdominal approach, as the pelvis is wider. Various techniques are now being introduced to enable anastomoses to be carried out at lower levels, thus increasing the possibility of preserving the anal sphincter mechanism for tumours situated in the middle third of the rectum. One such technique is described below. Though this makes it possible for nearly all tumours of the rectum to be removed with conservation of the anal sphincters, it must be stressed that this must not be done at the expense of the ultimate prognosis.

Indications

The patients must be carefully selected. There are three main criteria to be considered: the tumour must be mobile with no clinical evidence of extension into the perirectal fat; there should be no clinical evidence of enlarged lymph nodes as detected by careful palpation of the mesorectum through the posterior rectal wall; finally, on histological grading patients with anaplastic tumours should be excluded.

Pre-operative preparation

This is the same as for any restorative resection. It is essential that the colon be completely free of any faecal material.

Position of patient

The patient should be positioned on the operating table in the lithotomy-Trendelenburg position so that the subsequent colo-anal anastomosis may be performed using the per-anal route without moving the patient.

THE OPERATION

Mobilization of left colon

The sigmoid colon is an unsatisfactory part of the large intestine to anastomose to the anal canal as there is a tendency for it to undergo sudden necrosis 2–3 days postoperatively. The reason for this is not known, it may be due to sudden thrombosis in vessels affected with atheroma in which the blood pressure is reduced as a result of dissection. It is necessary therefore to use the upper descending colon or splenic flexure for the anastomosis, hence the distal transverse colon and the splenic flexure have to be mobilized and the blood supply of the colon will depend on the middle colic artery supplying the marginal arcade. The inferior mesenteric vessels may be divided close to their origin.

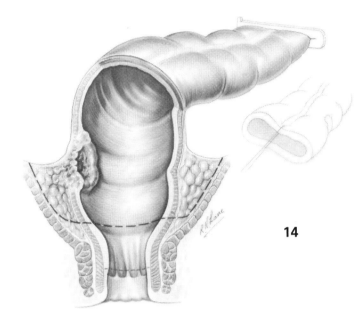

14

14

Rectal dissection

The rectal dissection is performed as for a low anterior resection. It is most important to identify the correct plane anteriorly. An incision is made in the peritoneum behind the bladder just above the peritoneal reflection and the plane between the seminal vesicles and Denonvillier's fascia identified. This plane is pursued by blunt dissection downwards behind the prostate. Blunt dissection laterally sweeps both the vas and the ureter away from the field of operation on each side and allows the lateral ligament to be divided without risk. Once the dissection has reached the lower part of the prostate, Denonvillier's fascia is divided and the dissection pursued to the upper part of the anal canal in the perirectal fat. The lateral ligaments are divided down to the levator ani muscles, the latter being displayed almost in their entirety. A clamp is placed across the rectum below the tumour and the anorectal stump is irrigated with a cytotoxic agent (such as 1:1000 mercuric perchloride, followed by sterile water). In the female the dissection is somewhat easier as the rectovaginal plane is found just below the cervix and can be readily opened up down to the anal canal. It is extremely important that the integrity of the vaginal wall is preserved, as, if it is divided and the mucosa of the vagina exposed, then a rectovaginal fistula may develop postoperatively. The rectum is divided below the clamp which may in some cases be at the junction of the rectum and the anal canal. After division of the rectum it is necessary to secure careful haemostasis in the pelvis so that the area is completely dry.

15

Removal of mucosa from anorectal stump

The surgeon then moves to the perineum to make the anastomosis. The retractor is passed into the anorectal stump. The submucosa above the dentate line is infiltrated with a solution of isotonic saline containing adrenaline (1:300,000). Using sharp pointed scissors the mucosa is excised between the dentate line and the cut end of the lower rectum usually in three or four strips. The excision is performed as close to the mucosa as possible to preserve the submucosal anastomosis. It is essential again to secure complete haemostasis.

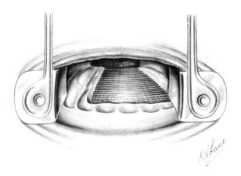

15

16

Delivery of colon through anorectal stump

From the abdomen the end of the colon is then passed down through the pelvis. Stay sutures are passed to the perineal operator who then gently draws the end of the colon into the anorectal stump.

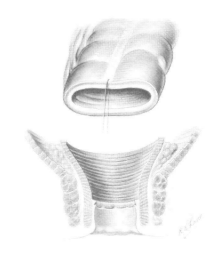

16

17

The anastomosis

An instrument with narrower blades attached is then passed into the colon which exposes the end of the colon in proximity to the cut mucosa. An anastomosis is carried out using interrupted non-absorbable sutures. Each stitch passes through the anal mucosa, then through a segment of the internal sphincter and then through full thickness of the terminal colon. About 20 such stitches are placed in position to complete the anastomosis.

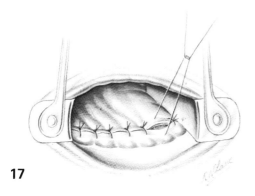

17

18

The final arrangement of the colon

The colon is arranged to the right of the small intestine and its mesentery and the mesocolon attached to the posterior abdominal peritoneum.

Conclusion of the operation

It is essential that good haemostasis is obtained in the pelvis, as the denuded pelvic cavity is an ideal place for the accumulation of blood and lymph. This may become infected and lead to a pelvic abscess which may discharge through the anastomosis. Not only will this increase the morbidity of the operation but, because of the subsequent fibrosis between the colon and the levator ani muscles, there will be impairment of sensation and deficient reflex linkage between the filling of the 'new-rectum' and the anal sphincters. It is therefore wise to place adequate suction drainage into the pelvic cavity.

It is also wise, particularly when the anastomosis is performed in the anal canal itself, to cover the whole procedure with a temporary loop transverse colostomy.

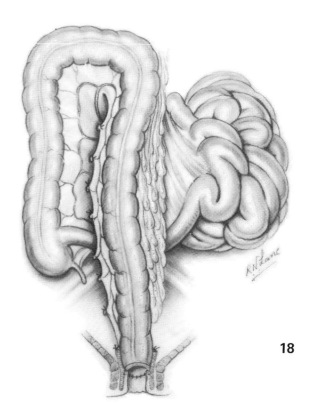

18

POSTOPERATIVE CARE

This in no way differs from that of a patient following an anterior resection. Once satisfactory healing of the anastomosis has occurred the colostomy may be closed and the sutures may be removed from the anal canal.

Functional results

The functional results of this operation are still being evaluated but whilst there may be some difficulty with control of loose stool initially after a few months satisfactory function is present in most patients. However, it is worth stressing that pelvic sepsis will lead to a less good functional result.

Reference

Parks, A. G. (1966). 'Benign tumours of the rectum.' In *Clinical Surgery,* Vol. 10, Abdomen and Rectum and Anus, pp. 541–548. Edited by C. Rob, R. Smith and C. Naunton Morgan. London: Butterworths

[*The illustrations for this Chapter on Per-anal Endorectal Operative Techniques were drawn by Mr. R. N. Lane.*]

Endo-anal Abdominoperineal Pull-through Resection with Colorectal Anastomosis

Daher E. Cutait, M.D., F.A.C.S.
Associate Professor of Surgery, Medical School of
the University of São Paulo, Department of Surgery,
Head of the Group in Charge of Colorectal Surgery

PRE-OPERATIVE

Choice of operation

Pull-through resections may be used for malignant as well as benign lesions of the rectosigmoid region. In cancer they are indicated mostly for tumours of the middle or upper rectum, in cases where it is technically difficult to perform safely an anterior resection. In the abdominal phase of these procedures, steps of the dissection and mobilization of the colon and rectum are identical to those of the Miles abdominoperineal excision. Re-establishment of the intestinal continuity, which is done in the perineal phase, may be executed in two different ways. Firstly, the anastomosis is made between the colon and the anal canal, as proposed by Hochenegg in 1888 and subsequently modified and popularized by many authors, as Babcock (1939, 1947); Bacon (1945) and Waugh and Turner (1958). Though this preserves the sphincter, it sacrifices the sensitive lower rectal mucosa, which is an essential mechanism of faecal control. Thus, patients may become incontinent. Secondly, the anastomosis is performed between the colon and a segment of retained rectum as proposed by Maunsell (1892) and Weir (1901) and modified by several surgeons, as Black (1948) for cancer and Swenson and Bill (1948) for Hirschsprung's disease. Preservation of a sufficient segment of rectum maintains the rectocortico-anal continence reflex, which is more comfortable for patients.

There are different methods of performing pull-through operations with a colorectal anastomosis. In this chapter account will be given only for two procedures. Firstly, the 'Endo-anal abdominoperineal pull-through resection with delayed colorectal anastomosis', a technique that was devised to prevent or lessen disruption of the anastomosis (Cutait, 1960, 1965, 1970; Cutait and Figliolini, 1961, 1962 *a, b*; Cutait *et al.,* 1965), which is a common complication after conventional immediate anastomosis. It is executed in two stages and is based on the principle of adhesion by contact between the muscular coat of the rectum and the serosal coat of the pulled-through colon in the first stage, and approximation of the mucosa of the rectum to the mucosa of the colon in the second stage. Secondly, the 'Endo-anal abdominoperineal pull-through resection with immediate colorectal anastomosis'.

Indications

Pull-through procedures may be used for several diseases and circumstances. (*1*) Tumours localized above the second Houston's valve ('plica transversalis of Kohlrausch'), which is situated at a distance of 8–9 cm from the anal verge. Lymphatic spread in these cases occurs mainly upwards through the superior haemorrhoidal pedicle. Anterior resection is adequate for the majority but a pull-through is a better procedure when technical difficulties do not permit the performance of a radical anterior resection with a safe low colorectal anastomosis. (2) Some special cases of benign lesions of the rectum, such as large villous adenomas occupying an extensive part of its wall, but sparing a sufficiently long segment of the distal rectum. (3) Hirschsprung's disease and acquired megacolon, in which the dilated sigmoid colon and most of the rectum are removed. (4) Some cases of inflammatory diseases of the bowel, such as ulcerative colitis and Crohn's disease, when distal rectum is normal or only slightly inflamed. (5) Congenital anorectal anomalies, particularly rectal atresia, where a pouch of normal rectum is present.

Pre-operative preparation

The patients should be submitted to a thorough physical examination and admitted to hospital at least 2 days before operation. Anaemia, protein deficit and hydroelectrolytic disturbances are corrected. A low-residue diet is recommended 4 or 5 days prior to the operation. A 15-mg dose of magnesium sulphate is given in the 2 days preceeding the operation. High colonic washouts are given twice a day for 2 or 3 days, until complete clearance of the bowel is achieved. Phthalylsulphathiazole, 2 g, and neomycin sulphate, 1 g, are given every 6 hr for 3 and 2 days, respectively, prior to the operation. As soon as the patient is anaesthetized a Levine tube is introduced into the stomach and a Foley catheter passed into the bladder. In males, penis and scrotum are strapped to the right thigh.

Anaesthesia

General anaesthesia is used for these operations in the majority of patients. Spinal or epidural anaesthesia is indicated only if general anaesthesia is considered harmful.

THE OPERATIONS

ABDOMINOPERINEAL PULL-THROUGH RESECTION WITH DELAYED COLORECTAL ANASTOMOSIS

The operation is performed in two stages.

FIRST STAGE

There are two phases, namely the abdominal and the perineal.

Abdominal phase

1

Incision and abdominal exploration

The patient is placed on the operating table in the lithotomy position, with moderate flexion of the legs to the pelvis. A long left paramedian incision is made extending from the pubis up to several inches above the level of the umbilicus. The abdominal cavity is explored thoroughly for the presence of intraperitoneal spread and hepatic metastases; the patient placed in Trendelenburg's position and the small intestine packed up away. The length of the colon and mesocolon and the vascular arrangement of the segment of the intestine to be used for the pull-through are carefully estimated. The procedure should be considered only when the colon and mesocolon are sufficiently long and the marginal arcade adequate.

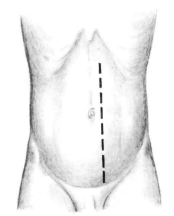

1

2

Dissection of the colon, ligature of the inferior mesenteric vessels and occlusive ligature of the colon

The peritoneum of either side of the colon is incised at its base, down to the bladder in the man or to the uterus in the female. The ureters are exposed, the left one being gently swept away from the base of the mesosigmoid. The inferior mesenteric vein is clamped, divided and ligated as high as possible, usually close to the duodenum or below the pancreas. The inferior mesenteric artery is ligated close to its origin from the aorta, or just below the left colic branch. If the artery is ligated close to the aorta, the blood supply of the sigmoid and descending colon may eventually become impaired. In this case it is necessary to dissect the entire left colon and to use the transverse colon for the pull-through. An occlusive ligature of heavy silk is applied to the bowel at the level of ligation of the marginal arcade. The length of colon necessary to extend beyond the anus is carefully estimated and additional length of the colon to facilitate the pull-through may be obtained by dividing and ligating some vessels of secondary arcades. In benign lesions it is not necessary to carry out a high ligation of the mesenteric vessels. In these cases a longer segment of mobile bowel may be obtained by ligating separately the sigmoid and left colon vessels.

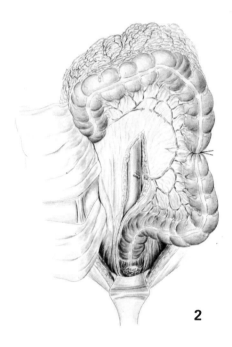

2

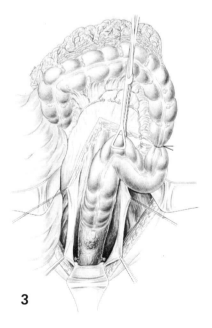

3

3

Dissection of the rectum

Dissection of the rectum is done as in Miles' operation: posteriorly to the level of levator ani muscles, anteriorly through Denonvillier's space in man and the rectovaginal space in women, and laterally to a corresponding level. The middle haemorrhoidal vessels are clamped, severed and tied. Upon completion of mobilization of the rectum, the colon prepared for the pull-through is carefully checked for its colour, pulsation of the smaller vessels and active bleeding of an epiploic appendage. When viability of this segment is doubtful, additional proximal mobilization is carried out.

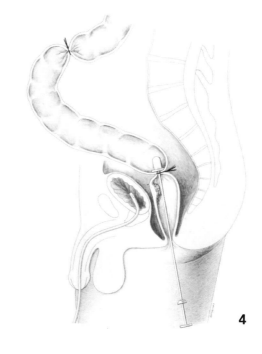

4

Perineal phase

4

Fixation of an obturator to the rectum

After gentle dilatation of the anal sphincter, an obturator of a sigmoidoscope is introduced through the anus to the proximal limit of the rectum and fixed at this level to the intestinal wall with a heavy silk ligature.

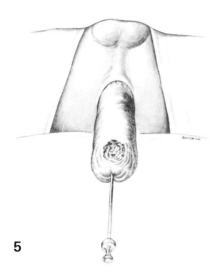

5

5

Intussusception of the rectum

Gentle downward traction of the obturator promotes eversion of the entire rectum and the pull-through of the lower portion of the sigmoid flexure.

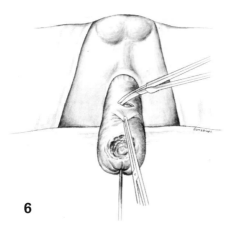

6

6

Incision of the rectum

The rectal wall is grasped with Allis' forceps and incised with scissors at approximately 4 cm from the pectinate line.

7a&b

Incision of the rectum completed

The incision is completed around the whole circumference of the rectum only, taking care not to incise the pull-through.

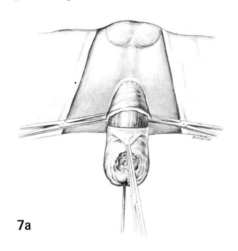

7a

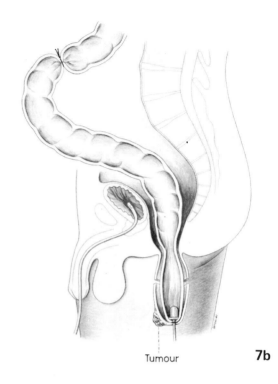

Tumour   **7b**

8

Pull-through and division of the colon

The bowel is drawn downward and out through the anus as far as the level of the occlusive ligature applied at the abdominal phase of the operation, exceeding by about 3 cm the border of the everted rectum. The colon is then clamped and divided distal to the ligature.

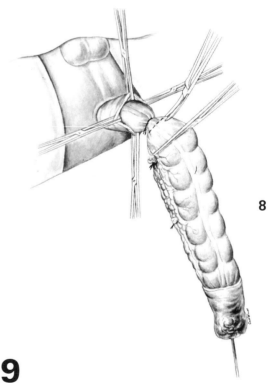

8

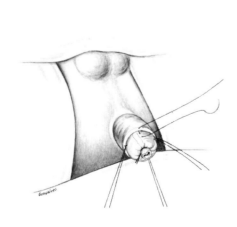

9

9

Fixation of the colon to the everted rectum

Four cotton stitches are applied to the seromuscular coat of the pulled colon and the border of the everted rectum, and tied.

10

Fixation of the colorectal stump to the perineal skin

The two lateral sutures are transfixed and attached to the perineal skin about 2 cm from the pectinate line. This prevents retraction of the colorectal stump. The stump is covered with Vaseline gauze.

While the perineal phase is being performed, assistants working in the abdomen proceed to reconstruct the pelvic peritoneal floor and close the abdomen. The pelvic cavity is drained by a Penrose drain or a rubber tube, or both, through a stab wound at the left or right lower quadrant of the abdomen. The occlusive ligature of the pulled-through colon is removed the day after operation, after which the pulled-through segment begins to act as a temporary perineal colostomy. The stitches fixing the bowel to the skin are removed 2 or 3 days after the operation.

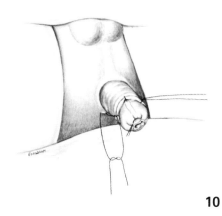

10

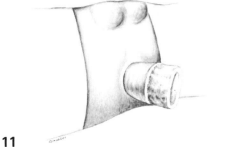

11

SECOND STAGE

This stage is performed about 10 days later, without anaesthesia.

11

Adhesion of the rectum to the colon

This period is sufficient to promote firm adhesion of the muscular coat of the everted rectum to the serosal surface of the pulled-through segment of the colon.

12a & b

Excision of the redundant colon

The colon is grasped with an Allis forceps and the seromuscular coat incised around the border of the everted rectum throughout the entire circumference. The mucosa is then dissected downwards for about 0·5 cm and divided with scissors around the entire circumference. This manoeuvre permits approximation of the colonic mucosa to the mucosa of the rectum without tension.

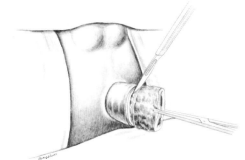

12a

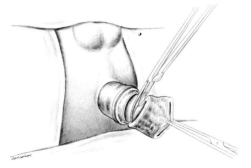

12b

13a & b

Suture of the mucosa of the rectum to the mucosa of the colon

Suture is done with interrupted fine cotton stitches.

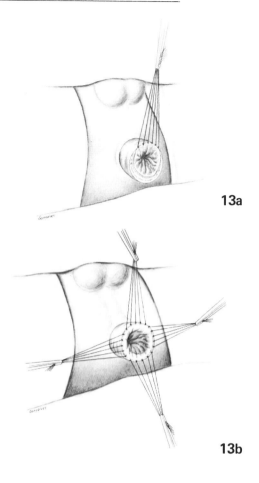

13a

13b

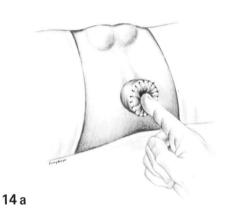

14 a

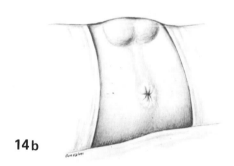

14 b

14 a & b

Reduction of the colorectal stump to the pelvic cavity

Upon completion of the suture, the colorectal stump is forced inside the pelvic cavity with the index finger. In some cases the use of a gauze facilitates this manoeuvre. The patient leaves the hospital after 2 or 3 days.

TUMOURS OF LARGE SIZE

In tumours of large size, due to the difficulty or impossibility of everting the rectum by the technique just described, the excision of the colorectal segment is done in the abdominal phase of the operation.

15

Excision of the rectum and colon

After completion of the colorectal mobilization, the rectum is clamped with a modified Wertheim clamp applied about 5 cm above the levator ani and incised, and the colon clamped and divided distal to the occlusive ligature.

16

Eversion of the rectum

After excision of the surgical specimen, an Allis forceps is introduced through the anal canal and grasps the cut edge of the rectum.

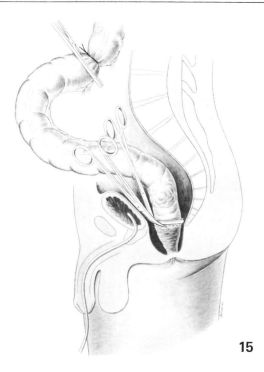

15

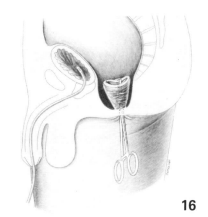

16

17a & b

Eversion of the rectum and pull-through of the colon

Gentle traction of the forceps promotes eversion of the rectum. Following this, a clamp introduced through the anus into the abdominal cavity grasps the occlusive silk ligature and pulls the colon through and out, exceeding by 3 cm the edge of the everted rectum. The operation is then completed in a similar manner to that already described.

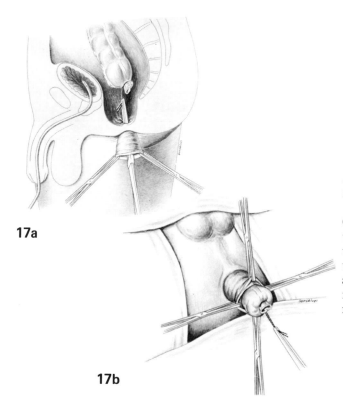

17a

17b

ENDO-ANAL ABDOMINOPERINEAL PULL-THROUGH RESECTION WITH IMMEDIATE COLORECTAL ANASTOMOSIS

The abdominal steps are identical to those described previously. The perineal phase is almost identical, the only difference being that the colorectal anastomosis is performed and completed in one stage.

18

Pull-through of the colon

After intussusception and division of the everted rectum, the colon is pulled down to the level where occlusive ligature exceeds about 3 cm the edge of the everted rectum.

19

Colorectal anastomosis — first layer

A two-layer colorectal anastomosis with interrupted cotton stitches is then performed. In the first, the stitches are applied through the muscular coat of the everted rectum and the seromuscular coat of the pulled-through colon.

20a & b

Colorectal anastomosis — second layer

In the second, which is made after division of the colon just distal to the first row of sutures, the stitches penetrate all coats of the rectum and colon. Upon completion of the anastomosis, the rectum is pushed up through the anus with the finger. A protective transverse colostomy should always be done when this method is used.

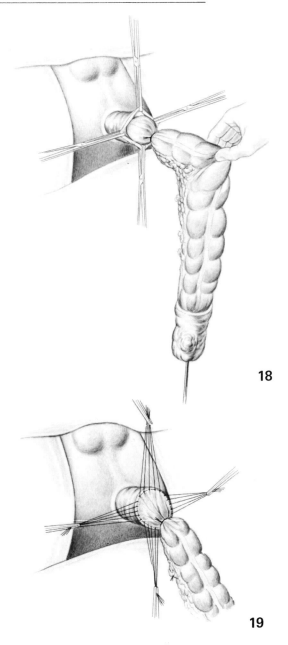

18

19

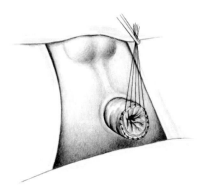

20b

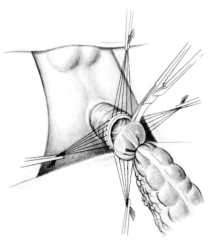

20a

POSTOPERATIVE CARE AND COMPLICATIONS

Oral feeding is restricted for 2 or 3 days. Fluid is given intravenously as required, and antibiotics are administered for 5 or 6 days. The gastric tube is removed as soon as flatus is passed. The urinary catheter is removed about the fifth day.

Necrosis of the colon

Necrosis occurs very occasionally after a pull-through procedure with a delayed colorectal anastomosis. It is not alarming provided it affects only the distal end of the exteriorized colon, but when intrapelvic colon is involved, an extensive pelvic abscess results. Sloughing is the result of a technical fault, being always due to a colon pulled down with an inadequate blood supply or under tension, or both. When extensive necrosis is diagnosed, a re-operation should be performed immediately, with the intention of pulling down normal proximal colon. However, when unfavourable anatomical conditions or severe infection are present, resection of the remaining rectum with establishment of a permanent colostomy must be considered.

Leakage of the anastomosis

This complication is common with immediate colorectal anastomosis, even when a covering colostomy has been performed, but is almost nil after a delayed colorectal anastomosis. It is usually followed by colorectal–perineal fistulae, infection and stenosis, but subsides with proper treatment in the majority of cases. In some instances, however, due to a persistence of these troubles, a colostomy will need to be instituted.

Retraction of the colorectal stump

This is a very rare complication of the delayed colorectal anastomosis. It may occur when dissection of the rectum is not carried down to the levator ani floor. In this case, much of the rectum lies inside the pelvic cavity and may thus suffer the influence of the negative pressure of the abdominal cavity during the inspiratory breath movements. As soon as this complication occurs, the colorectal stump should be grasped through a proctoscope with Allis' forceps and pulled down again. A strict vigilance should then be kept on the stump, which is covered with a thick Vaseline gauze dressing, until the date scheduled for the second stage of the anastomosis.

Pelvic infection

Infection of the presacral space follows leakage of the anastomosis, necrosis of the intrapelvic pulled colon or retraction of the colorectal stump. It may also occur when a large amount of serohaemorrhagic fluid collects in the pelvic cavity. Treatment consists in correction of the complication that caused the infection. Drainage of the pelvic cavity is recommended in all these cases, preferably by the perineal route.

Stricture

A slight stricture may be observed in the early postoperative days. It usually subsides spontaneously in a few weeks, but may persist when anastomotic leakage has occurred. Dilatation usually remedies this complication. In severe narrowing internal rectotomy is advised. A colostomy is needed in extreme cases.

Anal incontinence

Postoperative diarrhoea and pseudo-incontinence usually occur for 2–4 weeks, and subside spontaneously in the majority of cases. In some patients, however, normal continence is recovered only after several months have elapsed. Permanent impairment of continence is extremely rare.

References

Babcock, W. W. (1939). *Am. J. Surg.* **46,** 186
Babcock, W. W. (1947). *Surgery Gynec. Obstet.* **85,** 1
Bacon, H. E. (1945). *Surgery Gynec. Obstet.* **81,** 113
Black, B. M. (1948). *Proc. Staff Meet., Mayo Clin.* **23,** 545
Cutait, D. E. (1960). *I Congr. Lat. Amer.,* II Int., X Brasileiro de Proctologia **2,** 831
Cutait, D. E. (1965). *Dis. Colon Rectum* **8,** 107
Cutait, D. E. (1970). *Proc. R. Soc. Med.,* **Suppl 63,** 121
Cutait, D. E. and Figliolini, F. J. (1961). *Dis. Colon Rectum* **4,** 335
Cutait, D. E. and Figliolini, F. J. (1962*a*). *Rev. Ass. méd. bras.* **8,** 91
Cutait, D. E. and Figliolini, F. J. (1962*b*). *Rev. paul. Med.* **60,** 447
Cutait, D. E., Figliolini, F. J. and Branco, P. D. *et al.* (1965). *Rev. Ass. méd. bras.* **11,** 429
Hochenegg, J. (1888). *Wien klin. Wschr.* **1,** 254, 272, 290, 309, 324, 348
Maunsell, H. W. (1892). *Lancet* **ii,** 473
Swenson, O. and Bill, A. H., Jr. (1948). *Surgery* **24,** 212
Waugh, J. M. and Turner, J. C., Jr. (1958). *Surgery Gynec. Obstet.* **107,** 777
Weir, R. F. (1901). *J. Am. med. Ass.* **37,** 801

[The illustrations for this Chapter on Endo-anal Abdominoperineal Pull-through Resection with Colorectal Anastomosis were drawn by Mr. J. Gonçalves.]

Trans-sphincteric Resection

A. York Mason, B.Sc., F.R.C.S. (Ed.), F.R.C.S. (Eng.)
Surgeon, St. Anthony's Hospital (Medical,
Educational and Research Trust); Honorary
Consulting Surgeon, St. Helier Hospital and
Associated Hospitals; Late Honorary Consultant
Surgeon, Royal Marsden Hospital, London

INTRODUCTION

Sphincter division facilitates surgery for a variety of
rectal lesions, and there are essentially four variations
based on the trans-sphincteric exposure, described on
pages 396–404, which can be used to suit the individual patient.
   (1) Trans-rectal resection
   (2) Submucosal resection
   (3) Pararectal tube resection
   (4) Combined transabdominal and trans-sphincteric
       resection.
   Careful, detailed, pre-operative clinical assessment
of the pathology in every patient is essential in order
to select the appropriate resection technique. It is
not possible in a chapter devoted to surgical technique
to elaborate on this important aspect, but the author
has written previously about this problem (Mason,
1974, 1975, 1976) setting out the clinical staging of
rectal cancers, to which reference will be made during

description of techniques for selective restorative
surgery.

TRANS-RECTAL LOCAL EXCISION

Pre-operative bowel preparation

A clean bowel is essential and this can be achieved
by saline purgation and bowel washouts. The ideal
conditions can, of course, be obtained as described
in the previous chapter for the repair of a rectoprostatic fistula, by establishing a temporary defunctioning colostomy, but this is not necessary for
lesions which can be removed by simple local excision. It is not possible to sterilize the bowel before
operation, so pre-operative antibiotic preparation has
been abandoned; instead, a wide-spectrum antibiotic
is given intravenously at the start of the operation,
repeated towards the end, and continued for the first
four postoperative days.

TRANS-SPHINCTERIC EXPOSURE

The rectum and anal canal are opened up as described in the Chapter on 'Rectoprostatic Fistula' (*see Illustrations 6, 7* and *8*, pages 399–400). This provides an ideal exposure for the resection of a benign connective tissue tumour such as a leiomyoma.

1

This illustration shows the value of this exposure for excision of a large protuberant-type villous papilloma. Even although assessed pre-operatively as being a benign adenomatous lesion, full thickness excision is advisable because of the known high incidence of stalk invasion in large adenomatous polyps. The defect after this type of full thickness local excision is closed transversely, using a single layer of vertical mattress-type interrupted sutures of 3/0 chromic catgut. The flat, carpet-like villous papillomas can, if they are felt to be soft and velvety throughout, without any suspicious hard areas or surface ulceration, be treated by submucosal resection through the completely opened up rectum, and this technique is described later.

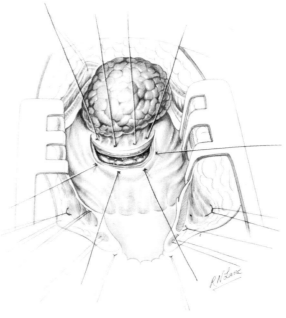

1

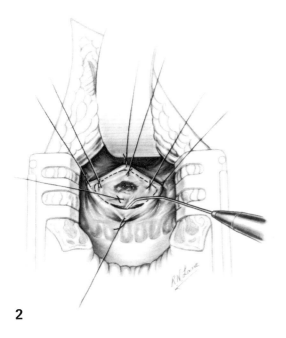

2

2

This illustrates local full thickness diathermy excision of a small freely mobile carcinoma sited on the anterior wall of the mid-rectum. The area to be excised is marked with paired sutures around the periphery, which help to keep diathermy excision 'on course,' holding the tissues taut. They also help to reduce bleeding. When elliptical excision has been completed, the resected tissue is lifted out, suspended by the inner circle of sutures.

3

The outer circle of sutures hold open the edges of the defect to provide clear vision of the extrarectal tissues. For a lowest third growth this would be vaginal wall in the female and prostatic capsule in a male patient. For higher placed growths (and even those in the upper third are accessible) an ellipse of peritoneum can be excised without danger because, with a patient in the prone jack-knife position, loops of small bowel slide away from the pelvic floor.

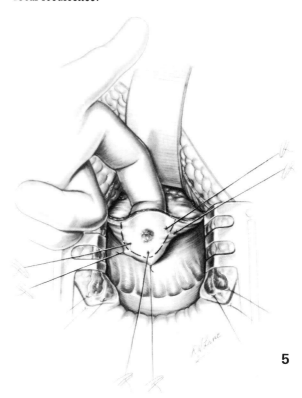

3

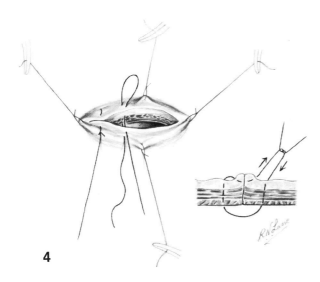

4

4

The defect is closed transversely by means of a single layer of interrupted vertical mattress sutures using 2/0 or 3/0 chromic catgut. This has proved to be a safe suture material and is preferred to non-absorbable sutures which may cause stitch granulomata and these may subsequently be mistaken for nodules of local recurrence.

5

This technique needs to be modified for posterior quadrant growths. Opening up of the anal canal and rectum should stop short of the lower edge of the growth. The rectum is then mobilized from the front of the sacrum and from the deep aspect of the levator ani. The mobilized posterior wall can now be prolapsed into the lumen of the rectum and the cancer seen face on. Full thickness diathermy excision is now carried out as described for anterior wall growths.

5

6

The result is a 'T' closure of the rectum, but if the corner stitches are placed accurately and not tied too tightly, there will be no healing problems at the junctional zone.

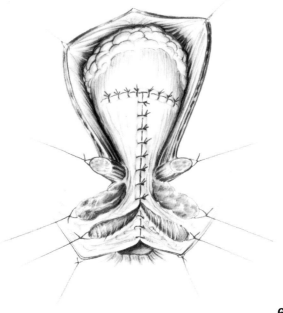

6

Washing out of all wounds with sterile water has proved sufficient protection from suture line implantation.

Closure of the trans-sphincteric exposure is carried out as described in the Chapter on 'Rectoprostatic Fistula' (*see Illustration 14,* page 402).

POSTOPERATIVE

There is no need to confine the bowels because wounds heal cleanly despite the passage of faeces. Defaecation occurs normally, without loss of normal sensation and without any impairment of anal continence.

SUBMUCOSAL RESECTION

7

The somatic tube has been opened up completely.
Division of the internal sphincter has been continued
up a short distance through the muscle wall of the
rectum to expose the submucosal plane. The 'water-
shed' at the level of the pectinate line can be seen
clearly.

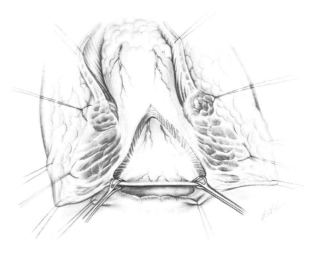

7

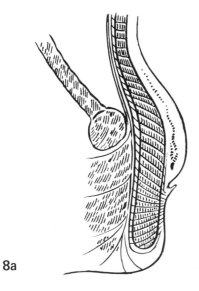

8a

8a

This sagittal section illustrates that below the level
of the pectinate line the lining of the anal canal is
tacked down to internal sphincter muscle by fibres
from the longitudinal coat passing inwards between
circular muscle coat bundles; above this level there
is a loose connective tissue space with a submucosal
vascular plexus.

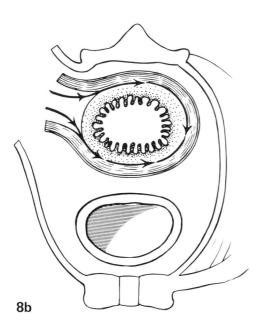

8b

8b

The arrows in this simplified diagram of a transverse
section through the pelvis indicate the convenient
plane through which a tube of rectal mucosa can be
resected after opening up the visceral muscle tube.

Indications

(*1*) Adenomatosis coli. The mucosa of the lower rectum can be removed through this plane after transabdominal colectomy, and the ileum brought down within the denuded muscle of rectum to be sutured to anal mucosa at the level of the pectinate line.

(*2*) In carefully selected patients with ulcerative proctocolitis a similar procedure can be used to restore continuity after total colectomy. This can only be done if the lower rectal mucosa is reasonably healthy and still mobile over the muscle coats.

(*3*) Benign villous papilloma carpeting the rectum.

PRE-OPERATIVE

Temporary deviation of faeces is advisable in these cases; a protective ileostomy in patients having a total colectomy or a left iliac colostomy in the case of extensive villous tumours carpeting the rectum. The presenting symptoms in some of these patients with extensive villous growths may be due to hypo-kalaemia, so correction of fluid and electrolyte imbalance is essential before surgery.

9

This illustrates submucosal resection of a large soft benign villous papilloma carpeting most of the rectum. Scissor dissection is shown proceeding around to the right side, keeping close to muscle and, throughout the course of this dissection, it is important to recognize feeding vessels which pass across the submucosal plane to join the plexus of vessels lying on the muscularis mucosae, and to diathermy these before division in order to maintain a clear field. Dissection around to the left is carried out in a similar manner and upwards to above the level of the villous carpet. Dissection continues around both sides to meet up in front. A closed mucosal tube containing the tumour can now be resected by proximal and distal transection. However, these tumours are often so soft that it is not possible to determine accurately by palpation alone that the lines of proximal and distal transection are well clear of the edges of the growth. It is usually necessary to open up the mucosal tube in order to visualize the edges of the soft carpet. In this illustration mucosa has been opened trans-versely at about the level of the pectinate line and for a short distance upwards through the tumour itself and, through this opening, the lower edge is seen clearly. For those growths which extend down to the pectinate line it is necessary to open up the anal canal completely in order to visualize the lower edge and, in some cases, the anterior part of the sub-mucosal resection can be carried out more easily from below upwards. Throughout the course of the submucosal resection it is essential to be on the alert for any loss of the clear submucosal plane which could be due to invasive carcinoma. Frozen tissue histology should be available and, if this confirms carcinoma, submucosal resection should be abandoned for more radical surgery.

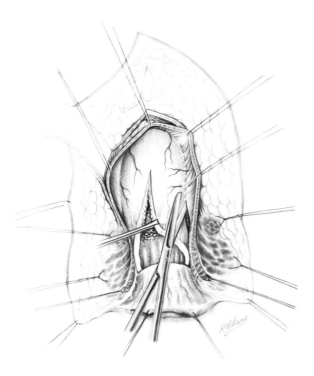

9

After submucosal resection, raw muscle defects of up to about 10 cm in length can be covered by suturing the upper and lower mucosal cuffs closely together with a few interrupted sutures, taking advantage of the natural tendency of the longitudinal coat to contract and 'concertina' the muscle wall of the rectum. This can be assisted by gently mobilizing the rectum from the front of the sacrum through the pararectal space. Complete coverage is not possible for defects longer than about 10 cm, but the mucosal cuffs can be drawn together and tacked to the underlying muscle to leave a smaller raw muscle defect. This will be covered first by granulation tissue and then re-epithelialized by growth of epithelium over the granulation tissue from the mucosal edges.

POSTOPERATIVE

Regular dilatation is essential to prevent stricture formation until the exposed muscle defect has been completely covered by new epithelium over matured granulation tissue. The temporary colostomy can, however, be closed before this stage, as soon as the trans-sphincteric exposure wound is cleanly healed, because the passage of faeces will not interfere with the growth of epithelium to cover raw muscle.

PARARECTAL TUBE RESECTION

A complete tube of rectum can be dissected out and resected through the pararectal space.

Indications

(1) *Rectal prolapse.* Tube resection is easy in patients with rectal prolapse because of the abnormal mobility of the rectum. Redundant bowel can be resected with ease if this is considered advisable and continuity restored by end-to-end anastomosis. However, if it is decided that resection of redundant bowel is not necessary, the mobilized rectum can be replaced at a higher level and secured by sutures placed between the deep aspect of the levator and the pararectal tissues. Overlapping of the cut ends of the puborectalis restores the anorectal angle and this, together with reefing of the levator ani to restore a posterior shelf, has cured the associated incontinence in these patients.

(2) *Low segment Hirschsprung's disease.*

(3) *Benign fibrotic strictures* can be resected through this space, but for postirradiation strictures, a combined procedure is preferable in order to bring down healthy non-irradiated colon for anastomosis to the anal canal.

(4) *Tube resection* has proved to be adequate curative surgery for patients with small mobile cancers of the lower two-thirds of the rectum.

PRE - OPERATIVE

A temporary defunctioning colostomy is advisable. For benign lesions this can be established at a preliminary operation and, for patients with low segment Hirschsprung's disease, it is better to defer resection for several weeks in order to clear impacted faeces and to give time for the dilated bowel above the stricture to return to a more normal diameter. For patients with carcinoma, however, there is evidence to suggest that it is probably better not to subject them to a preliminary operation so the procedure would be: (1) examination under general anaesthesia to obtain an accurate clinical assessment of the primary growth; (2) laparotomy, which provides valuable additional information; (3) the establishment of a temporary defunctioning colostomy of the type described on page 397; (4) closure of the laparotomy wound; (5) cleansing of the rectum by irrigation through the catheter sited in the distal limb; and then (6) repositioning of the patient for trans-sphincteric tube resection.

10

The somatic tube is shown opened up to expose the posterior pararectal space. White fascia propria covering the lower rectum is easily recognized and superior haemorrhoidal vessels can be seen emerging from under cover of the pararectal fat. Lymphatic vessels can usually be seen lying on the fascia propria and pararectal lymph nodes can be palpated through the fat. Upward exposure is improved by division of lower fibres of the gluteus maximus, and then by extension upwards of the incision through the levator ani. Posteriorly the rectum is mobilized from the front of the sacrum up to the level of the promontory. Mobilization is carried out around both sides, using a combination of blunt finger and sharp scissor dissection, to meet up in the mid-line anteriorly.

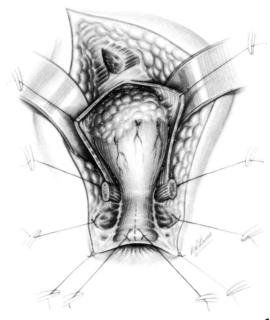

10

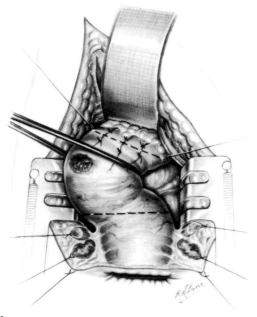

11

11

Peritoneum of the rectovesical or rectovaginal pouch is opened freely and the fully mobilized rectum can now be delivered out of the wound, held up by tapes or rubber tubing, and the appropriate length resected as a closed tube. Two details in this illustration need explanation; a mid-third carcinoma is depicted on the external surface of the rectum but this growth would not, of course, be visible on this aspect. Also, the proximal line of transection is shown passing across clearly visible, doubly ligated superior haemorrhoidal vessels but, at this level, they lie hidden in pararectal fat. Dissection should be carried out close to the deep aspect of the outer tube, so that the resected closed tube of rectum, with its contained growth, would have a covering of pararectal fat. The line of distal transection is shown at 1 cm above the level of the puborectalis.

12

Continuity is restored by end-to-end rectorectal anastomosis. The bowel ends are shown correctly aligned for anastomosis by lateral stay sutures. The posterior half of each end is retracted by similar stay sutures in order to provide clear vision of the anterior wall. A single layer of interrupted vertical mattress, mucosa inverting sutures of 2/0 chromic catgut is used for the anastomosis.

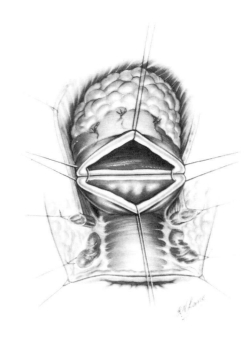

12

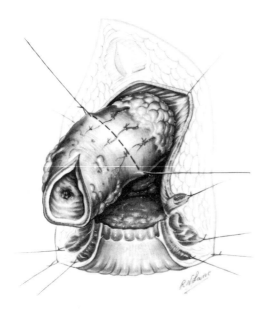

13

13

This technique needs to be modified for low-sited cancers. The anal canal is opened up (*see* dotted line in *Illustration 10*) in order to visualize the lower edge of the growth and so to make sure that the line of distal transection will be well clear of this lower edge. A better exposure is provided for upward dissection in the case of anterior quadrant growths. The partially opened up anorectal tube can now be resected.

14

Continuity is restored by recto-anal anastomosis. The anterior half of the opened-up anal canal is correctly aligned to the rectum by stay sutures. The first stitch for the anastomosis is placed in the mid-line anteriorly, subsequent sutures being placed to either side of the first stitch, so restoring the flat opened-up anal canal back to a tube as the sutures continue around both sides towards the mid-line posteriorly. It is sometimes possible to match the different circumferences of rectum and anal canal by crimping the former and stretching the latter but, to equalize the two ends, it may be necessary to cut away a wedge (the shaded area) in order to equalize the circumference of the two bowel ends.

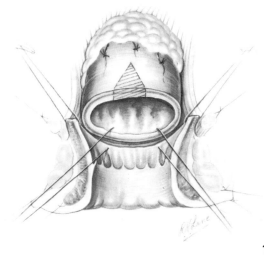

14

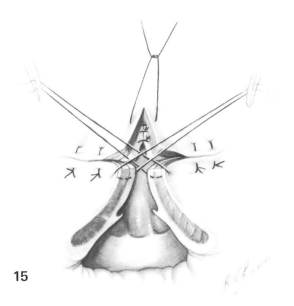

15

15

The anastomosis is nearing completion and, because a wedge of rectum has been excised, there will be a cross junction.

16

The recto-anal anastomosis has now been completed. Vertical closure of the anal canal is carried out as described in the Chapter on 'Rectoprostatic Fistula', pages 396–404. Two Shirley sump drains are placed in the pararectal space before closure of the outer somatic tube. Citrate solution is run in through one of these and suction applied to the other, until the returning fluid is clear. This has proved to be the most effective way to prevent haematoma formation in the presacral space.

POSTOPERATIVE

The temporary colostomy should not be closed until both the anastomosis and the trans-sphincteric exposure wound are cleanly healed and pliable. It may be advantageous to allow the patient to have a spell at home before re-admission for formal closure of the colostomy, and one of the main advantages of the end colostomy described in the Chapter on 'Rectoprostatic Fistula', pages 396–404, is that it is a comfortable one, easily managed and well tolerated by the patient for as long as may be necessary. If closure of the colostomy is deferred until the sphincters have become pliable, the patient will enjoy a normal pattern of defaecation with full anal continence from the time of the first bowel action.

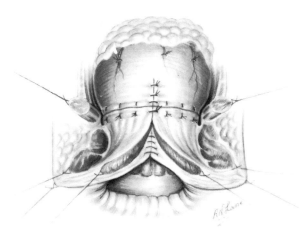

16

COMBINED TRANSABDOMINAL AND TRANS-SPHINCTERIC EXPOSURE FOR RESECTION AND LOW ANASTOMOSIS

Indications

The use of this combined procedure for patients with adenomatosis coli and for some patients with ulcerative proctocolitis has already been mentioned. It has proved to be very successful in the treatment of strictures and fistulae following irradiation for gynaecological cancers. This combined procedure can be used for operable cancers of the rectum, considered suitable for restorative surgery, but sited too low for transabdominal anastomosis after resection.

With the patient supine, a full length paramedian incision is used for the transabdominal part. The nature and extent of the abdominal resection will vary with the pathology.

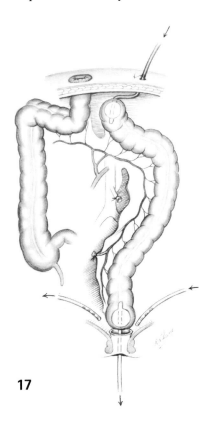

17

17

As an example, this diagram illustrates its use for a mid-third carcinoma of the rectum. A temporary defunctioning right transverse colostomy has been established. Distal large bowel has been mobilized and the rectum dissected out down to the pelvic floor. Proximally, the colon has been transected at a carefully selected site, distally the rectum has been transected at the level of the pelvic floor, well clear of the lower edge of the mid-third rectal cancer. The intervening bowel has been removed. The proximal colon has been drawn down by means of a Foley catheter to lie abutting the rectal stump, correctly orientated and free from tension. A pair of Shirley sump drains, one for irrigation and the other for suction, are shown placed in the pelvis. The abdomen is now closed and the patient repositioned prone for trans-sphincteric anastomosis.

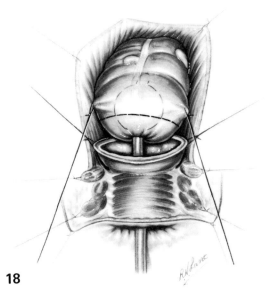

18

18

The somatic tube has been opened up to provide an ideal exposure for low anastomosis. The invaginated end of colon is now trimmed away to release the balloon catheter. An end-to-end anastomosis is carried out with ease and safety under direct vision, using a single layer of interrupted catgut sutures as described and illustrated previously (*see Illustration 12*).

19

This technique needs to be modified for bulky growths because it may not be possible to visualize the rectum clearly enough for transection between clamps below the lower edge of the growth, or to complete dissection satisfactorily via the abdominal exposure. In these patients the mobilized bowel is left in the peritoneal cavity, the chosen site for proximal transection being marked with orientating stitches, the abdomen is closed and the patient then repositioned prone for the trans-sphincteric part. Both the somatic and visceral tubes are opened up. The lower edge of growth can be clearly visualized and the anal canal transected well clear of this lower edge. Any further necessary dissection can be carried out via this wide exposure from below upwards, and this is particularly valuable for low-placed anterior wall growths. The completely freed bowel can now be drawn gently down through the widely opened-up sphincters until the marking sutures come into view. The colon is transected at this level. Colo-anal anastomosis is carried out with ease and clear vision as described previously, after resection of a partially opened-up tube of rectum (*see Illustrations 14–16*).

This is a combined sequential procedure which necessitates repositioning of the patient for the second part of the operation. However, if this is carried out correctly and gently, it causes minimal disturbance. The need to reposition the patient is more than compensated for by the excellence of the exposure afforded for both parts of the operation. The main postoperative complication is presacral haematoma formation and subsequent infection of this collection of blood. The most significant advance in the prevention of presacral haematoma formation has been the use of Shirley sump drains for combined irrigation and suction.

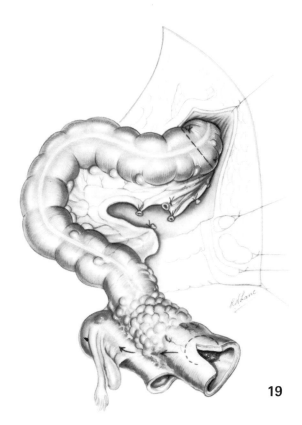

19

POSTOPERATIVE

Irrigation and suction via the Shirley sump drains is continued until the returning fluid is clear and this is usually necessary for only a few hours. The defunctioning colostomy should not be closed until the anastomosis can be seen and felt to be cleanly healed and pliable. In most cases the patients will welcome a short period at home before returning for formal closure of the colostomy (*see Illustrations 15–18, pages 403–404*).

Functional results

Although defaecation and anal control in the healthy adult is dependent on a highly complex neuromuscular mechanism, experience with low trans-sphincteric anastomosis has shown that patients will all regain an acceptable pattern of defaecation and of anal control, provided they retain the essential stretch receptors in a healthy, pliable levator ani–puborectalis sling, and the fine sensory receptors in the mucosa of the sampling zone of the anal canal. Stretch reception is impaired by inflammation and subsequent fibrosis in the levator ani–puborectalis complex. This is minimized by routine use of a completely defunctioning colostomy and the avoidance of presacral haematoma formation. The greater the length of colon lost, the greater the problem patients will experience initially in having to pass liquid stools frequently. Codeine phosphate is the most effective constipating drug, but reassurance that there will be progressive improvement over the course of the next 2 years is necessary.

References

Mason, A. Y. (1974). 'Trans-sphincteric surgery of the rectum.' In *Progress in Surgery*, Vol. 13, pp. 66–97. Basle: S. Karger
Mason, A. Y. (1975). 'Malignant tumours of the rectum: local excision.' *Clins Gastroent.* 4, 582
Mason, A. Y. (1976). 'Rectal cancer: the spectrum of selective surgery.' *Proc. R. Soc. Med.* 69, 237

[*The illustrations for this Chapter on Trans-sphincteric Resection were drawn by Mr. R. N. Lane.*]

The Kraske, Sacral or Posterior Approach to the Rectum

Max Pemberton, M.B.E., T.D., F.R.C.S.
Consulting Surgeon, Chase Farm Hospital, and
Enfield War Memorial Hospital

The sacral or posterior route to the rectum is usually associated with the name of Kraske who described his technique for excision of the rectum in 1885. An abdominal phase was later added to constitute a combined type of operation for a sphincter-saving resection and was called an abdominosacral resection.

Neither the abdominosacral procedure nor the sacral approach to the rectum have been popular in the English-speaking countries. Many surgeons still think that when an anastomosis is made by this route, there is a high incidence of a persistent faecal fistula through the posterior wound. In addition, incisions in this situation have a notorious reputation for impaired healing.

Dehiscence of an anastomosis accomplished by this approach is probably associated with inadequate exposure and it is interesting that most of the breakdowns which occurred in Localio and Baron's cases (1973) were in younger men with a small pelvis which led to technical difficulties in performing the anastomosis. Excision of the coccyx and lower part of the sacrum alone gives insufficient access; a transverse incision with the removal of the coccyx and transverse division of the levator ani muscles (Localio, 1971) also appears restrictive.

An anastomosis which can be achieved easily and without the need of traction or instrumental handling of the bowel should unite more certainly than one made during a low anterior resection at some awkward distance from the surgeon.

The technique described here provides adequate access and space; and the method of repair of the wound ensures sound healing *per primam*.

ANATOMY AND PRINCIPLE

1

The rectum extends for approximately 15 cm from the middle of the third piece of the sacrum to the anal canal. Ideally, a surgical exposure should give access to the whole length of a viscus without inflicting permanent damage on important structures.

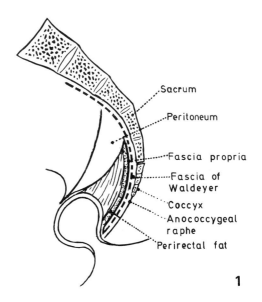

1

2

Ligaments of the pelvis viewed from behind

It is clear that the basal attachments of the sacro-
tuberous and sacrospinous ligaments to the sides of the
last two sacral and first coccygeal vertebrae must be
divided if the lower two pieces of the sacrum and
coccyx are removed. This procedure does not cause
any disability.

When these vertebrae are removed and the
anococcygeal raphe is divided longitudinally as far
forward as its anterior termination at the junction of
the rectum and anal canal, the full extent of the
dorsal aspect to the rectum is directly accessible.

The freeing of the iliococcygeus and pubococcygeus
muscles from their attachments to the coccyx and the
anococcygeal raphe disconnects the insertions of
these two parts of the levator ani muscle. With the
division of the fascia of Waldeyer, the rectum can be
mobilized and a space opened up in three dimensions
to give generous access for any required procedure on
the rectum.

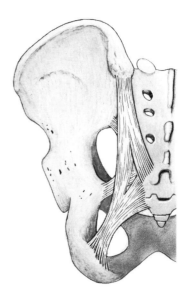

2

PRE-OPERATIVE

Indications

The sacral approach has many advantages for the
treatment of benign lesions of the rectum which
cannot be excised *per anum* or through an operating
sigmoidoscope. It is particularly useful for dealing
with extensive villous adenomas. Large leiomyomas
arising in the muscular wall of the rectum have been
removed (Norbury, 1934) by this route.

The sacral or abdominosacral approach may be
necessary for extrarectal tumours situated posteriorly;
teratomas and dermoid cysts are the commonest of
these retrorectal lesions.

It is the operation of choice for cases of benign
strictures of the rectum. A complete stricture following the breakdown of the anastomosis after an
anterior resection of the rectum can be successfully
managed by abdominal mobilization of the proximal
segment followed by a sacral excision of the stenotic
area and axial anastomosis; the antecedent transverse colostomy would have defunctioned the distal
colon.

Successful results with local destruction or local
excision to treat carefully selected cases of invasive
adenocarcinoma of the rectum have been reported in
recent years. The Kraske procedure may, therefore,
prove to be of value for resecting small, mobile,
low-grade, malignant lesions of the rectum through

the opened-up rectum or for performing a segmental
resection in slightly larger lesions.

At the present time, carcinomas of the middle
third of the rectum which are not high-grade lesions
or fixed to adjacent structures such as the vagina, are
treated in the hands of experienced surgeons by a low
resection; the anastomosis is performed by several
different methods; but the sacral route gives the most
direct access.

A low anterior resection has a high frequency of
dehiscence but Localio and Baron (1973) of New
York City have practised 'abdominotrans-sacral'
resection for these mid-rectal cancers with a com-
paratively low incidence of anastomotic breakdown.

Localized recurrences following a restorative
resection for rectal cancer can often be treated
satisfactorily by a further sphincter-saving procedure,
particularly if the original lesion was found after the
first operation to be a Duke's A or a Duke's B case; a
recurrent lesion follows the pattern of the original
growth (Pemberton, 1972). The sacral approach has
been used successfully by the author for resection of
recurrent rectal carcinoma (Darke, 1973).

The abdominosacral operation may also be used
to effect a low anastomosis subsequent to a
Hartmann excision of the rectum.

Rectal prolapse

For the management of this condition, the sacral approach has special merit. With this access, the puborectalis muscles can be readily approximated anterior to the rectum to control a complete rectal prolapse (Davidian and Thomas, 1972). However, it is easier and more expeditious to employ this route for performing one of the various methods of rectopexy with the use of synthetic materials. Ripstein's second technique (Ripstein, 1972) can easily be carried out but the sling may cause a mechanical obstruction. A procedure using Ivalon sponge is recommended. It has proved particularly useful in frail subjects unfit for an abdominal operation. A low epidural or caudal anaesthetic can be used in patients rejected for a general anaesthetic. This procedure avoids the complications which may follow the implanting of a Thiersch wire and would seem preferable to the high or supralevator Thiersch operation (Notaras, 1973) or other recent modifications of the Thiersch operation (Plumley, 1966). Indeed, the author now considers it the operation of choice for all cases of complete rectal prolapse.

Contra-indications

A sacral bedsore will prevent the use of a sacral incision; however, excoriation of skin due to excessive discharge of mucus from a permanently prolapsed rectum is not a contra-indication. The excoriation heals when the mucous discharge ceases. For malignant lesions which lie in the upper third of the rectum an anterior resection should always be employed and not an abdominosacral procedure. Further, the sacral approach should not be used for palliative treatment or for the treatment of lesions which are invading another viscus.

Pre-operative preparation

The colon and rectum should be cleansed by a mechanical and dietary regime which ensures that the colon and rectum are empty of faeces. When the bowel is to be opened or an anastomosis performed, oral antibacterial agents, e.g. Sulfathalidine, should be given before operation. A self-retaining catheter is passed into the bladder in the operating theatre and connected to a closed drainage system. A Silastic catheter is preferable if the period of catheterization is likely to be prolonged.

Position of patient

There are a number of choices. The patient may be placed in the prone position with the chest and pelvis supported and the abdomen free. The 'right lateral' position is preferred by some surgeons and Localio uses this position to gain simultaneous access to the abdomen and sacral region; in this way, the need to reposition the patient is avoided.

An exaggerated lithotomy position can also be used for the combined abdominosacral resection.

3

However, for the sacral incision, most surgeons will probably feel more comfortable sitting with the patient in the familiar 'left lateral' position. A pillow is placed under the upper knee (not shown) of the patient. Waterproof plastic adhesive strapping is attached to the upper buttock and used to open up the intergluteal crease and tilt the pelvis slightly anteriorly.

When performing an abdominosacral resection, it will be necessary to turn the patient into this position after completing the abdominal phase. Although this technique lacks the advantage of synchronous access, the preliminary dorsal position allows the use of a long, paramedian incision extending down to the pubis and will facilitate mobilization of the splenic flexure and give safer access to the depths of the pelvis.

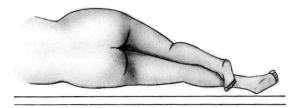

3

THE OPERATION

4

The anus is gently dilated and a small antiseptic gauze roll is placed in the lower rectum and anal canal. The skin of the sacral area and perineum is prepared with Hibitane and Spirit and drapes are adjusted to leave sufficient space on either side of the proposed incision for deep tension sutures and a drainage tube. When the skin is quite dry, a Steridrape is applied over the whole area, sealing off the anus.

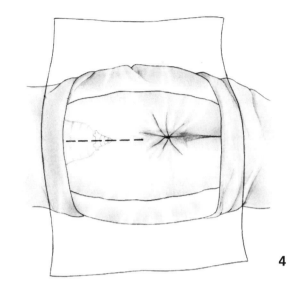

4

5

The sacral incision is made in the mid-line from the level of the spinous process of the third sacral vertebra to just behind the anus. It is deepened to the fascia overlying the sacrum. The anococcygeal raphe is defined; the lateral muscular and ligamentous attachments to the sides of the coccyx are then divided. The thick anococcygeal raphe is incised throughout its length from the tip of the coccyx to the external anal sphincter. Some fibres of the puborectalis will be seen deep to the external sphincter. A finger can now be inserted and the fascia of Waldeyer separated from the coccyx.

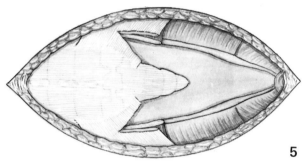

5

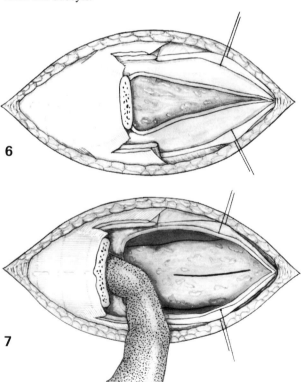

6

7

6 & 7

The coccyx is removed with powerful, double-action, rongeur forceps. The exposed fascia of Waldeyer is divided in the mid-line as far forward as the puborectalis. The rectum can now be separated easily from the hollow of the sacrum. To obtain more space, the fascia of Waldeyer is freed from the anterior surface of the lower sacrum; the fifth sacral segment is excised and, if necessary, the body of the fourth sacral vertebra medial to the fourth sacral foramina is nibbled away; the lateral masses are usually left. The third sacral nerves must not be damaged. The median sacral vessels are identified and ligated; bleeding from the divided bone can be controlled with bone wax (Ethicon), or by stitching a fold of fascia over the end of the bone.

8

In order to expose completely the posterior aspect of the rectum, all that remains is division of the thin fascia propria and separation of the fat in the mid-line between the terminal branches of the superior haemorrhoidal vessels.

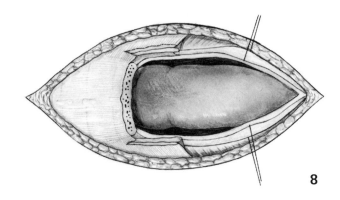

8

9

Procedure for the removal of a benign lesion

If mobility is required, the bowel should be dissected free from the bladder and prostate and seminal vesicles in the male, and from the vagina in the female; the peritoneum may be separated by blunt dissection or opened if required. A villous adenoma of the rectum is often very extensive and may form a complete circumferential carpet. If possible, the rectum should be opened between stay sutures where it is not involved by the lesion. It is an advantage to lift a villous adenoma off the circular muscle coat by injecting saline with adrenaline (1:300,000). The tumour can then be dissected off the underlying muscle with scissors. It is often possible to close the defect in the mucosa with interrupted sutures of fine catgut inserted from within the lumen. However, a large denuded area may be created which is impossible to repair, but such defects may be left and will heal in time.

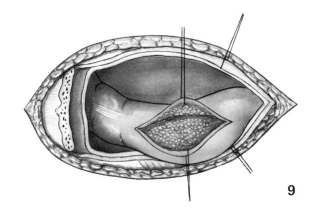

9

10

The sacral approach for the treatment of complete rectal prolapse

It is not necessary to open the peritoneum but the rectum is mobilized and an estimation made of that part of the rectum which can be drawn firmly upwards and applied to the hollow of the sacrum. This part of the posterior aspect of the rectum is then cleared down to the muscle of the rectum prior to the application of a patch of synthetic mesh or Ivalon sponge; usually, an area 6 cm long by 3 cm wide is prepared. (A 5 cm × 3 cm patch of Ivalon sponge has been used in the author's cases.) It is cut to size and softened in water and then stitched with superficial bites to the muscle of the rectum using interrupted atraumatic sutures of Ethiflex. The sponge must not encircle more than two thirds of the bowel: the anterior one-third of the circumference is left free.

Four sutures of 1/0 Ethiflex or Prolene (polypropylene) are then inserted from above down through the presacral fascia on the hollow of the

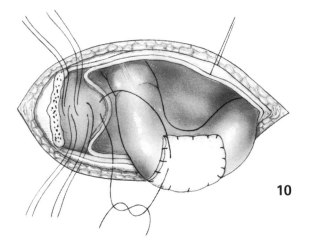

10

sacrum. The median sacral vessels should be carefully avoided. Each of these four sutures is taken in turn and passed through the middle of the patch of Ivalon. The rectum is now lifted upwards and the sutures are tied from above down. The lower rectum should be reasonably taut when all the sutures are tied.

If plastic materials are being used, it is especially important to avoid infection. As an additional precaution, 1 g of cephaloridine powder has been inserted into the wound before starting the closure.

Technique for a low rectal anastomosis using the abdominosacral approach

In the abdominal phase, thorough mobilization of the colon is essential as a transverse colostomy will almost always have been constructed either prior to the operation or as the first step in the procedure; the colostomy tethers the colon.

It is important when mobilizing the colon prior to resection and anastomosis to free a longer loop than would appear necessary to reach the floor of the pelvic cavity: any excess colon can be trimmed later before the anastomosis from below.

For a carcinoma of the middle third of the rectum, the colon is divided using Cope's clamps; with a small pelvis it is better to close the colon stump for use in the anastomosis with an inverting (Mikulicz) suture so that it can be delivered without any difficulty or trauma from below.

Orientation of this colon loop to avoid twisting when it is drawn down will be assured by the placing of a coloured stitch on the left side of the bowel with a differing one on the right. The rectum with its tumour is dissected free from surrounding structures as in the conventional restorative procedure and divided, if possible, between clamps not less than 5 cm below the lower end of the growth. The pelvic peritoneum is left open and the abdomen closed.

When a very low anastomosis is required, the procedure is different. The colon is not divided during the abdominal stage, nor is the dissected rectum transected or removed. A site on the colon is selected which is considered more than adequate to reach the anus. The mesocolon is divided; and the marking stitches are placed on the bowel within the area of viability.

During the perineal phase, the rectum is ligated with strong linen below the tumour and then, after the usual preparation, divided at a suitable distance below the ligature. This allows the surgeon to grasp the proximal end of the transected rectum and ease it down through the posterior incision with the distal colon following.

When the level of the colon selected for the anastomosis is lined up with the rectal stump, the colon is clamped and divided.

For a very low anastomosis, it will be necessary to sever the puborectalis sling between paired marking sutures. An anastomosis even to the anorectal junction is then possible. The author uses one layer of interrupted Dexon (polyglycolic acid) sutures which are gently tied with the knots inside the lumen. These do not vitiate the blood supply of the bowel ends.

The 'abdominotrans-sacral' method used by Localio allows the advantage of synchronous access to the abdomen and the sacral region so that there is the guarantee of accurate mobilization of the colon, but the posterior approach in this method gives less room for work on the anastomosis than in the method just described.

Closure

11

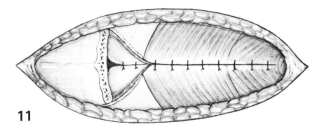

11

Redivac wound suction is ideal for drainage. The fascia of Waldeyer is approximated by interrupted sutures of Dexon. The anococcygeal raphe is repaired using interrupted sutures of stainless steel wire; if the puborectalis sling has been divided, it is carefully sutured with wire. Reef knots are used and the ends are cut separately flush with the knots so that practically no ends of wire project; the tissue will not be strangulated because the second throw when tied firmly does not tighten the first throw. These knots never untie and when the suture finally fragments, it does so opposite the knot.

12

A 90 mm atraumatic curved cutting needle (Colts) with strong nylon is used to insert deep tension sutures. Usually four or six of these are required and they pass through the skin, subcutaneous tissues, and the fascia overlying the sacrum or through the anococcygeal raphe. The skin is then approximated with vertical mattress sutures of fine nylon lightly tied.

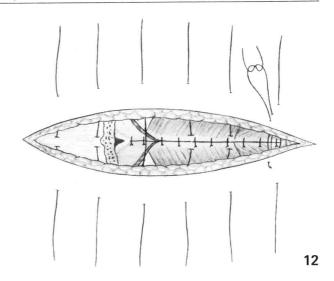

12

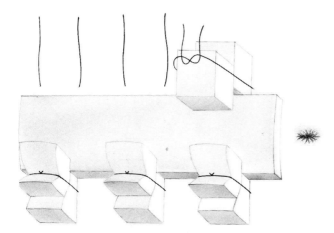

13

13

Finally, the deep tension sutures are tied over at least two Lyo foam preparation swabs. Two ipsilateral adjacent sutures are first tied together and then the corresponding ends are pulled reasonably taut and tied together over Lyo foam swabs on the other side of the wound. A Lyo foam dressing is usually applied to the wound and a large amount of sterile gauze is placed over the Lyo foam dressing. The whole is held in position with micropore tape. Suction is finally applied when the dressings are in place.

POSTOPERATIVE CARE AND COMPLICATIONS

The patient is kept on his back for a few hours to exert gentle compression on the wound. Thereafter, the most comfortable position for these patients is a lateral one and the position should be changed from one side to the other every 3 or 4 hr until the patient is mobile.

Redivac suction is maintained until there is no discharge. When an anastomosis has been made, the Redivac tube is kept in place for 6 days. The vertical mattress sutures of fine nylon can be removed about the fifth or sixth day without disturbing the deep tension sutures and usually Steristrips are applied across the wound as alternate sutures are removed. The deep tension sutures are maintained for at least 14 days; this time is needed for the subcutaneous tissues to become firmly adherent to the deeper, less vascular tissues. Conventional deep tension sutures are usually removed on the seventh or eigth day owing to their tendency to cut into the tissues. The urethral catheter is removed on the fifth day; the bowels are usually confined for at least 6 days by a low-residue diet. Thereafter, the patient is given a bulking agent and if the bowels do not open normally washouts of dioctyl sodium sulphosuccinate are given.

Complications

There is often some infection of the sacral wound when this approach is used in the presence of pelvic infection, e.g. when treating a rectal stricture. Delay in wound healing may occur and almost always affects the upper part of the wound overlying the sacrum.

The author has not noted a faecal fistula as a complication, but prior to every low anastomosis he has always established a defunctioning transverse colostomy. Should a fistula occur and persist, then an efficient defunctioning transverse colostomy should be performed.

Incontinence may be present for some time in those patients in whom the colon has been anastomosed to the rectum just above or at the anorectal ring; but treatment with Imodium (Loperamide) or other agents which increase intestinal transit time, and thickening of the stool with Metamucil (psillium) or Celevac (methyl cellulose) helps such patients to gain acceptable control of bowel function. In a few cases, this may take 6–12 months.

A bulge or impulse on straining may be observed at the posterior part of the wound where the coccyx and segment or segments of the sacrum were removed. This does not, however, cause any symptoms. Anaesthesia of the skin overlying the region of the former coccyx due to injury to the coccygeal plexus may occur but the affected area is always small.

Infrequently, patients complain that it is uncomfortable to sit on a hard chair, the discomfort being felt in the region of the divided end of the sacrum.

References

Darke, S. G. (1973). *Proc. R. Soc. Med.* **66**, 678
Davidian, U. A. and Thomas, C. G. (1972). *Am. J. Surg.* **123**, 231
Donaldson, G. A., Rodkey, G. V. and Behringer, G. E. (1966). *Surgery Gynec. Obstet.* **123**, 571
Edwards, F. S. (1908). *Diseases of the Rectum, Anus and Sigmoid Colon.* London: Churchill
Jackman, R. J. (1961). *Dis. Colon Rectum* **4**, 429
Jenkins, S. G. and Thomas, C. G. (1962). *Surgery Gynec. Obstet.* **114**, 381
Kraske, P. (1885). *Verh. dt. Ges. Chir.* **14**, Part 2, 464
Localio, S. A. (1971). *Surgery Gynec. Obstet.* **132**, 123
Localio, S. A. and Baron, B. (1973). *Ann. Surg.* **178**, 540
Marks, G. (1973). *Dis. Colon Rectum* **16**, 378
Mason, A. Y. (1972). *Proc. R. Soc. Med.* **65**, 974
Mason, A. Y. (1975). *Clinics Gastroent.* **4**, 582
McLean, D. W. and Arminski, T. C. (1959). *Dis. Colon Rectum* **2**, 534
Norbury, L. E. C. (1934). *Proc. R. Soc. Med.* **27**, 930
Notaras, M. J. (1973). *Proc. R. Soc. Med.* **66**, 684
Pemberton, M. (1972). *Proc. R. Soc. Med.* **65**, 663
Plumley, P. (1966). *Br. J. Surg.* **53**, 624
Ripstein, C. B. (1972). *Dis. Colon Rectum* **15**, 334

[*The illustrations for this Chapter on the Kraske, Sacral or Posterior Approach to the Rectum were drawn by Mr. F. Price.*]

Hartmann's Operation

J. D. Griffiths, M.S., F.R.C.S.
Consultant Surgeon, St. Bartholomew's Hospital, and
The Royal Marsden Hospital, London

PRE-OPERATIVE

Introduction

The principle of Hartmann's operation is the excision of the upper two-thirds of the rectum and sigmoid colon with the construction of a left iliac colostomy and closure of the lower third of the rectum which is left *in situ*, along with the pelvic floor. This operation was first described by Hartmann in 1923 and was the operation of choice for carcinoma of the upper and middle thirds of the rectum before anterior resection became a safe procedure. Hartmann's operation need rarely be performed in modern practice — now being the operation of choice only where anterior resection or abdominoperineal resection are contraindicated.

Indications

Hartmann's operation is indicated in two main groups of patients:

(*1*) Those patients with carcinoma of the upper two-thirds of the rectum who are either: (*a*) bad risk patients in whom excision of the pelvic floor would add to the mortality or morbidity of the operative procedure without subsequent benefit to the patient; (*b*) patients in whom carcinoma of the upper two-thirds of the rectum has perforated with associated peritonitis or with diffuse metastatic pelvic floor seedling, in whom anterior resection is unwise.

(*2*) Some patients with diverticulitis. The operation has been used in recent years as the initial stage in cases where there has been perforation and peritonitis or gross pelvic inflammation which make primary anastomosis a hazardous procedure.

Advantages

The advantage of Hartmann's operation in diverticulitis is that it enables removal of the diseased area of bowel which allows inflammation to settle before performing an end-to-end anastomosis. It has advantages over the staged operation in which the transverse diversionary colostomy leaves the affected bowel *in situ*. This procedure is often followed by attacks of infection which delay excision of the area and subsequent anastomosis.

This operation may also be performed with safety when the bowel has not been prepared.

Contra-indications

This operation should not be performed if:

(*1*) The patient is fit for either an anterior resection or abdominoperineal resection.

(*2*) There is carcinoma of the lower third of the rectum. Removal of the pelvic floor is a necessary part of curative excision of this lesion.

(*3*) There has been perforation with peritonitis in a case of diverticulitis and the toxaemic state of the patient indicates that a transverse colostomy, as a quick, safe procedure, is the method of choice.

THE OPERATION

Position of patient

The patient should be in an extended lithotomy-Trendelenburg position (Lloyd-Davies). It is often necessary, especially in cases of carcinoma of the rectum for a rectal washout to be performed, using a cancericidal agent, before closure of the rectal stump.

Incision

A long left paramedian incision, as for anterior resection or abdominoperineal resection, should be made.

PROCEDURE

1

Mobilization

The sigmoid colon and rectum should be mobilized as described for anterior resection. The inferior mesenteric artery pedicle should be ligated appropriately. Care should be taken that the left ureter is identified.

Ligation of superior rectal artery

The superior rectal artery should be ligated on the rectal stump.

Clamping

A clamp should be placed between the upper two-thirds and lower third of the rectum. A rectal washout below the clamp is advised using a cancericidal agent or antiseptic solution as required.

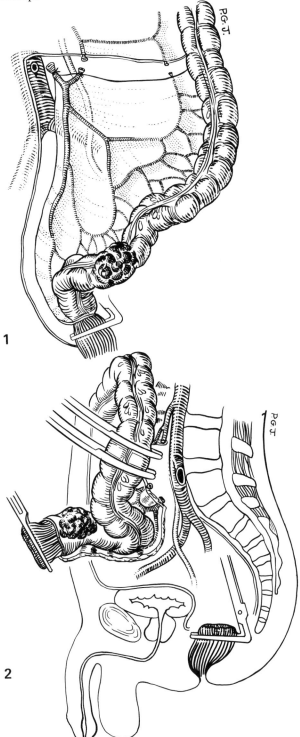

2

Division of the rectum

The rectum is divided and the rectal stump oversewn with chromic catgut as the division is made. It is better to avoid unabsorbable suture material. If possible the stump is covered with peritoneum.

Division of the sigmoid colon

The sigmoid colon should be divided at an elected site — in cases of diverticulitis above the affected area and in cases of carcinoma at a convenient site, allowing a colostomy to be constructed without tension.

Construction of left iliac colostomy

A separate incision should be made in the left iliac fossa at a point equidistant from the anterior iliac spine, the umbilicus and the pubic tubercle, as in the case of abdominoperineal excision of the rectum. The bowel should be brought through this incision, and the lateral space between the peritoneum and mesentery closed with a continuous thread stitch to prevent herniation of bowel on the lateral side of the colostomy (*see* Chapter on 'Abdominoperineal Excision of the Rectum', pages 118–132).

The colostomy should remain clamped until the abdominal wound is closed.

Suturing the abdominal wound

The abdominal wound should be closed in layers. The pelvis is drained through a stab incision using a Redivac or corrugated drain. The incision should be sealed.

Fixture of the colostomy

The colostomy should now be unclamped and the wall of the colon stitched to the skin using interrupted chromic catgut sutures around its circumference.

Anal sphincter

It is important at the end of the operation to dilate the anal sphincter or to insert a large soft rubber tube drain to prevent retention of secretions and blood in the rectal stump.

POSTOPERATIVE CARE

Patients should be managed as for an anterior resection or abdominoperineal excision.

Drains

The pelvic drain should be shortened after the first 24 hr then shortened each day for 4 days and then removed. The rectal tube should be removed after 48 hr.

Complications

Pelvic abscess

A pelvic abscess may develop and may discharge spontaneously through the rectal stump. In such cases gentle irrigation of the stump with normal saline is indicated.

Small bowel obstruction

Small intestine can enter the pelvis and become attached to the rectal stump by adhesions. This may produce intestinal obstruction postoperatively or at any time subsequently. It is one of the main disadvantages of this operation.

Reference

Hartmann, H. (1923). *Congre's Fr. Chir.* **30,** 411

[*The illustrations for this Chapter on Hartmann's Operation were drawn by Mr. P. G. Jack.*]

Fulguration of Malignant Rectal Tumours

John L. Madden, M.D.
Clinical Professor of Surgery, New York Medical College

Introduction and indications

During the past 20 years, electrocoagulation in the treatment of cancer of the rectum has been of proved merit. Accordingly, its continued use is recommended. Although many will use this technique for polypoid lesions, they consider it contra-indicated for ulcero-cancers. In our own experience, it is used for both types of lesions. In fact, the more ideal the tumour is for treatment by abdominoperineal excision, the more suited it is for treatment by electrocoagulation.

This method of treatment is limited to lesions located 10 cm or less from the anal orifice. A limit is not placed on the size of the lesion except that, in the presence of completely encircling lesions, abdominoperineal excision is preferred.

Electrocoagulation in the treatment of cancer of the rectum should always be done in the hospital and not as an office procedure. Spinal anaesthesia is preferred, and the position of the patient depends upon the location of the lesion. In posterior wall tumours, the lithotomy position is used and when the tumour is anterior, the patient is placed in the prone position. Dependent upon the size of the tumour, both the lithotomy and prone positions may be used in the same session.

The initial period of stay in hospital varies from 18 to 20 days. Ten to fourteen days after the operation, the patient is again taken to the operation room and, under spinal anaesthesia, the site of the original tumour is inspected and a biopsy for routine documentary study is taken. The area is again treated thoroughly by electrocoagulation. The results under this regime have proved better than if only one procedure is undertaken at the first hospital admission.

Patients are seen once a month for the first 6 months after the operation, during which time one or more admissions for repeat electrocoagulation may be necessary for the treatment of residual tumour. If at the end of 6–8 months the tumour is not completely eradicated, abdominoperineal excision is advised.

Results justify the further evaluation of this method of treatment.

TECHNIQUE

1

Under satisfactory spinal anaesthesia, the patient is placed in the prone position and the cancerous lesion in the anterior wall of the rectum is exposed by retraction of the adjacent walls.

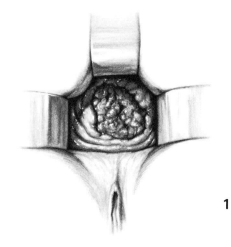

1

2

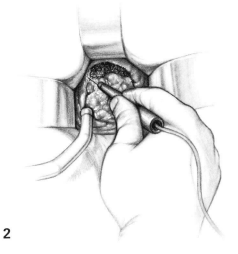

2

Using the needle-point electrode and with the dial of the coagulation current set at 50, the margins of the tumour are first defined and 1 cm of the normal surrounding mucosa is included in the electrocoagulation. The electrocoagulation proceeds from the elevated periphery to the central crater. The coagulation of normal tissue is indicated by a visible 'bubbling'. The suction tip in the field is indispensible in the aspiration of the smoke to maintain a clear visual field.

3

The coagulation completed, a uterine curette is used to scrape off the coagulum and expose the underlying untreated area of the tumour. The sequence of coagulation and curettage may be repeated five to six times to obtain the desired effect. Digital palpation after each curetting is most important in the detection of residual areas of tumour.

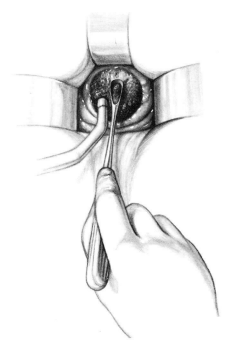

3

4

Upon the completion of each curetting, the treated area is irrigated with copious quantities of warm saline solution to wash away the tissue debris.

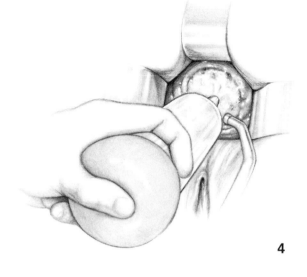

4

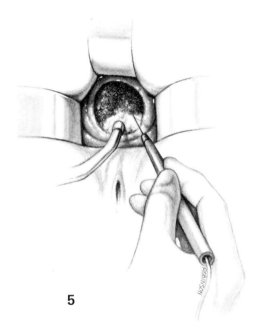

5

5

The final electrocoagulation is being completed. The small greyish–white 'islands' visible in the coagulated area are representative of the underlying muscle layer and indicate that the depths of the tumour have been penetrated. In posterior wall lesions, the extent of the electrocoagulation, if required, may penetrate the whole thickness of the rectum and expose large areas of retrorectal fat without untoward complications.

6

The electrocoagulation is completed and three dry gauze strands are inserted into the rectal lumen to effect a soft tamponade. They are removed in 3 hr.

In the primary treatment of a rectal lesion, the duration of the operation will vary with its size and may take as long as 2 or 2·5 hr. Postoperatively, mild catharsis and a regular diet are prescribed. Antibiotics are used only for specific indications and not as a routine.

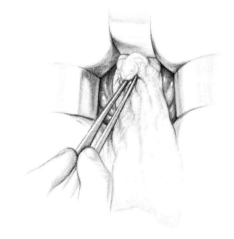

6

[*The illustrations for this Chapter on Fulguration of Malignant Tumours were drawn by Mr. F. Robinson.*]

Tube Caecostomy

James P. S. Thomson, M.S., F.R.C.S.
Consultant Surgeon, St. Mark's Hospital, London

At the present time tube caecostomy is not a very commonly-performed procedure. Its indication is to decompress the distal bowel but in order to ensure that it succeeds in this purpose a considerable amount of nursing care is required. It is thus a less efficient method of defunctioning the distal bowel than a transverse loop colostomy. Its principal use is to decompress the colon proximal to a newly constructed anastomosis but, on occasions, particularly in a seriously ill patient, it may be used to relieve a large bowel obstruction. From time to time a large bowel obstruction results in caecal perforation. Under these circumstances a caecostomy may be necessary, but a transverse loop colostomy should always be performed in addition.

PRE - OPERATIVE

Pre-operative preparation

Caecostomy is usually performed as a concomitant procedure and thus the preparation of the patient will be that for the other procedure. When, however, it is used in a patient with a large bowel obstruction it is important that the patient be fully resuscitated prior to operation with the institution, if indicated, of intravenous therapy.

Anaesthesia

The operation is best performed under general anaesthesia, although in a seriously ill patient it may be done under local infiltrative anaesthesia.

Principle of technique

A large bore rubber tube, such as a 30 French-gauge Foley catheter, is inserted and secured in the caecum with its distal end directed towards the hepatic flexure. The caecum in turn is fixed to the anterior abdominal wall. It is usual to remove the appendix as it is theoretically possible for its opening into the caecum to become obstructed by the tube.

There is no place for performing a caecostomy with a mucocutaneous suture. The effluent from such a stoma would be very difficult to control and would cause considerable skin excoriation. Furthermore, it would require a formal closure whereas with a tube caecostomy the fistula between the caecum and the skin will close spontaneously provided there is no distal obstruction.

THE OPERATION

1

The incision

When a tube caecostomy is constructed in association with a colonic anastomosis a stab incision is made in the right iliac fossa. If the caecostomy is performed on its own then a small oblique incision some 6 cm in length is made over the caecum.

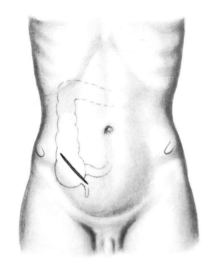

1

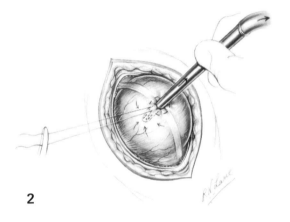

2

2

Opening the caecum

A purse-string suture of chromic catgut is placed in the caecum at the site of the anterior taenia. The caecum is incised and, if necessary, its contents are emptied with low pressure suction.

3

Insertion of caecostomy tube

The Foley catheter is inserted into the caecum through the incision which was used to empty its contents, its distal end advanced towards the hepatic flexure and the purse-string suture secured. The balloon of the Foley catheter is then inflated. A second chromic catgut purse-string suture is placed outside the original one, taking a small bite of the wall of the tube. When this is tied it has the effect of inkwelling the catheter into the caecum.

   This is a convenient time to perform the appendicectomy if this has not already been done. This operation is carried out in the usual way. It is unwise to try to insert the caecostomy tube through the appendix stump as this faces inferiorly and is not the best position for getting apposition of the caecum to the anterior abdominal wall.

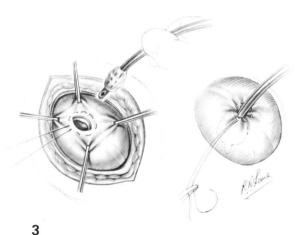

3

4

Securing the caecum to the anterior abdominal wall

A series of non-absorbable sutures are placed around the caecostomy to ensure that the caecum is held to the parietal peritoneum. Some surgeons also use a purse-string suture to close the lateral space.

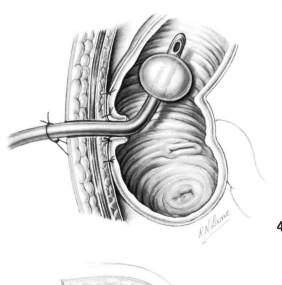

4

5

Closure of the wound

If an incision in the right iliac fossa was made then it should be closed in layers using chromic catgut.

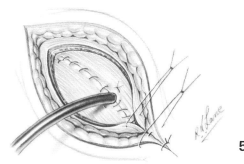

5

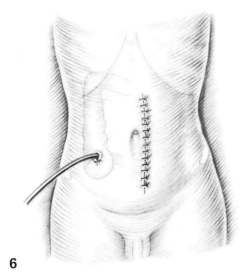

6

6&7

Securing the tube to the anterior abdominal wall

The tube is primarily secured by a suture to the anterior abdominal wall. A convenient way to avoid the tube being pulled on is to attach Elastoplast to it as indicated. The small tab placed distally on the caecostomy tube may be pinned to the flange, thus transmitting any traction on the tube to the Elastoplast and the abdominal wall rather than to the tube in the caecum and the stitch holding it. The tube is usually attached to a urine drainage bag, thus creating a closed system.

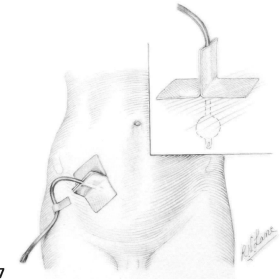

7

POSTOPERATIVE CARE

Care of the tube

After 36 hr the caecostomy tube is washed through every 6 hr with 100 ml of physiological saline warmed to body temperature. Water should be avoided as its use can lead to water intoxication. The same volume of fluid should then be syphoned from the caecum.

Removal of the tube

A fistula between the caecum and anterior abdominal wall should be well established by the seventh post-operative day. The anterior abdominal wall stitch holding the catheter should be removed on this day and the balloon of the Foley catheter released. The tube usually falls free spontaneously by the ninth day and, provided there is no distal obstruction in the bowel, the opening will close. Only very rarely is formal closure required.

Laxatives

It is preferable to use a bulk laxative as mineral laxatives acting on the small intestine will increase the faecal fluid content and so tend to keep this temporary fistula open.

[*The illustrations for this Chapter on Tube Caecostomy were drawn by Mr. R. N. Lane.*]

Colostomy

James P. S. Thomson, M.S., F.R.C.S.
Consultant Surgeon, St. Mark's Hospital, London

PRE-OPERATIVE

Indications for the construction of a colostomy

The construction of a colostomy to divert the faecal flow on to the anterior abdominal wall may be either temporary or permanent. A temporary colostomy is often constructed as an emergency measure in patients with a left-sided large intestinal obstruction due to carcinoma, or because of complicated diverticular disease of the left colon. The left colon may also be defunctioned to allow a distal anastomosis to heal, or to allow certain anal operations, such as those for complicated fistula or an anal sphincter repair, to be carried out in the absence of faecal matter. A permanent colostomy is performed in association with operations to excise the rectum.

Types of colostomy

The four main types of colostomy are: (*1*) loop colostomy (*2*) double-barrelled colostomy (*3*) divided colostomy (Devine) (*4*) terminal colostomy.

Loop colostomy

This is the most usually formed temporary colostomy. Its site depends on the reason for its construction and it may be either in the transverse colon or sigmoid colon. In principle a loop of colon is brought to the surface and held there by a glass rod or rubber tube. In addition, it is now usual for these colostomies to be opened at the time of operation and for a mucocutaneous suture to be performed. As most loop colostomies are constructed during an emergency laparotomy the colon is usually unprepared. However, if the operation is being performed as a planned procedure it is desirable to prepare the colon in a way similar to that for an anterior resection.

Double-barrelled colostomy

This is the type of colostomy used in the Paul Mikulicz operation. A spur is constructed between the two limbs of the colostomy which can subsequently be necrosed by the application of a crushing-enterotome. Theoretically this type of colostomy should close spontaneously after the spur is crushed but usually a formal closure is required. Whilst this operation was originally described for treating patients with complicated diverticular disease of the colon or carcinoma, its use now is confined to the treatment of patients with acute sigmoid volvulus.

Divided colostomy

This colostomy is constructed with a bridge of skin between each of the two limbs of the stoma. It was thought that this defunctioned the distal bowel more efficiently than a loop colostomy. However, this is not the case and as a loop colostomy is more satisfactory to close, a divided colostomy has little place in current surgical practice.

Editorial comment.   Though the formal Devine colostomy probably has no place in modern surgical practice, a divided loop sigmoid colostomy may sometimes be useful. The operation is carried out in the usual way except that a tongue of skin taken from the edge of the incision is passed through the mesentery beneath the rod and sutured into a small V-incision cut on the opposite side. After a week the mucosal bridge over the rod may be divided, the rod removed and the two ends of the bowel will be separated by a small skin bridge. This manoeuvre is helpful where the operation may be considered semipermanent.

Terminal colostomy

This is constructed in association with operations to excise the rectum and Hartmann's procedure. The colostomy is usually formed from the sigmoid or lower descending colon, which is brought to the surface through a trephine in the left abdominal wall. At the conclusion of the operation a direct mucocutaneous suture is performed.

There is some debate, which is unresolved, as to whether the trephine should be made through the left rectus muscle, with the operation being performed using a right paramedian incision, or through the oblique muscles in association with a left paramedian incision. With the latter situation the colon may be placed either intraperitoneally or extraperitoneally. If the intraperitoneal position is chosen then the space between the colon and the abdominal wall (lateral space) will have to be closed as this is a potential site for internal herniation of the small intestine.

This procedure will be referred to only briefly in this chapter as it is also referred to in the Chapter on 'Abdominoperineal Excision of the Rectum' (*see* pages 118–132).

Anaesthesia

General anaesthesia is to be preferred as traction on the mesentery causes pain and nausea. However, it is possible to undertake this operation under local field anaesthesia.

THE OPERATIONS

LOOP COLOSTOMY

1

Incision

The sites of the incision for a transverse colostomy and a left iliac fossa sigmoid colostomy are shown in the accompanying illustration. The ideal siting for a transverse colostomy is in the right upper abdomen mid-way between the umbilicus and the costal margin placed over the rectus abdominis muscle and extending just lateral to the lateral border of the rectus abdominis muscle. It is usually 6 cm in length.

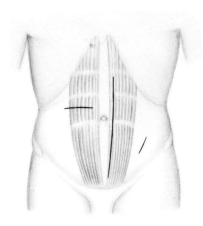

1

2

Division of rectus abdominis muscle

The incision is deepened through all the layers of the anterior abdominal wall. The muscle fibres of the rectus abdominis are divided as indicated.

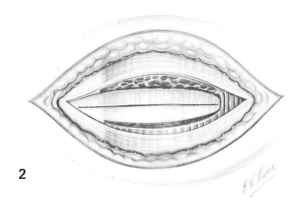

2

3

Preparation of the colon

The transverse colon is prepared for delivery through the anterior abdominal wall, either by incising the greater omentum, as shown, or by bringing it below the free border of the greater omentum. A small hole is made in the transverse mesocolon by the edge of the bowel wall and a rubber tube placed through it to facilitate delivery of the colon through the anterior abdominal wall.

Editorial comment.   If a sigmoid loop colostomy is to be made, the sigmoid is identified. It has no omentum, but has appendices epiploicae and taeniae.

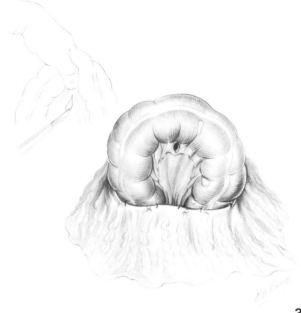

3

4

Securing the colostomy

Once the colon has been delivered through the anterior abdominal wall, it is held on the surface, either with the aid of a glass rod, or rubber tubing. This latter method allows easier application of the colostomy appliance. The colon may be opened longitudinally as indicated but some surgeons prefer to open the colon transversely as this damages fewer of the encircling vessels in the colonic wall. Transverse opening also facilitates mucocutaneous suturing and probably subsequent closure also.

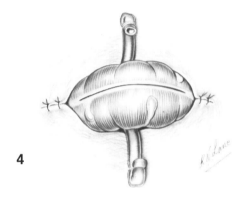

4

5

Mucocutaneous suture

Once open the colostomy is sutured to the skin using a chromic catgut suture. Tincture benzoin co. is then applied to the skin around the colostomy and an appliance immediately fitted.

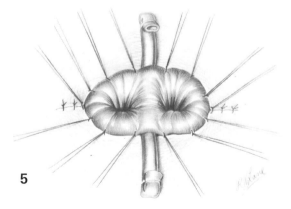

5

TERMINAL COLOSTOMY

6

Removal of skin disc

The exact site for the colostomy, whether it is to be made in the region of the left rectus muscle or the oblique muscles, should be selected pre-operatively to ensure that an appliance will fit satisfactorily away from the umbilicus and the anterior superior iliac spine. A disc of skin approximately 2 cm in diameter is excised. This may be done using a cruciate incision and excising the four pieces of skin with curved scissors. A more satisfactory trephine is obtained if it is made prior to the main laparotomy incision.

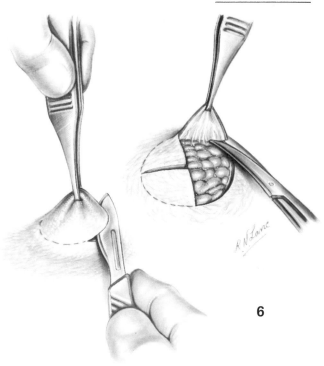

6

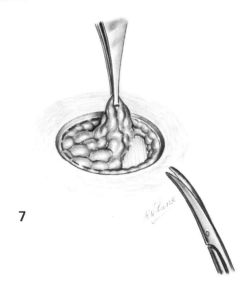

7

7

Removal of cylinder of superficial fascia

A cylinder of superficial fascia is removed, care being taken to obtain good haemostasis.

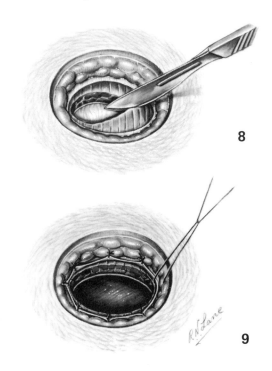

8

8 & 9

Division of muscle layers

A disc of the external oblique or anterior rectus sheath is excised in the line of the trephine and the underlying muscle divided. The peritoneum is also divided. There is a potential space between the fibrous layer of the superficial fascia and the external oblique or anterior rectus sheath. It is in this space that the considerable bulge of a colostomy hernia occurs. This space may be obliterated by a series of sutures joining these two layers.

9

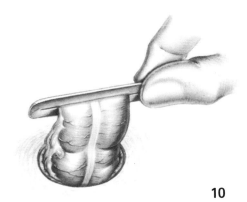

10

10 & 11

Mucocutaneous suture

After the lateral space has been obliterated and the main abdominal wound has been closed and dressed, the clamp on the distal colon is removed and a mucocutaneous suture performed with 3/0 chromic catgut. It is important to ensure that by adequate mobilization of the colon there is no tension on this suture line.

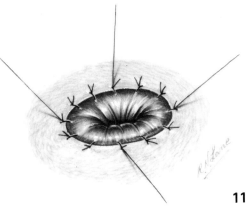

11

POSTOPERATIVE CARE

General management

The general care of the patient will be largely determined by the indication for performing the colostomy. It is generally wise for the patient to be maintained on intravenous fluids until such time as the colostomy has discharged some flatus and the bowel sounds are well established.

It is important to check the viability of the colostomy in the early postoperative period and also to make certain that it has not retracted.

Care of the colostomy

It is usual to apply an appliance as soon as the colostomy has been constructed. As the effluent from a transverse colostomy is somewhat liquid some protection for the skin ought to be provided and Stomahesive or a Karaya gum washer is very useful in this respect as it can be shaped to the colostomy. Loose colostomy effluent may be considerably helped by hydrophilic substances or codeine phosphate taken orally.

COMPLICATIONS

Loss of viability

This will occur early in the postoperative course if the blood supply to the colostomy has been compromised. It necessitates re-formation of the colostomy with viable colon.

Separation of the colostomy

This is usually the result of tension at the muco-cutaneous junction and if this occurs circumferentially the colostomy will have to be re-established. Partial separation may also occur either due to tension or infection and will usually heal spontaneously provided less than half the circumference is involved.

Infection

Although working in a potentially septic field it is very rare for sepsis to complicate the construction of a colostomy. This does, however, occasionally happen with surrounding cellulitis and there may be some separation of the edge of the colostomy. An haematoma surrounding the colostomy is a possible predisposing factor and this emphasizes the importance of good haemostasis in the colostomy wound. Provided there is adequate drainage the colostomy will heal but subsequent scarring might lead to some stenosis at the mucocutaneous junction.

Stenosis

Stenosis of a colostomy usually occurs at the muco-cutaneous level but is unusual when direct muco-cutaneous suture has been performed provided there has been no sepsis. To correct this complication the colostomy needs to be refashioned after excising a disc of skin and any scar tissue that might be present. Whilst this is best carried out under general anaesthesia it may be performed under local anaesthesia.

Hernia

Some degree of herniation is very common with a terminal colostomy. It usually takes the form of an interstitial bulge between the muscle layer and the superficial fascia. Occasionally it results from considerable widening of the trephine in the muscle layer. The former is usually best treated initially by wearing a belt. If, however, it is large or the belt is unsatisfactory, the excess colon may be excised after mobilizing the colostomy. The space between the muscle layer and the superficial fascia will also need to be closed.

The latter type of colostomy hernia is best treated by resiting the colostomy and closing the defect by direct suture or by inserting a piece of synthetic mesh.

Prolapse

Prolapse may occur with either a transverse colostomy where it more commonly involves the distal limb, or a terminal colostomy. As a transverse colostomy is usually a temporary measure prolapse is relatively unimportant, although occasionally if the viability of the prolapse is in question re-operation may be needed. With prolapse of a terminal colostomy if it troubles the patient and causes colostomy dysfunction then it will have to be reconstructed and possibly resited.

[*The illustrations for this Chapter on Colostomy were drawn by Mr. R. N. Lane.*]

Closure of Loop Colostomy

James P. S. Thomson, M.S., F.R.C.S.
Consultant Surgeon, St. Mark's Hospital, London

PRE - OPERATIVE

Indications

A temporary loop colostomy is closed when there is no longer a need to defunction the distal bowel. If a colostomy has been constructed to cover a healing anastomosis then it is essential that total healing of the anastomosis has occurred before undertaking the colostomy closure. This may be assessed either endoscopically with the sigmoidoscope or radiologically using a barium enema, when two films in planes at right angles (anteroposterior and lateral) should be taken. The position of the anastomosis is more readily judged on the radiograph if two silver clips have been placed on the outer layer of sutures at the time the anastomosis was performed. In addition, the colostomy itself must be suitable for closure in that it should be pink in colour and not cyanosed or oedematous. It is unlikely that the local conditions for closure will be ideal until after 3—4 weeks from the time of construction of the colostomy (Thomson and Hawley, 1972).

Preparation of patient

The proximal bowel is prepared by placing the patient on fluids only for the 2 days prior to the operation and by proximal colonic washouts. Oral purgatives should be avoided as uncontrollable diarrhoea may occur.

The distal bowel is washed through with normal saline. This is especially important when a barium enema has been performed as, if the barium remains in the bowel, it may solidify and act as an intraluminal obstructing agent. Some surgeons advocate the use of antibiotics such as neomycin or phthalylsulphathiazole in the preparation of the distal bowel.

Anaesthesia

The operation is best performed under general anaesthesia.

Principles of technique

A loop colostomy may be closed using one of two techniques: (*1*) *simple closure*—where after mobilization of the colon the opening is sutured (half-anastomosis); (*2*) *excision of the colostomy and anastomosis*—where the site of the colostomy is excised and the continuity of the colon restored by end-to-end anastomosis.

In both these instances the operation is conducted so that the colon is returned to within the peritoneal cavity. So-called extraperitoneal closure of the colostomy is seldom performed and is unsatisfactory. This is because there is inadequate mobilization of the colon which leads to an unsatisfactory anastomosis, almost invariably under tension.

THE OPERATION

1

Mobilization of the colostomy

Eight strong silk sutures are placed around the mucocutaneous junction of the colostomy. This allows good control of the colon during mobilization. The incision is made around the edge of the colostomy taking a small fringe of skin approximately 2 mm wide. If necessary the incision may be enlarged at either end of the colostomy in the transverse plane.

1

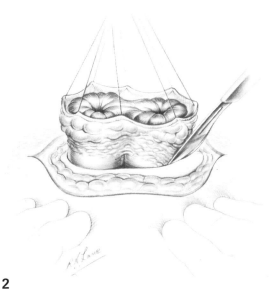

2

2

Separation from the anterior abdominal wall

With traction applied to the colostomy using the stay sutures the tissue of the anterior wall are freed from the colon. Great care must be exercised to remain in the correct plane and avoid damage to the colon. There is usually little blood loss during this procedure. If there is haemorrhage this suggests the surgeon is in an incorrect plane.

3

Removal of the skin edge and unrolling of the colostomy edge

The rind of skin is removed and the edge of the colostomy unrolled. When all the scar tissue has been removed the colon is then ready for closure.

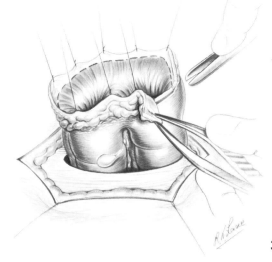

3

4&5

Simple closure of the colon

This is usually done in two layers. A layer of chromic catgut sutures, often performed using the Connell stitch and taking all layers, are inserted first. Then an outer layer of interrupted fine silk seromuscular Lembert sutures are inserted. If the colostomy has been excised an end-to-end anastomosis is performed in the same way as this operation would be performed during the course of a transverse colectomy. It should be added that some surgeons advocate using a single layer of sutures for this closure.

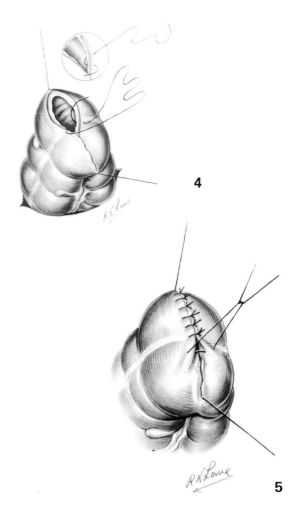

4

5

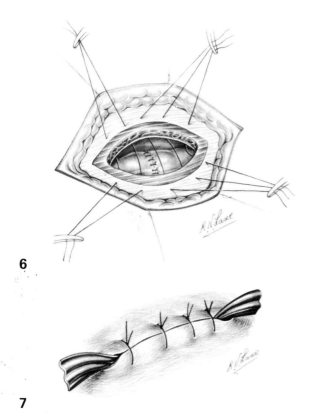

6

7

6&7

Closure of the abdominal wound

A single layer of monofilament nylon sutures are inserted into all layers taking large bites of tissue on either side of the wound. After all the sutures have been placed they are tied so that the edges of the abdominal wall are closely, but not tightly, applied. The skin wound is loosely closed over a corrugated drain which is placed from one end of the wound to the other. This is a potentially infected wound and this loose suturing of the skin is to allow any haematoma to drain and thus avoid wound infection.

POSTOPERATIVE CARE AND COMPLICATIONS

General

It is unusual for the patient to require a nasogastric tube. The patient is maintained on intravenous fluids until good bowel sounds are established and the patient has passed flatus. Oral fluids are then started and gradually increased. Milk of magnesia is a useful laxative if there is some delay in establishment of the bowel movements once oral feeding has begun. The drain is usually removed after 48 hr.

Complications

At the site of colostomy closure

Wound infection.   This is usually avoided if the skin has been loosely sutured and a wound drain is used.

Wound hernia.   There is a definite incidence of hernia in these wounds and occasionally this is complicated by strangulation.

Breakdown of the colonic suture line.   This either results in a faecal fistula, which usually closes spontaneously, or peritonitis, which will require re-establishment of the colostomy.

At the site of the distal anastomosis

If the colostomy is closed before satisfactory healing of the anastomosis has occurred then an abscess may develop at this site. This may also necessitate re-establishment of the colostomy. However, if the proper indications for performing colostomy closure have been observed this complication should not occur.

Reference

Thomson, J. P. S. and Hawley, P. R. (1972). 'Results of closure of loop transverse colostomies.' *Br. med. J.* **3**, 459

[*The illustrations for this Chapter on Closure of Loop Colostomy were drawn by Mr. R. N. Lane.*]

Complete Rectal Prolapse: Ivalon Sponge Repair

Nigel H. Porter, F.R.C.S.
Consultant Surgeon, Brighton and Lewes Group
of Hospitals

PRE - OPERATIVE

Rectal prolapse presents a formidable triad of symptoms—namely, the obvious anatomical displacement of the rectum, coupled with an intractably disordered bowel habit in 80 per cent of cases and some degree of distressing faecal incontinence in 80 per cent of cases (Morgan, Porter and Klugman, 1972). The symptoms are beyond control until the prolapse is corrected. If the best results are to be obtained, bowel habit and continence demand careful attention and management postoperatively and, on occasion, may require a subsidiary minor operative procedure.

A multiplicity of operations have been designed for the treatment of complete prolapse, which serves to emphasize the difficulty of the problem. Reviews conducted by Hughes (1949) and Porter (1962) indicate the very unsatisfactory results of most of the traditional operations, particularly rectosigmoidectomy. The addition of a pubococcygeus repair to rectosigmoidectomy failed to improve the poor results. However, the Roscoe Graham operation as popularized by Goligher (1958), and an extension of this—the combined repair practised by Hughes, Gleadell and Turner (1957)—and of anterior resection (Muir, 1955), have all shown improved results. The first two operations require a great deal of technical expertise for success, as does the latter which also entails a large bowel anastomosis deep in the pelvis with its known attendant risks. For these reasons, and the additional one that the results are excellent, the use of a polyvinyl alcohol sponge implant to fix the rectum, as described by Wells (1959) and by Naunton Morgan and Wells (1962) is favoured. This operation is safe and, above all, simple in its execution. The results are excellent (Morgan, Porter and Klugman, 1972). In a series of 150 cases there have been only three complete recurrences. Continence shows an improvement of up to 50 per cent and bowel function is therefore much more easily managed.

IVALON SPONGE IMPLANT

Postoperative cineradiological studies confirm the excellent rectal fixation into the hollow of the sacrum and the improved position of the levator shelf (Fry, Griffiths and Smart, 1966).

Polyvinyl alcohol sponge (Ivalon), like other plastic materials, carries the risk of inducing neoplasia. In experimental animals, sarcomata were reported in rats following the implantation of Ivalon (Oppenheimer, Oppenheimer and Stout, 1948). In clinical practice, however, no case of sarcoma has been reported in the human subject. A careful study by Walter and Chiaramonte (1965) confirming the incidence, although low, of rat sarcoma in response to Ivalon implants, relates this to the thickness and bulk of the implant and, what is more, suggests that there is a species susceptibility to the induction of neoplasia by a variety of implants, even stainless steel. Their conclusions are that Ivalon sponge is carcinogenic to the rat but not necessarily to man. Clinical use over the last 25 years bears out this conclusion.

Indications

The occurrence of 'complete' rectal prolapse in a patient fit to undergo laparotomy. In poor risk patients the Thiersch wire operation is sometimes advocated.

Pre-operative investigation and preparation

Sigmoidoscopy is vital to exclude the presence of a carcinoma, large polyp or villous tumour which may have induced tenesmus and straining, resulting in the development of a prolapse. This is not a common cause of prolapse, but must always be excluded.

Prior to operation the bowel must be emptied by aperients from above and bowel washouts from below. These patients are rarely able to retain an enema. As a precaution against infection occurring within the sponge, Sulfathalidine is given pre-operatively for 5 days and a full course of a suitable antibiotic is also given postoperatively. In addition the pelvic cavity is dusted with 1g of chloramphenicol powder at the time of operation.

THE OPERATION

Care must be taken to ensure adequate sterilization of the Ivalon sponge implant. This should be auto-claved and then moistened in sterile normal saline before implantation to make it pliable and easier to handle.

1

Position and incision

The patient lies supine in 15°–20° of Trendelenburg tilt. The bladder should be catheterized and any residual urine expressed. A left paramedian incision is made extending from the pubis to 3 inches (7·5 cm) above the level of the umbilicus.

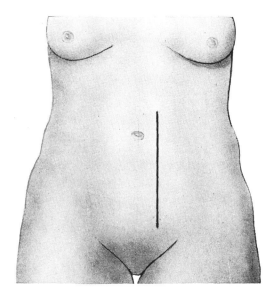

1

2

Laparotomy

A careful laparotomy is performed; not infrequently a small hiatus hernia is found. The small and large bowel are packed off into the upper abdomen. At this stage the operation is greatly facilitated by introducing a self-retaining retractor with a median blade to retain the packs and viscera in the upper abdomen.

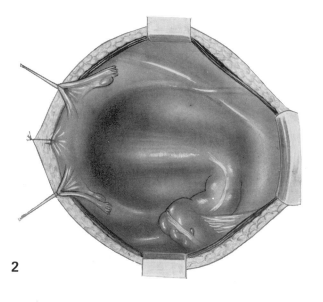

2

3

Incision in peritoneum

The peritoneum is incised on both sides of the pelvic mesocolon, the incisions commencing about 5 cm above the pelvic brim. They are eventually prolonged down into the pelvis and joined in front of the rectum on the anterior wall of the pouch. The left peritoneal incision is made first, the left ureter is identified, and gently brushed laterally to avoid injury when this incision is carried down over the pelvic brim.

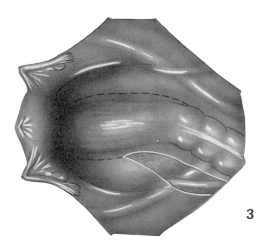

3

4

Opening of the areolar plane

The index finger of the left hand is inserted beneath the inferior mesenteric artery, just proximal to the sacral promontory, the vascular pedicle hooked forward and, using blunt-ended scissors together with gentle dissection with the fingers, the loose areolar plane between the rectum and sacrum is opened up. Bleeding points are diathermied as this part of the dissection progresses, to ensure haemostasis. It is unwise at this stage to insert a hand behind the rectum to elevate it forcefully from the pelvis. This may result in troublesome haemorrhage which will hinder the rest of the operation. The posterior and posterolateral dissection should extend downwards beyond the tip of the coccyx, as far as the anorectal junction, until the upper surfaces of the levatores ani are seen.

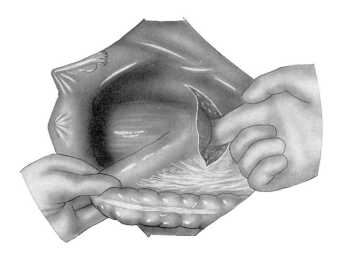

4

5

Division of lateral ligaments

The posterior plane of dissection is carried forward on either side. Strands of areolar tissue often containing accessory haemorrhoidal vessels are found, the so-called lateral ligaments. These are carefully divided and all bleeding points secured. The rectum must be adequately mobilized down to the pelvic floor. Failure to do this will leave redundant bowel below the point of fixation and this redundant bowel will prolapse. Although mobilization of the prolapsed rectum is not a difficult procedure it must be carried out with strict attention to haemostasis. The presence of a large pelvic haematoma invites bacterial colonization and disastrous infection.

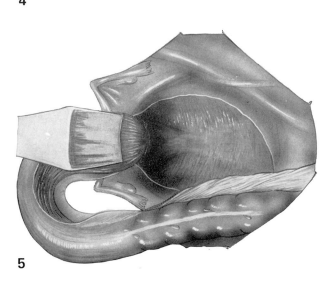

5

6

Mobilization of rectum

This is completed by joining the lateral peritoneal incisions in front of the rectum just anterior to the deepest part of the pouch. There is no need to attempt extensive dissection in this anterior plane as the presence of the deep peritoneal hernial sac will have completed this. Dissection of the plane between rectum and structures anterior to it is greatly facilitated if the posterior lip of this peritoneal incision is grasped with a long haemostat and retracted upwards by the surgeon, whilst the assistant exerts firm traction on the anterior viscera. It is sufficient to expose the vault of the vagina in the female and the seminal vesicles in the male. Diathermy should be used with care in the region of the vaginal vault owing to the risk of necrosis and consequent infection.

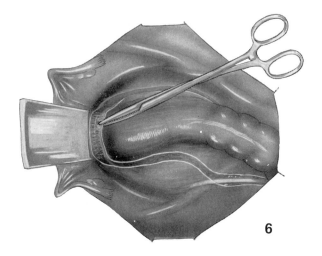

6

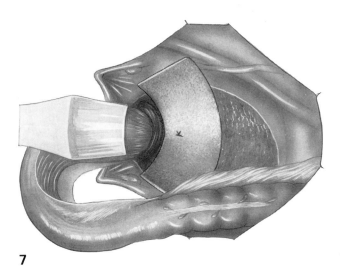

7

7

Insertion of Ivalon sponge

The Ivalon sponge should be sutured as low down as possible in the pelvis. One piece is used, measuring 8 cm wide, 20 cm long and 3 mm thick. With the rectum retracted forwards, one suture of 2/0 linen thread is passed through the centre of the Ivalon sheet and is then placed in the loose fascia in front of the coccyx in the mid-line. The Ivalon is now 'railroaded' down into the pelvis. This is sufficient to anchor the Ivalon in position until the fibroblastic reaction it excites fixes it in place.

Editorial comment

Some people believe that the Ivalon stops the prolapse by preventing the rectum intussuscepting by forming a rigid cuff at the bottom of the rectovaginal pouch, rather than causing adhesion to the sacrum. The positioning of the sponge half above and half below the reflexion is thus important. Some surgeons also add a tail to the Ivalon implant making it T-shaped so that the tail lies below on the divarication of the pubococcygeus muscles.

8

Positioning of sponge

The rectum is now allowed to fall back into the concavity of the sacrum and the Ivalon foam sheeting loosely wrapped around it to enclose about five-sixths of its circumference. It is important to leave a gap in front to avoid any possibility of rectal stricture. The inferior edge of the Ivalon is placed at the level of the vaginal vault or vesicles, secured anteriorly by an atraumatic linen suture which passes from the inferior corners and lightly picks up the fascia on the extraperitoneal aspect of the anterior wall of the rectum. The superior corners of the Ivalon 'gutter' are then loosely secured with a linen suture. The pelvic cavity is sprayed with an antibiotic powder.

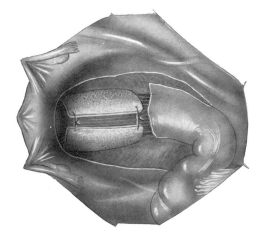

8

9

Closure

The final stage is important as the Ivalon must be completely extraperitonealized. The lateral flaps of peritoneum are mobilized from the pelvic walls and the peritoneal floor reconstituted at the level of the brim of the true pelvis using a 3/0 atraumatic Mersilene inverting suture. In the final closure of the peritoneal floor it is important to attach the edge of the peritoneum to the wall of the rectum above the Ivalon. In reperitonealizing the mesentery of the sigmoid colon the base of the sigmoid loop should not be narrowed. The abdomen is closed in layers without drainage.

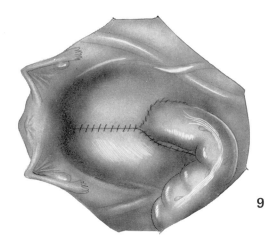

9

POSTOPERATIVE CARE

This usually presents no difficulty. There is no need for intravenous infusion or nasogastric suction unless postoperative ileus occurs, which is unusual.

It is important, however, to keep the rectum empty. The patient commences an aperient regime on the second postoperative day, and if the bowels have not been opened by the third day an enema is given. Digital rectal examination is carried out daily to be sure that faecal impaction does not develop. After the first week an attempt should be made to find a suitable aperient to produce, if at all possible, a regular bowel habit. If this cannot be achieved, the use of glycerine or bisacodyl suppositories is often helpful in keeping the rectum empty. When satisfactory evacuation can be achieved, the patient is less likely to suffer from postoperative incontinence and leakage.

Functional improvement may be surprisingly satisfactory following the operation. In those patients still remaining incontinent to some degree, an expectant policy should be pursued, as improvement is not infrequently gradual and the patient should be persuaded to wait a year before any secondary procedure with regard to continence is considered, since many of them will not require it after this interval. It must be emphasized that very careful follow-up and attention to bowel habit is necessary to achieve the best results. Residual mucosal prolapse may be cured by ligature and excision, or injection.

References

Fry, I. K., Griffiths, J. D. and Smart, P. J. (1966). *Br. J. Surg.* **53**, 784
Goligher, J. C. (1958). *Br. J. Surg.* **45**, 343
Graham, R. R. (1942). *Ann. Surg.* **115**, 1007
Hughes, E. S. R. (1949). *Proc. R. Soc. Med.* **42**, 1007
Hughes, E. S. R., Gleadell, L. W. and Turner, J. (1957). *Br. med. J.* **2**, 179
Morgan, C. N. and Wells, C. (1962). *Proc. R. Soc. Med.* **55**, 1084
Morgan, C. N., Porter, N. H. and Klugman, D. J. (1972). *Br. J. Surg.* **59**, 841
Muir, E. G. (1955). *Proc. R. Soc. Med.* **48**, 33
Oppenheimer, B. S., Oppenheimer, E. T. and Stout, A. P. (1948). *Proc. Soc. exp. Biol. N.Y.* **67**, 33
Walter, J. B. and Chiaramonte, L. G. (1965). *Br. J. Surg.* **52**, 49
Wells, C. (1959). *Proc. R. Soc. Med.* **52**, 602

[*The illustrations for this Chapter on Complete Rectal Prolapse: Ivalon Sponge Repair were drawn by Mr. F. Price.*]

Complete Rectal Prolapse : Ripstein Operation

Robert Britten-Jones, M.B., B.S., F.R.C.S., F.R.A.C.S.
Senior Visiting Surgeon, Royal Adelaide Hospital,
South Australia

PRE - OPERATIVE

A simple procedure to treat rectal prolapse in which the rectum is retained in the hollow of the sacrum by a plastic-mesh sling, has been described by Ripstein (1965). It is based on the fact that, in this disease, the rectum is unusually mobile and easily displaced forward from the sacral concavity to form a straight tube. In this position when the patient strains, all the intra-abdominal forces act in the long axis of the tube, favouring prolapse. By means of this operation the sacral curve of the rectum is restored and maintained when straining, so that the intra-abdominal forces tend to push the rectum backwards against the hollow of the sacrum rather than vertically downwards. The sling can be made of Mersilene, Teflon or Polypropylene (Marlex) mesh. The latter is now favoured because it excites less tissue reaction and is a little more rigid than the other materials (Ripstein, 1976).

Personal experience with this operation has proved it to be safe, simple and effective. The Lahey Clinic figures reported by Jurgeleit *et al.* (1975) confirm this view, with no deaths in 55 patients undergoing Teflon-sling repair over 10 years and 7 per cent recurrence rate. Morgan (1975), in a similar number of operations, reports one postoperative death and no cases of recurrent complete prolapse. Ripstein is quoted by Morgan (1975) as having only two cases of recurrence after 500 sling operations.

Indications

An advantage of the operation is that only minimal mobilization of the rectum is necessary. The lateral ligaments are not divided and no dissection is required anteriorly, thus blood loss is very slight and there is no risk of postoperative impotence in the occasional male patient. The frail and aged, in whom prolapse is relatively common, withstand the operation well. All patients with complete rectal prolapse who are fit to undergo laparotomy are suitable for the procedure.

Contra-indications

Partial or 'mucosal' prolapse is better treated by ligature and excision of the prolapsing mucosa.

Investigations and preparation

Sigmoidoscopy is essential to exclude the occasional case of associated carcinoma, villous tumour or polyp which, by inducing constant straining, may precipitate prolapse. A barium enema to exclude any other lesion, particularly diverticular disease, is advisable. It is most important to empty the large bowel before surgery. This is achieved by oral aperients, low-residue diet and colonic lavage daily for 4 days prior to operation. Phthalylsulphathiazole 8 g daily is given orally in divided doses during this period; anaemia is corrected and perineal sphincter exercises with faradic stimulation if necessary, are commenced. If incontinence is a problem, as it often is in cases of long standing, the patient should be warned that, although the bowel will no longer protrude after the operation, continence may not be restored completely.

Anaesthesia

A general anaesthetic with muscular relaxation is essential.

THE OPERATION

1

Incision and laparotomy

The patient is placed supine, the bladder catheterized and any residual urine expressed. Fifteen to
twenty degrees of head-down tilt facilitates exposure
of the rectum. A left paramedian incision is made
extending from the pubis to the level of the umbilicus
with the operator, if right handed, standing on the
left side of the patient. Laparotomy is carried out,
carefully palpating the intraperitoneal organs and
looking particularly for any co-existent large bowel
pathology. A self-retaining retractor is placed in the
wound and the colon and small bowel pushed into
the upper part of the abdomen and held out of the
pelvis by packs. In the female, the uterus is held
forward by stay-sutures passed through the broad
ligaments.

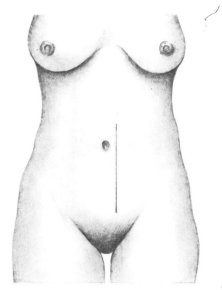

1

2

Left lateral peritoneal incision

After freeing the congenital adhesions between the
sigmoid mesocolon and the parietes, the peritoneum
and subperitoneal tissue on the left side of the
mesorectum are incised with dissecting scissors from
the level of the promontory of the sacrum as far down
as the peritoneal reflection. Diathermy is used to
coagulate any small vessels divided. The ureter must
be recognized crossing the pelvic brim at the level of
the common iliac artery bifurcation and avoided.

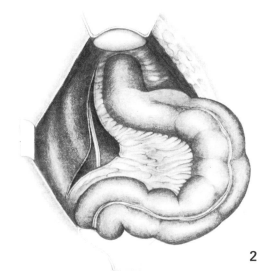

2

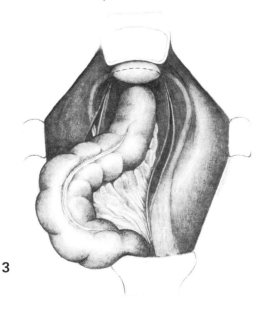

3

3

Right lateral peritoneal incision

A similar incision is made in the peritoneum on the
right side of the base of the mesorectum. The peritoneum on the anterior surface of the rectovesical
pouch, about 3 cm above its deepest point, is divided
transversely to join the lower ends of the two lateral
incisions.

4

Opening of the areolar plane

With the left hand holding the rectosigmoid junction forward, the operator's right index finger is introduced into the loose areolar plane between the rectum and the sacral promontory, behind the inferior mesenteric artery at the upper end of the right lateral peritoneal incision. The left index finger is then substituted, holding the mesorectum with the inferior mesenteric vessels forward and introducing dissecting scissors to open the areolar plane until the four fingers of the right hand can be gently inserted between the presacral fascia and the upper half of the rectum. This must be carried out with care to avoid rupturing small presacral veins. The rectum is not mobilized further and the lateral ligaments are left undivided. Anterior to the rectum, below the peritoneal reflection, only sufficient dissection is done to take up the slack of the lower rectum. In many cases this can be carried out without dissecting at all in this plane.

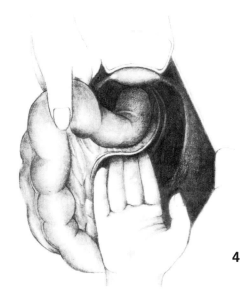

4

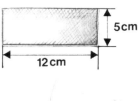

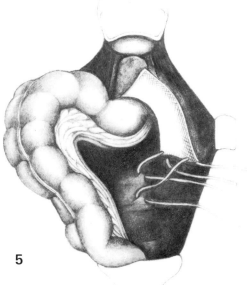

5

5

Fixation of sling to sacrum

A piece of presterilized Teflon or Marlex mesh is cut to form a rectangle, measuring 12 cm × 5 cm. The rectum is held forward to expose the anterior surface of the sacrum. One of the two narrower edges of the rectangular plastic mesh is then sutured to the sacrum 5 cm below the promontory, using four non-absorbable sutures threaded on a small Mayo needle. Deep bites are taken of the presacral fascia and periosteum with each stitch about 1 cm to the right of the mid-line, carefully avoiding presacral blood vessels as haemorrhage here may be difficult to stop. The sutures are left loose and untied until all four have been inserted. (For purposes of clarity only two of these sutures are shown in the accompanying illustrations.)

6

Encircling of rectum with sling

The opposite short edge of the plastic-mesh sling is then carried around the rectum anteriorly and similarly sutured to the sacrum just to the left of the mid-line. Before tying these sutures the surgeon must ensure that the sling is sufficiently lax. This is checked by pulling both ends of the sutures taut and, with the sling thus held temporarily in position, it should be possible to insert two fingers easily behind the rectum. If it is too tight, faecal impaction may result.

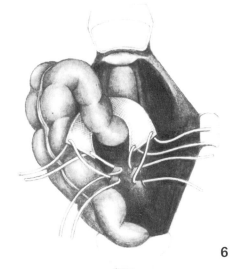

6

7

Fixation of sling to rectum

The rectum is pulled upwards and rendered taut. The upper and lower borders of the sling are then attached by fine non-absorbable sutures to the seromuscular layer of the rectum at about the level of the peritoneal reflection. Wrinkling of the sling is avoided by spreading the plastic mesh in the vertical plane over the anterior surface of the rectum before inserting the sutures in the anterior and lateral rectal wall. If angulation of the rectum by the sling is apparent, a 'hitch' suture of non-absorbable material can be placed between the anterior surface of the lumbo-sacral disc and the mesorectum. In the occasional case, resection of grossly redundant sigmoid colon may be necessary.

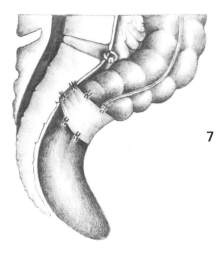

7

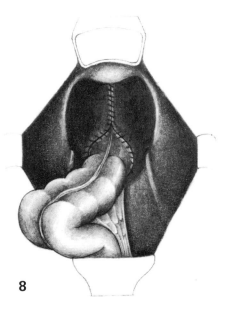

8

8

Closure

If Teflon is used, the sling should be buried beneath the pelvic peritoneum to avoid the possibility of small bowel adhering to it, by a running suture of chromic catgut closing the anterior and lateral peritoneal defects. However, using Marlex with its minimal tissue reaction, adherence to small intestine is most unlikely and the peritoneal defects may be left open. If they are closed, it is most important that a sump drain be placed in the presacral space and brought out through a stab incision in the anterior abdominal wall. The abdominal wound is then closed in layers.

POSTOPERATIVE CARE AND COMPLICATIONS

Oral feeding may commence early and intravenous infusion and nasogastric suction are unnecessary. Prophylactic antibiotics are a wise precaution as the plastic mesh is a foreign body and, as such, predisposes to infection, and also because the bowel may be inadvertently punctured by a suture. Aqueous penicillin 1,000,000 I.U. and Streptomycin 0·5 g are given by intramuscular injection immediately before operation and continued postoperatively for 3 days. A soft-formed daily bowel action should be induced by administering lubricant aperients from the second day after operation and if no bowel action has occurred by the third day, a tap water enema is given. Thereafter, to ensure that faecal impaction does not occur, daily rectal examination is performed until normal bowel actions are established. If it should occur it must be broken up by manipulation and enemata. The patient whose bowel habit hitherto has been faulty, is encouraged to develop a satisfactory bowel action with the aid of adequate roughage in the diet and added daily bran or bulk-forming laxatives. Perineal sphincter exercises are continued.

Persisting incontinence especially for flatus, occurs in a number of patients but they can be encouraged, as improvement is often gradual and may take many months. If the patient's bowel can be managed adequately after the operation so that he normally has a soft-formed stool, continence is considerably better (Hawley, 1975).

Residual mucosal prolapse is best treated by ligature and excision.

Faecal impaction should not occur if care is taken to make the sling around the rectum sufficiently loose, if angulation is avoided, and soft faecal consistency maintained.

Abscess formation is rare but if it occurs, drainage with removal of the sling and transverse colostomy is essential.

References

Hawley, P. R. (1975). *Dis. Colon Rectum* **18,** 461
Jurgeleit, H. C., Corman, M. L., Coller, J. A. and Veidenheimer, M. C. (1975). *Dis. Colon Rectum* **18,** 465
Morgan, B. P. (1975). *Dis. Colon Rectum* **18,** 468
Ripstein, C. B. (1965). *Dis. Colon Rectum* **8,** 34
Ripstein, C. B. (1976). Personal communication

[*The illustrations for this Chapter on Complete Rectal Prolapse: Ripstein Operation were drawn by Mrs. H. Lillecrapp.*]

Mucosal Prolapse: Ligature and Excision

Nigel H. Porter, F.R.C.S.
Consultant Surgeon, Brighton and Lewes
Group of Hospitals

PRE - OPERATIVE

Indications

Mucosal prolapse presents, broadly speaking, in two types. First, there is simple uncomplicated mucosal prolapse with adequate sphincters and no incontinence. Secondly, the mucosal prolapse is complicated in some degree by faecal incontinence in 60 per cent of patients (Porter, 1962). Examination in these cases reveals a variable degree of anal laxity.

Surgical treatment in both groups entails ligature and excision of the prolapsing mucosa provided the surgeon is absolutely sure that it is a mucosal and not in fact, a complete prolapse.

In the second group some ancillary procedure or treatment may be necessary to correct the laxity of the sphincters and the resulting faecal incontinence. It is this latter symptom that determines the need for a second procedure.

THE OPERATION

Position of patient

Lithotomy position.

1

Marking of redundant mucosa

The redundant mucosa is drawn down and gripped with three artery forceps, sited in left lateral, right anterior and right posterior quadrants—the sites of the three primary haemorrhoidal areas.

At this stage it is essential to differentiate with certainty between a mucosal and a full thickness rectal prolapse. Feeling the prolapsing mucosa between finger and thumb will reveal the presence or absence of full thickness rectal wall. If the latter is present the operation of ligature and excision must be abandoned.

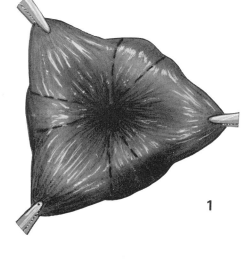

2

Division of mucosa

The mucosa is divided by scissor cuts into three portions, corresponding to the three primary haemorrhoids. Skin and mucosal bridges must be left between each portion to allow healing without stricture formation.

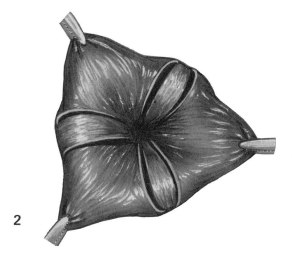

3

Division of mucocutaneous junction

The mucocutaneous junction at the base of each section is divided with scissors and, by further dissection, the lower border of the internal sphincter is demonstrated. This completes mobilization of the prolapsing mucosa.

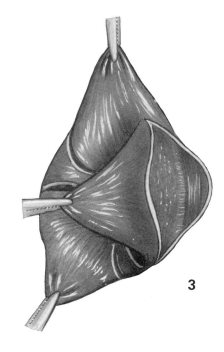

4

Ligation and excision of pedicles

Each pedicle is then transfixed and ligated with 2/0 chromic catgut and the redundant tissue excised. If any of the pedicles is exceedingly bulky, and this is often so in the left lateral quadrant, it is a useful technique to use Goodsall's stitch. Two needles threaded on a long length of 2/0 chromic catgut are passed from without inwards, dividing the pedicle into three equal parts. When the needles are cut off the operator is left with three transfixing ligatures to tie. This effectively divides a large bulky pedicle into three smaller and thus safer bundles. After proctoscopic examination has shown satisfactory ligation of the pedicles and haemostasis, flat Vaseline gauze dressings are applied to the anus but not tucked into the lumen.

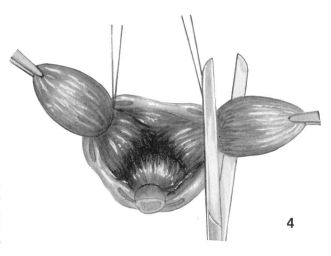

4

POSTOPERATIVE CARE

Suitable aperients are given and the patient is allowed to sit in the bath twice a day from the first postoperative day. After the bath the parts are dabbed dry and a Vaseline gauze dressing, gauze and T bandage applied. There is no need to tuck dressings into the anal canal—this only causes pain.

On the sixth postoperative day a finger is inserted gently into the anal canal to ascertain that healing is progressing satisfactorily and, most important, that anal stenosis is not imminent. If there is evidence of impending stenosis the patient should be instructed to use an anal dilator daily for 1 month, However, if there is no evidence of a stricture there is no need to pass an anal dilator.

Postoperatively a certain number of patients will continue to complain of anal leaking and will have obviously incompetent anal sphincters. Two methods of treatment may be used to correct this. First, a Thiersch wire may be inserted. Secondly, the patient may use an external anal stimulator (Hopkinson and Lightwood, 1966). This is applied with the object of producing continuous faradic stimulation to the lax sphincters to increase their resting contraction and thus improve sphincter tone, although it must be admitted that this type of faradic stimulation is only of help in about 20 per cent of patients.

RECTAL PROLAPSE IN CHILDREN

The majority of cases of rectal prolapse in infancy recover spontaneously without treatment (Jackman and Cannon, 1949). Recovery may be aided by submucosal injections of 5 per cent phenol in almond oil, or alternatively in severe cases by means of a Thiersch type of operation using catgut instead of silver wire (Stephens, 1958).

Abdominal operations are absolutely contraindicated. Only very rarely is it necessary to perform rectosigmoidectomy for irreducible gangrenous prolapse.

In those cases of rectal prolapse that are complete or persist after infancy in association with lax sphincters, there may be either a congenital neurological defect responsible or a gross functional defect of the megarectum type. Attempts at operative correction in these patients, without the most careful investigation and assessment, are to be strongly deprecated and they are much better managed in special centres.

References

Hopkinson, B. R. and Lightwood, R. (1966). *Lancet* **2,** 297
Jackman, R. J. and Cannon, E. E. (1949). *Surg. Clins N. Am.* **29,** 1215
Porter, N. H. (1962). *Proc. R. Soc. Med.* **55,** 1087
Stephens, F. D. (1958). *Med. J. Aust.* **1,** 244

[The illustrations for this Chapter on Mucosal Prolapse: Ligature and Excision were drawn by Mr. F. Price.]

Ribbon Dacron Mesh Encirclement

M. J. Notaras, F.R.C.S., F.R.C.S. (Ed.)
Consultant Surgeon, Barnet General Hospital;
Honorary Senior Lecturer and Consultant Surgeon,
University College Hospital, London

INTRODUCTION

Where an abdominal repair of a rectal prolapse is contra-indicated due to the high risks to the patient because of their age and general condition then most surgeons prefer the Thiersch method (Kirschner, 1933). A wire ring is placed around the anus so that it acts as an obstruction to an intussuscepting rectal prolapse. This wire is rigid and is at the anal verge. There is no lateral support to the anal canal. There are also the problems of fracturing of the wire and faecal impaction if too tight.

1

To overcome the disadvantages of the Thiersch method another useful perineal technique (Notaras, 1973) is to place a ribbon of Dacron mesh (Mersilene or Marlex) around the anal canal and anorectal musculature at the level of the puborectalis muscle thus supporting the anorectal angle and the length of the anal canal. The mesh becomes incorporated with the anorectal musculature and as it is not rigid will move with these muscles when they are contracted. Breakage and cutting through does not occur.

This method is also useful for the treatment of large anterior wall mucosal prolapse and certain types of anal incontinence associated with weak pelvic floor muscles.

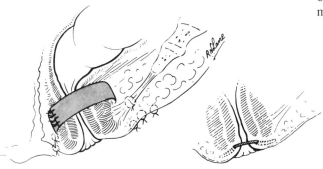

1

TECHNIQUE

Before operation it is essential to clear the lower bowel of faeces by enemas. The operation is performed with the patient in the lithotomy position. The patient is catheterized. A swab is inserted into the anal canal and rectum to prevent leakage of mucus and descent of the prolapse. A stitch to close the anus over the swab is occasionally necessary.

2

A transverse incision is made anterior to the anus and perineal body. With scissor dissection the recto-vaginal space is entered to a level well above the pelvic floor muscles.

A sagittal incision is then made posterior to the anus to enter the retrosphincteric space and the dissection is continued towards the coccyx.

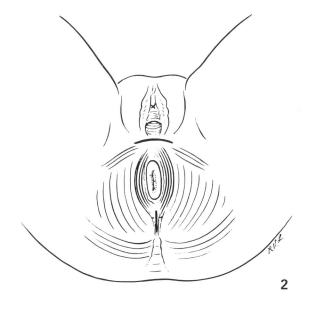

2

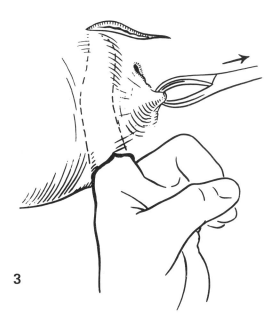

3

3

The index finger is then inserted through the posterior skin incision and by blunt dissection is pushed forwards and laterally towards the ischial tuberosity. The finger which is now high in the ischiorectal space is then hooked medially until it meets the levator muscles which form the roof of the space and which prevents the finger from entering the recto-vaginal or supralevator space.

4

A large curved artery forceps is then introduced through the anterior incision and the forceps tip directed in a posterolateral direction towards the finger in the ischiorectal space. It is then pushed through the levator muscles (mainly the puborectalis muscle where it fuses with the perineal body) and thus passes from the supralevator (rectovaginal) space on to the tip of the finger in the infralevator (ischiorectal) space which then acts as a guide and is withdrawn with the forceps passing through the posterior incision. (This part of the technique is important as it safeguards against accidental perforation of the rectum.) The procedure is repeated on the opposite side.

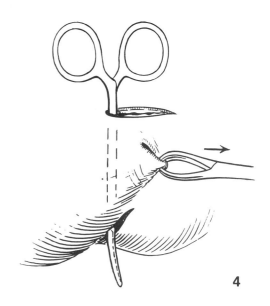

4

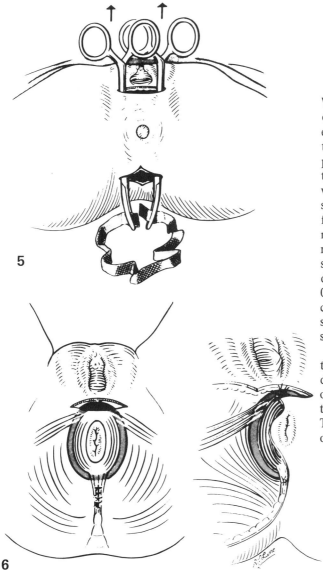

5

6

5&6

With the two forceps surrounding the anus a ribbon of mesh (approximately 4 cm wide) is grasped at its ends by the forceps which are then withdrawn pulling the mesh into a position where it surrounds the posterior and lateral aspects of the anorectal musculature. The mesh is then double-breasted in the rectovaginal space and sutured together with interrupted synthetic (Mersilene or Marlex) suture materials. A further stitch is placed to bring the puborectalis muscles together and at the same time to include the mid-anterior part of the mesh ring. This important stitch helps to pull the mesh as a sling in a forward direction and helps to fix it to the perineal body. 0/0 Dexon sutures are then used to close the subcutaneous space and to bury even further the synthetic sutures. The skin is closed with 0/0 Dexon sutures.

With regard to the diameter of the circle of mesh, there are various methods used: the mesh may be double-breasted over a standard sized proctoscope or as the author prefers two fingers are inserted into the anal canal and the diameter assessed digitally. This latter method requires frequent glove changing over the original surgeons gloves.

POSTOPERATIVE CARE

It is important for the patient to be established on a suitable bowel regime to ensure regular emptying of the rectum. Suppositories may be necessary in addition to stool softeners.

On rectal examination the mesh is felt as a cord around the anorectal junction. If it proves to be too tight or loose then it is a simple matter to resuture the mesh through the anterior incision under local anaesthesia.

References

Kirschner, M. (1933). *Operative Surgery*, p. 63. Philadelphia: Lippincott
Notaras, M. J. (1973). *Proc. R. Soc. Med.* **66,** 684

[*The illustrations for this Chapter on Ribbon Dacron Mesh Encirclement were drawn by Mr. R. N. Lane.*]

Pelvic Floor Descent

C. N. Hudson, M.Chir., F.R.C.S., F.R.C.O.G.
Reader in Obstetrics and Gynaecology,
Medical College of St. Bartholomew's Hospital, London

PRE - OPERATIVE

Posterior colpoperineorrhaphy is a standard gynae-cological operation commonly performed for laxity and overstretching of the vaginal introitus following childbirth. This laxity is often, though not invariably, accompanied by an anterior bulge of the middle third of the posterior vaginal wall termed rectocele. The latter is often made larger as well as more prominent by deficiency of the fibromuscular perineal body.

This state of affairs to a minor degree is very common in parous women and often requires no treatment. Symptoms attributable to it are a feeling of perineal insecurity, a palpable bulge, ineffective coital performance, and occasional difficulty in faecal evacuation overcome by digital pressure on the posterior vaginal wall during defaecation. Backache and perineal pain should not be regarded as features of rectocele; the former alone may occasionally be ascribed to second-degree uterine prolapse with obvious stretching of the posterior limb of the cardinal ligaments (uterosacral ligaments). Dyschezia is not a feature and tenesmus rarely so, except when a prolapsing retroverted uterus presses on the anterior rectal wall producing a sensation reminiscent of that induced by a descending fetal head in labour. These symptoms are elaborated as they must be distinguished by rectal surgeons dealing with problems of excessive pelvic floor descent, and indeed of rectal prolapse.

Gynaecological displacements and their corrective surgery may actually aggravate problems of defaecation. Over-acute angulation at the anorectal junction may prevent adequate descent of the faecal bolus, over-stretching and impairment of the 'levator sling' may render incompetent the pelvic floor elevation necessary to complete evacuation, and alteration of the anatomy of the uterosacral ligaments and pouch of Douglas may facilitate invagination of the anterior rectal wall into the anal canal with the formation of a solitary rectal ulcer and indeed the formation of actual intussusception which may develop into rectal prolapse.

Many patients with rectal prolapse give a history of straining at stool with consequent inhibition of the pelvic floor muscles leading to traction neuropathy and eventually incontinence. This sequence may sometimes be secondary to some of the above circumstances, together with the excessively deep pouch of Douglas which is or becomes a regular feature.

The need for a modified form of gynaecological pelvic floor repair is nevertheless apparent in some women whose symptoms may be primarily rectal. If the associated or indeed underlying cause of straining is uterine prolapse, the pelvic floor repair operation may conveniently be accompanied by vaginal hysterectomy. If, however, uterine removal is inappropriate but there is significant uterine descent posterior sacral hysteropexy may be preferable. Manchester repair, on the other hand, may aggravate the rectal situation because plication of the cardinal ligaments in front of the cervix inevitably opens the gap between the uterosacral ligaments and predisposes to vaginal enterocele or rectal prolapse in a susceptible patient if appropriate additional steps are not taken.

Objectives of the operation

(1) Excision of a redundant pouch of Douglas (enterocele).

(2) Reduction by 'keel' repair of redundant rectal wall, which has previously constituted either a high rectocele or anterior rectal wall prolapse (with or without solitary ulcer).

(3) Reduction of the overstretched urogenital hiatus by artificially approximating the puborectalis and pubococcygeus muscles to form a new apex to the perineal body together with such supralevator fascia as may be obtained.

Indications

These objectives which may be achieved vaginally roughly correspond to those of the abdominal Roscoe-Graham operation and are subject to the same limitations.

The operation should be considered as a second stage if a standard operation for rectal prolapse (e.g. Ivalon sponge repair) has not been completely successful. Its main place is, however, in the treatment of early rectal prolapse and pelvic floor descent, associated with a degree of vaginal rectocele and enterocele. It can be combined with transperineal anterior plication of the anal sphincter muscle.

In cases of solitary rectal ulcer the operation is unlikely to be successful if persistent mucous discharge remains.

Special contra-indications

(1) Anal incontinence associated with loss of the anorectal angle, and gross pelvic floor neuropathy. Some such cases may respond better to a postanal repair.

(2) Intrinsic rectal disease responsible for local ulceration, including lymphopathia venereum.

(3) Habitual anal coitus.

Special pre-operative preparations

The general evaluation and care of any patient undergoing vaginal surgery is necessary. Special packs and douches are not usually necessary. Special attention must be paid to the following:

(1) Elimination of intrinsic bowel disorders by sigmoidoscopy and, if appropriate, barium studies.

(2) Evaluation of the degree of genital prolapse, coital status (actual or prospective) and future reproductive requirements.

(3) Evaluation of associated general pathology such as chronic bronchitis and obesity.

(4) Examination, including cervical cytology, to exclude any associated gynaecological pathology, particularly that which would suggest hysterectomy and which might thus determine an abdominal approach. Local vaginal pathology and infections may require topical treatment including oestrogen creams. Some surgeons advocate a short course of systemic oestrogen but the possible increased risk of thrombo-embolism has to be balanced against the therapeutic advantage.

The presence of stress incontinence may be a factor requiring additional individual evaluation and attention.

(5) Thiersch wires should be removed and the bowel emptied.

THE OPERATION

1

The standard lithotomy position is used. Caudal or lumbar epidural anaesthesia as an adjuvant is often helpful.

Bimanual examination should be performed, and traction applied to the cervix with a vulsellum to assess descent. On this may depend a decision whether to proceed first to vaginal hysterectomy. In any event diagnostic curettage should be carried out. The labia should be distracted.

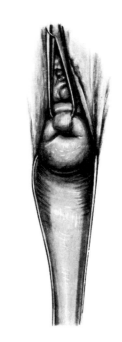

1

2a & b

An individual decision should be made as to the approach to the perineal body. If the introitus is lax a measured standard transverse incision should be used. Otherwise, if subsequent coital performance is desirable, a mid-line episiotomy is preferable.

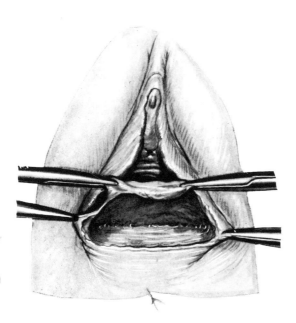

2a

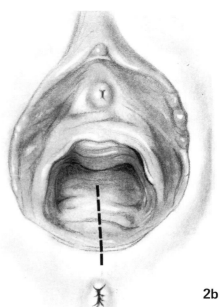

2b

3

The cut edges of the mid-line incision must be elevated with small clips and dissected free from the perineal body and above this the underlying rectum. It is helpful to keep an index finger in the vagina against the flap so that the correct thickness of flap may be judged.

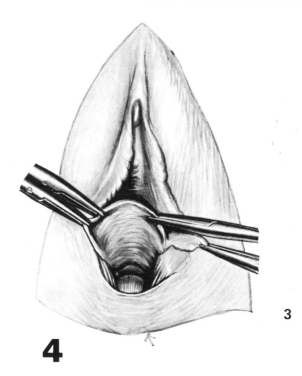

3

4

Once the attachment of the prerectal fascia to the apex of the perineal body is passed a plane of cleavage may be established as far as the peritoneal attachment of the pouch of Douglas to the anterior rectal wall. The vagina should be incised up to the back of the cervix or the equivalent, and the pouch of Douglas opened.

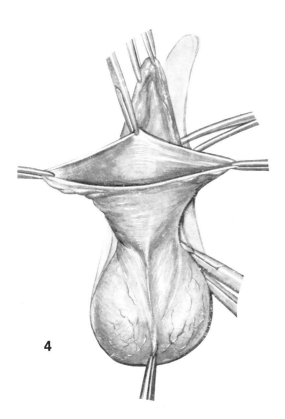

4

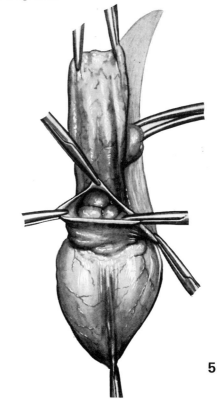

5

5

At this stage a finger should be inserted into the pouch of Douglas to palpate for ovarian or other pathology and then to evaluate the size of the redundant sac as in any other hernia repair. When freed right to the rectal attachment the sac should be transfixed closed and excised.

6

If the uterus has been removed it is desirable to approximate the uterosacral ligaments with one or two interrupted catgut sutures. Caution should be exercised because the ureter may have been drawn down by peritoneal mobilization.

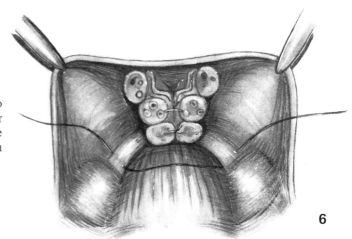

6

7

The redundant infraperitoneal rectal wall should now be infolded in a manner comparable to the 'keel' repair of abdominal wall herniae. Full thickness wedge excision of the rectal wall has been advocated but this is not usually regarded as necessary. A continuous suture of polyglycolic acid is suitable.

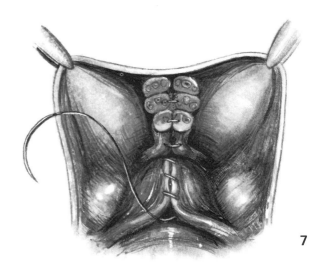

7

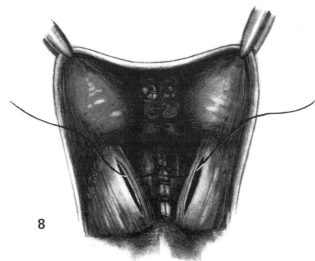

8

8

At this stage further mobilization of the rectal wall from the levator muscles and pelvic side-walls may be necessary. When these are clear, a stab incision with scissors is made under the fascia on the superior surface of the pubococcygeus muscle. This layer may be united with its fellow in front of the rectum without producing too much vaginal constriction and hopefully joining with the posterior uterosacral stitch.

9

Thereafter two or three interrupted sutures can be placed in the puborectalis/pubococcygeus muscles to approximate them at the apex of the new perineal body, a position which they do not normally occupy. It is most important to insert two fingers into the vagina to test whether an undue 'hourglass' constriction has been induced. 1/0 Chromic catgut is suitable for the sutures although some surgeons have used unabsorbable wire or nylon sutures but there are inherent risks of sinus formation and strong catgut seems preferable.

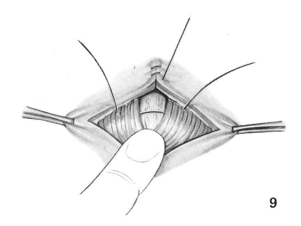

9

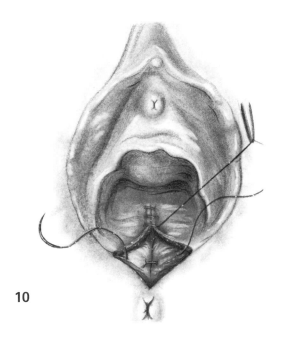

10

10

Once these sutures have been checked they can be tied. It then remains to build up a new perineal body in such a way that the vaginal lumen re-forms in a tubular rather than a 'hourglass' fashion. Buried sutures are best inserted from within outwards into the halves of the recently or previously divided perineal body.

11

It should be noted that unless there is significant redundant vaginal skin over a rectocele, there need be no trimming of the vaginal wall incision. Merely opening and closing such an incision reduces the available lumen slightly, and coital function can as easily be impaired by excision of too much vaginal skin as by over-zealous suture of the pubococcygeus muscle.

The original episiotomy should be repaired with subcuticular polyglycollic acid sutures.

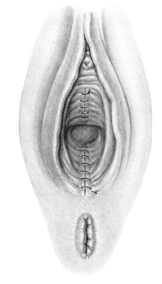

11

POSTOPERATIVE CARE

In view of the fairly extensive infraperitoneal dissection, haematoma formation from branches of the internal pudendal vessels is common. A vaginal pack for 24–48 hr is prudent, and indeed suction drainage through a perineal stab has much to recommend it.

Even without anterior repair, many of these patients will have retention of urine and an indwelling catheter is required for a few days, covered by prophylactic nitrofurantoin. If there is extensive bruising, antibiotic cover is preferable.

Gentle digital examination prior to discharge from hospital is desirable, to break down any soft adhesions.

Care of the bowels is important. Constipation and straining is most harmful but liquid paraffin as a laxative is unsatisfactory. Early resort to bran or its substitutes is recommended. Coitus should be avoided until after a postoperative visit at 6 weeks.

[*The illustrations for this Chapter on Pelvic Floor Descent were drawn by Mr. P. A. Darton and Mr. R. N. Lane.*]

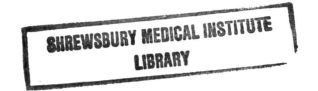

Surgical Repair of Anal Sphincters following Injury

A. G. Parks, Ch.M., F.R.C.S., F.R.C.P.
Consultant Surgeon, St. Mark's Hospital, London
and The London Hospital

and

J. F. McPartlin, F.R.C.S.
Consultant Surgeon, Ashford General Hospital,
Royal Victoria Hospital, Folkestone and
Buckland General Hospital, Dover

INTRODUCTION

Normal anorectal control is automatically maintained by the reflex activity of the anal sphincter muscles. The sphincter ring has two components, the internal sphincter which is a continuation of the circular muscle of the rectum, and the external sphincter composed of striated muscle. The external sphincter surrounds the internal at all levels. The internal sphincter is composed of smooth muscle which has a constant tone holding the anal canal closed and preventing the seepage of mucus and flatus. It is not capable of controlling stool. Fortunately, the external sphincter and puborectalis muscles have a constant tone (unlike most skeletal muscle) and it is this tone, re-inforced by reflex action, which enables the normal person to maintain faecal control effortlessly. The puborectalis muscle passes from pubic arch to pubic arch, describing a $\frac{5}{8}$ circle behind the anorectal junction. By its contraction the junction is drawn upwards and forwards, maintaining closure of the upper anal canal and creating a right angle between the axis of the anal canal itself and the lower rectum. It is this angulation which establishes a flap valve, now thought to be such an important factor in automatically sealing the anorectal junction.

The severity of the incontinence produced by division of the sphincter muscles depends on the site and the amount of muscle divided. Anterior rupture, almost always the result of childbirth, causes less severe incontinence than lateral or posterior injuries, since the puborectalis sling remains intact. However,

with severe injuries at other points of the anal ring the puborectalis is also divided; in these cases all the muscles of continence are severed, and severe incontinence ensues. Most of these injuries are due to surgical treatment of fistula-in-ano. Less commonly the sphincter may be divided by direct trauma or by severe pelvic injuries.

Complete division of the sphincter ring is followed by retraction of the cut ends to about half a circle. During the subsequent healing the gap is filled by fibrous tissue which only contracts a little and leaves a long non-contractile segment. The aim of surgical repair is to remove this segment and to recreate a long anal canal surrounded by active sphincter muscle.

General considerations

Age and prolonged incontinence are not barriers to a successful outcome. As long as about half the sphincter ring remains active there is a good chance of restoring satisfactory control.

Pre-operative bowel preparation

If a colostomy has already been established it is only necessary to ensure that the distal loop of colon and the rectum is empty by giving a distal loop irrigation. In other cases the colon is prepared in the standard fashion to ensure that it is completely empty. A temporary transverse colostomy is carried out at the time of the surgical repair.

245

THE OPERATION

1

A general anaesthetic is administered and the patient is placed in the lithotomy position. The illustration shows the appearance before operation, the anal canal is gaping and there is a healed wound with extensive scarring.

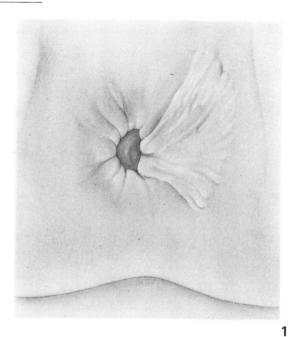

1

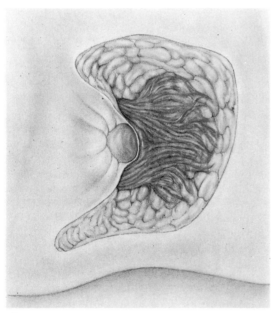

2

2

Through a generous incision scarred skin with its underlying fibrous tissue is removed and the ischiorectal fat exposed. The muscle ends will not be seen at this stage though the scar tissue between them will be obvious as well as the strands of fibrous adhesions extending out in to the ischiorectal fossa. The skin incision will need to be a long one extending from a point anterior in the perineum to well behind the anal canal in order to allow adequate mobilization of the muscles.

3

After the scarred tissue has been excised a considerable cavity is created in the ischiorectal fossa. The muscle ends are identified, but an effort is made to leave some scar tissue attached to them to hold the sutures which will be needed for the repair, as stitches placed in bared muscle ends will tend to cut out.

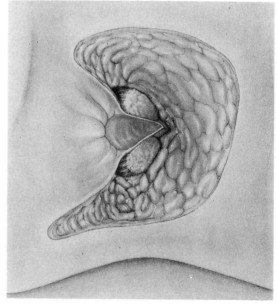

3

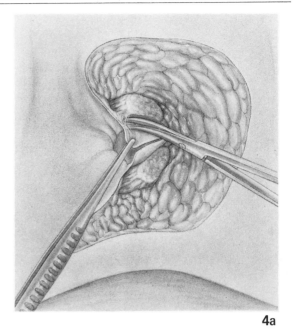

4a

4a & b

The skin of the lower anal canal together with the upper anal epithelium is now mobilized from the inner surface of the sphincters for about 1 cm, and the free edges are sutured together with a continuous stitch of 2/0 chromic catgut (*Illustration 4a*). This results in the closed anal canal as shown (*Illustration 4b*).

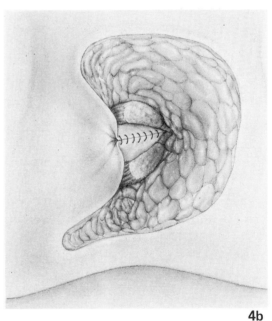

4b

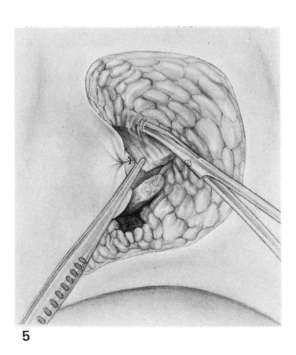

5

5

Perhaps the most important and most difficult manoeuvre of the entire operation is the liberation of the outer surface of the sphincters from fibrous adhesions. A delicate balance has to be struck between sufficient mobilization to allow repair without tension, and at the same time avoiding excessive division of blood vessels with possible necrosis of the muscle. Posteriorly, it is helpful to divide the insertion of all the muscles attached to the coccyx to allow the posterior limb of the sphincter to be lifted forwards without tension. This leaves a cavity between the coccyx and the rectum.

6

The mobilized ends of the sphincters can now be overlapped for about 2 cm which will create a snugly closed anal canal. Two layers of monofilament stainless steel wire (gauge 4/0), which cause no tissue reaction and seldom result in tissue infection, are used. Multifilament wire is less satisfactory in this respect. The first layer consists of approximately five mattress sutures which pass through the full thickness of both muscles. It is essential that these sutures are tied with no tension, to avoid necrosis of muscle. Another layer of stitches is placed between the end of the limb of muscle which is uppermost and the surface of the partially covered limb.

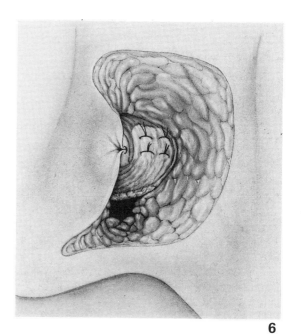

6

7

The free edge of the mucosa is then sutured back on to the muscle with a few fine chromic catgut sutures. This diagram also clearly illustrates the effect of dividing the muscles attached to the coccyx with the creation of a cavity posteriorly.

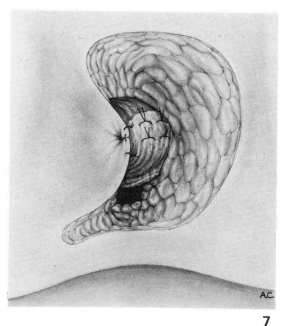

7

At the end of the operation the anal canal should be tightly closed; indeed it will feel almost stenosed. Over the next 10 days however, the tissues will become somewhat more lax, resulting in a canal which both feels normal and will function normally. No attempt is made to close the large defect in the skin and ischiorectal fat. The cavity is lightly covered with gauze soaked in dilute hypochlorite and is allowed to granulate. In fact, healing of this defect occurs with great rapidity. The colostomy which may have been carried out at the same time as the repair can usually be closed 3—4 weeks later.

[Twenty-one cases of lateral or posterior sphincter division, all of whom suffered severe incontinence, have been treated with this technique. Only one has had an unsatisfactory result.]

[The illustrations for this Chapter on Surgical Repair of the Anal Sphincters following Injury were drawn by Mrs. A. Christie.]

Postanal Pelvic Floor Repair (and the Treatment of Anorectal Incontinence)

A. G. Parks, M.Ch., F.R.C.S., F.R.C.P.
Consultant Surgeon, St. Mark's Hospital, London
and The London Hospital

INTRODUCTION

Anorectal incontinence is not a common condition but it is so distressing to the patient that every attempt to relieve it must be made. Although it is found in all age groups, it is very rare until the middle years, when its frequency rises. In the elderly person it is doubly unfortunate in that it may lead to rejection by the family. Women are affected ten times more commonly than men. Patients with this condition may be divided into two main groups, those whose symptoms are preceded by the development of a large rectal prolapse, and those in whom prolapse is minimal. In all cases there is profound weakness of the musculature of the pelvic floor, including the anal sphincters. Recent evidence has strongly suggested that this weakness is due to degeneration of the nerves supplying the pelvic floor muscles, a condition similar to an ulnar nerve neuropathy at the elbow. In those with rectal procidentia it is probable that the neuropathy is caused by the massive descent of the pelvic floor with consequent traction on the nerves.

In the second, or idiopathic group, other factors may be at work, including traction nerve injury during difficult labour. The median in this group is at an earlier age than the previous one.

It is important to examine patients carefully in order to eliminate other causes of muscle weakness, such as dehiscence during childbirth or injury from fistula operations, etc. These are best treated by direct muscle suture as described on pages 245–248. Investigations which may prove helpful are electromyography, anal pressure measurements and lateral radiography of the lower rectum to demonstrate the presence or absence of normal anorectal angulation. However, simple digital examination will usually provide as much information about muscle function as is necessary. In particular, an assessment of the resting tone is made and the power developed on voluntary contraction is determined. In most patients the resting tone will be minimal or absent entirely; good contraction of the puborectalis muscle on voluntary effort is the most hopeful prognostic sign.

1

Any operation designed to relieve this condition must take into account the fact that the muscles are already partially degenerate; the aim is to make residual function maximally effective. One of the most important features in the maintenance of continence is the valve effect caused by the double right-angle which normally exists between the anal canal, the lowermost rectum and the mid-rectum. The force of abdominal pressure acts upon the anterior rectal wall, thrusting it on to the closed anal canal and so effectively blocking it. The valve action is normally overcome by the passage of faeces through the viscus, propelled by contraction of the rectal muscle itself. The puborectalis muscle, by its sling-like action, normally maintains the necessary angulation.

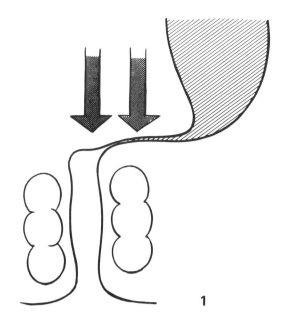

1

Patients with incontinence have either lost this normal angulation, so that the anal and rectal axes are nearly in a straight line, or else this occurs under stress, such as coughing or walking, due to a drop of the pelvic floor. An essential part of any therapeutic procedure must therefore be the reconstruction of the anorectal angulation, with the restoration of a reliable flap-valve mechanism which does not give way under stress. The pelvic floor sphincters, including the puborectalis, are circular and, when they weaken, the diameter of the circles they describe enlarges. It is necessary therefore to narrow this diameter, at the same time reducing the circumference of the circle which the sphincters make. A method by which this is achieved can best be understood by imagining a circle and then pinching or constricting it at its mid-point so that the remaining circle has half the diameter and a quarter of the area. To achieve this in the case of the pelvic floor muscles, it is necessary to approach them from their inner surface, that is within the circle. There are two reasons for this; the first is that stitches can be placed across from one side of the circular muscle to the other, in this way imbricating the muscle and reducing the diameter

and area which it describes. The second reason is that neither nerves nor important blood vessels reach the muscles from this aspect; they enter from the outer surface. The anatomical approach itself is an interesting and not a difficult one provided the basic anatomy of the region is understood. The only structures which pass through the pelvic floor muscles and are therefore in contact with their inner surface are the terminations of the intestinal and genito-urinary viscera. All that is required therefore is to displace these viscera forwards to obtain access to the posterior and lateral inner surfaces of the external sphincter, puborectalis and levator ani muscles. The approach is made behind the viscera because it is here that the muscles must be approximated to narrow their fields of action and to restore the normal anorectal angulation.

Pre-operative preparation

The colon and rectum must be completely evacuated during the 48 hr prior to operation.

THE OPERATION

2

The patient is placed in the lithotomy position (although the jack-knife would be equally suitable). After routine skin preparation, a solution of saline containing 1:300,000 adrenaline is injected into the fat and subcutaneous tissue around the posterior part of the anal canal. This cuts down capillary bleeding and enables the operator to differentiate between the internal and external sphincters, a vital first stage in the dissection.

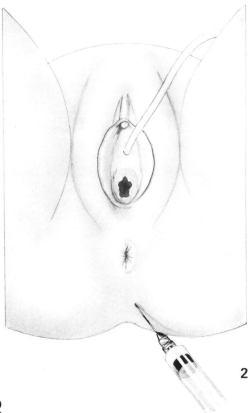

2

3

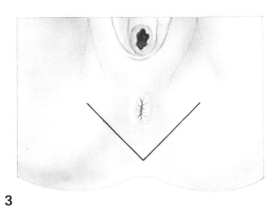

3

A V-shaped incision is made in the perineum about 6 cm behind the anal canal. The reason for placing the wound so far behind the anus is that in the course of repair the skin of the anal region is drawn into the canal itself; if the wound were put too close, it would be pulled into the anal canal and infection would result. The skin anterior to the incision is then raised with scissor dissection until the anal verge is reached.

4

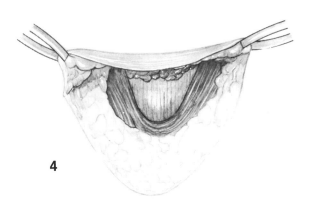

The posterior half of the external sphincter and the lower border of the internal sphincter are exposed. The plane between the two is relatively bloodless and can be identified anatomically; the longitudinal fibres guide the operator to the correct site. The external sphincter is usually red and easily identified, whereas the internal sphincter is white. However, if the external sphincter is degenerate, then the distinction between the two muscles becomes blurred, but stimulation of the tissue with diathermy current will usually cause contraction in the external sphincter. By gentle scissor dissection the internal sphincter is displaced off the lower part of the external sphincter over about half its circumference.

5

As the dissection progresses, the viscus is lifted off the upper part of the external sphincter, progressively onward and upward until the puborectalis is reached. It is necessary to avoid straying from this plane as it is not difficult to enter the rectum and somewhat easier to dissect through the external sphincters into the ischiorectal fat. Throughout the dissection the separation between the two layers is carried as far forward on each side of the anal canal as possible. Above the puborectalis muscle Waldeyer's fascia is encountered and is divided, exposing the mesorectal fat.

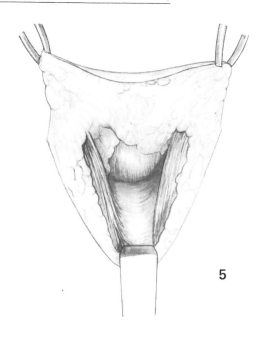

5

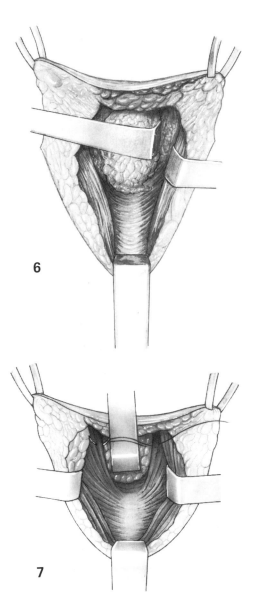

6

7

6&7

A deep retractor is then placed into the pelvis to hold the rectum forwards so that the origin of the levator ani muscles on both sides can be seen. Sutures of floss or braided nylon are placed across it. The highest and most lateral point of the levator group is identified with blunt dissection, close to the spine of the ischium which is readily palpable. A small curved needle is then passed under a fairly large bundle of the levator on one side. The retractor is then moved to expose the exactly equivalent site of the muscle on the other side. The needle containing nylon then picks up an exactly similar bundle of muscle on the other side. About three sutures are placed at this topmost level and are tied only lightly, without tension, to form a lattice across the pelvis. The next layer of sutures is placed in the upper part of the pubococcygeus muscle and again each is tied only lightly with the formation of a lattice. The lower part of the pubococcygeus, however, is a stronger bar of muscle and its origin is much nearer the midline on the pubic arch. Sutures are placed as close to its origin on each side as possible and again about three are used.

8

The most important layer of all is that put into the puborectalis. The muscle is the strongest and thickest of all those encountered and can be seen with ease. Once more the sutures are placed as near to the origin on the pubis as possible. Each is tied so that the muscle is approximated but a small gap is left to take into account swelling which may occur in the tissues postoperatively. Another layer of sutures is placed in the external sphincter below the puborectalis and finally, at the anal margin, a layer of catgut stitches is used to avoid putting nylon too near the skin. A Redivac drain is placed in the pelvis.

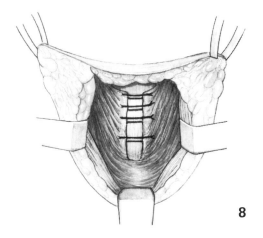

8

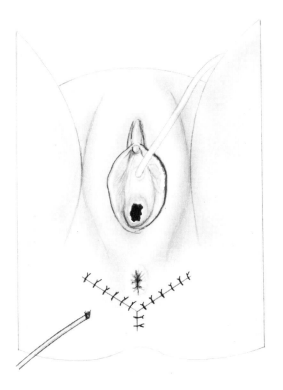

9

9

As a result of the repair, the anterior skin flap is drawn forwards and cannot be resutured to the posterior skin edge without undue tension. The wound is therefore reconstituted in the shape of a Y. It is not uncommon for local necrosis to occur at the apex of the anterior flap but this always heals uneventfully.

POSTOPERATIVE CARE

A catheter is placed into the bladder for 2–3 days. Were the patient to strain in the immediate post-operative period and to pass a large stool through the anal canal, it would disrupt the whole repair. The two ways of avoiding this are either to fashion a temporary colostomy or to create a state of permanent diarrhoea for about 12 days. Neither alternative is pleasant but the diarrhoea regime is preferable and to this end magnesium sulphate is prescribed in sufficient doses to maintain about three semiformed stools a day. Once this period has passed, the chance of doing sudden damage to the muscles by defaecation straining is over. However, it is essential that straining habits are not resumed, because in that case the repair will gradually weaken, or more likely the muscle itself, will weaken over months and symptoms recur. The patient must therefore steer a mean course between hard stool which cannot be expelled easily and diarrhoea which may only be controllable with difficulty. To accomplish this, a sufficiency of a simple laxative, such as paraffin emulsion or one of the hydrophilic group, is given by mouth and each morning two glycerine suppositories are inserted routinely. The latter induce rectal contraction so that the stool is expelled by the *vis a tergo* of the rectal wall rather than by abdominal straining. This regime is continued indefinitely and it is necessary to reiterate this to the patient on several occasions. Only too frequently do they feel that there is now no longer a problem and they can give up using the suppositories. The result may be either intermittent impaction of faeces or gradual resumption of straining efforts.

RESULTS

In general the best results are obtained in the younger patient, those who still have good powers of voluntary contraction and in whom the muscle degeneration seen on histological appearance is minimal. In patients who have a complete rectal procidentia the first step is to perform an abdominal rectopexy. This will relieve the incontinence in about half the patients, the remainder will then require a postanal repair about 3 months later. The functional results in this group are not quite as satisfactory as in those without an initial major prolapse.

Intelligent co-operation in the postoperative regime is essential and the operation should be avoided in a patient who is unlikely to follow instructions conscientiously. Patients above the age of seventy also tend to do less well, as there is more muscle degeneration and again unfortunately co-operation in continuing care after operation tends to be less forthcoming. However, in the case of a woman in her mid-seventies who is thin and retains full mental faculties the chance of restoration to normal should not be withheld.

It must be emphasized that, in a situation where the muscles are partly degenerate, it is unlikely that any operative procedure can restore total normality. The majority have some difficulty in controlling flatus and may have soiling if affected with an attack of diarrhoea. However, to keep matters in proportion, even a normal person can have problems under such circumstances. Generally speaking, these patients are transformed from being social recluses to people who can once more live a normal active life.

[*The illustrations for this Chapter on Postanal Pelvic Floor Repair (and the Treatment of Anorectal Incontinence) were drawn by Mr. F. Price.*]

Thiersch's Operation

Ian P. Todd, M.S., M.D. (Tor.), F.R.C.S., D.C.H.
Consultant Surgeon, St. Bartholomew's Hospital, St. Mark's Hospital
and King Edward VII Hospital for Officers, London

and

Nigel H. Porter, F.R.C.S.
Consultant Surgeon, Brighton and Lewes
Group of Hospitals

PRE - OPERATIVE

Indications

This operation should probably never be used for the primary treatment of complete rectal prolapse, as even the very old and infirm are probably fit for an Ivalon sponge wrap or the Ripstein operation using an abdominal approach or the modified Kraske procedure (*see* pages 191–198). It is, however, a satisfactory operation for mucosal prolapse in the elderly or as a secondary operation, following a major procedure, to narrow the outlet when anal tone has not been regained and where a postanal repair (*see* pages 249–254) seems unnecessary.

Pre-operative investigations and preparation

Careful investigation of the intestine with barium studies and sigmoidoscopy should be carried out, as manipulations to remove something such as a polyp may be difficult once the anal orifice is narrowed. As re-establishment of its function may be difficult after the procedure, the bowel should be emptied beforehand.

Anaesthesia and position of patient

General, caudal or epidural anaesthesia may be used. Local anaesthesia is probably unwise as infection around the foreign body is the main risk of the operation. The patient is placed in the lithotomy position. The skin around the anus is carefully cleansed and the area towelled up, using mastisol or something similar to prevent the towels slipping. Strict attention to asepsis is essential and the wire, nylon or Silastic should not be allowed to touch skin at any stage.

THE OPERATION

1

The incision

Two tiny (0·5 cm) incisions should be made approximately 2 cm from the anal verge anteriorly and posteriorly. A small space is made subcutaneously within the posterior wound so that the 'knot' may be adequately buried, as this can be uncomfortable to sit on.

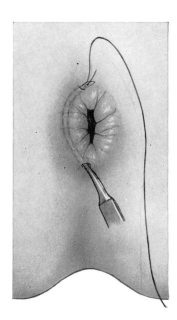

1

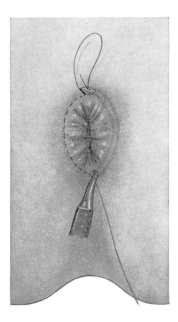

2

2

Introduction of needle

A curved Doyen needle is introduced into the posterior incision. The point first aims towards the coccyx; when it has passed upwards about 4 cm, the point is turned outwards towards the ischiorectal fossa. As it enters this, it will be found to give in the softer tissues; it should be swept around in this layer well outside the sphincter mechanism, high in the fossa and brought out in the firmer anterior structures as far forwards as possible. No. 20 silver wire, No. 1 nylon or Silastic rod is threaded into the needle which is then withdrawn, carrying the circlage material with it. The needle is then passed around the other side of the anus, threaded and withdrawn in a similar manner.

3

Completion of encirclement

In the case of silver wire, the wire is tightened and twisted equally three times upon a No. 19 Hegar dilator held in the anal canal. The ends are then cut flush and bent upwards. Other forms of wire, mono-filament and braided, are less successful. If nylon is used, it should be monofilament and it has been found more successful to encircle the anus three times, using the same piece, introducing it with the same technique. It should be tied, using a double-throw surgeon's knot, around a No. 18 Hegar dilator, as though it tends to stretch on being pulled up, the three throws seldom pull up equally. Silastic rod is very elastic and is probably best tied around an index finger to make sure it is not too tight, as in all cases, if the ring is too tight, the operation is likely to fail because of repeated faecal impaction. The problem with Silastic is, though theoretically much superior, it is difficult to tie. The ends are best overlapped and then a ligature whipped around them. If used, the hole in the Doyen needle will need to be enlarged.

Both incisions are then sprayed with an anti-biotic powder, closed with Michel clip or Dexon and sprayed with a sealer (Octaflex, Nobecutane). Alternatively a soluble suture may be used.

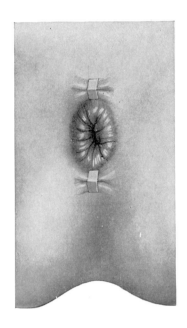

3

POSTOPERATIVE CARE

Only a dry dressing is needed and the clips may be removed on the third postoperative day. Faecal impaction is very probable and must be anticipated. The faeces should not be allowed to become hard. A paraffin emulsion should be given, 10 ml three times a day immediately following operation with a larger dose on the second evening postoperatively. Once the bowel is open, hydrophilic bulking agents (methyl cellulose, psillium) or bran should be given. If impaction occurs with leakage, bearing down discomfort or pain, it is confirmed with the finger, broken up and evacuated with the help of suppo-sitories and enemas. Until the bowel habit is well regulated a careful follow-up is needed. Most patients require bulk and some mild laxative (senna, bisacodyl) continuously, for prolapse is probably secondary to a disorder of defaecation with inadequate rectal sensation and dyschezia. Occasionally a suppository regime is the best way to establish a reasonable bowel function if a balance cannot be struck between constipation with impaction and diarrhoea with incontinence.

[The illustrations for this Chapter on Thiersch's Operation were drawn by Mr. F. Price.]

Operations for Diffuse Diverticular Disease of the Colon

W. W. Slack, M.Ch., F.R.C.S.
Consultant Surgeon, The Middlesex Hospital, London

Operations for diffuse diverticular disease are rare events as the vast majority of operations are for disease of the sigmoid colon alone. When diverticula of the colon are present in the sigmoid colon, in about 15 per cent of cases they can be found throughout the length of the colon, usually asymptomatic, but the complications that can occur are: perforation, bleeding and obstruction.

PRE - OPERATIVE

Indications for operation

Perforation

As a rule the perforation is localized and abscess formation may occur, thereby allowing time for bowel preparation, but if there is an acute perforation into the peritoneal cavity, then immediate laparotomy is necessary.

Caecal diverticula when inflamed may simulate appendicitis and the true diagnosis is only established at operation. Unless such a diverticulum has perforated nothing further than the insertion of a drain is necessary.

Haemorrhage

Rarely in diverticular disease does this occur, but it can be profuse. The patient is frequently elderly and hypertensive. Initially simple causes such as tumours, gastroduodenal lesions and bleeding disorders should be excluded. Sigmoidoscopy should always be attempted and angiography in rare instances has shown the source of the bleeding. Conservative management should be attempted first, but if bleeding continues for more than 24 hr then operative intervention is advisable.

Obstruction

Obstruction from diffuse diverticular disease is even rarer than in sigmoid diverticular disease. The appropriate treatment for large intestinal obstruction is instituted.

Pre-operative preparation

In cases where the patient has been having recurrent episodes of symptoms attributed to either right-sided diverticula or diverticula elsewhere in the colon a full bowel preparation should be carried out if possible. In an acute situation either from perforation or bleeding the usual resuscitative measures are carried out prior to laparotomy.

THE OPERATIONS

1 & 2

Perforation

If the perforation has sealed itself off or there is only local inflammation present, drainage is all that is necessary (*see Illustration 1*). If a frank perforation has occurred then simple suture and drainage may be possible. Frequently the lesion can be mistaken for a carcinoma of the caecum and a right hemicolectomy is performed. A finger invaginating the anterior caecal wall may feel the mouth of a diverticulum elucidating the diagnosis.

If a diverticulum in the transverse colon or descending colon perforates, a local resection should be performed. A primary end-to-end anastomosis can be carried out with a proximal defunctioning colostomy (or caecostomy) or else the two bowel ends can be exteriorized. In performing any operation in diverticular disease it is important that the bowel should be anastomosed so that the anastomosis is not made through a diverticulum (*see Illustration 2*).

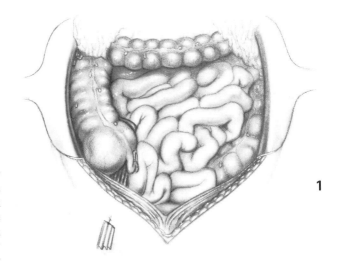

1

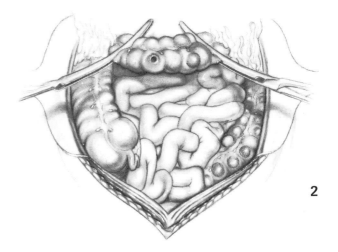

2

Haemorrhage

If pre-operative selective angiography has diagnosed the bleeding point, vasopressor agents may be tried; if they are unsuccessful then a local resection of the area containing the bleeding point is performed.

If the bleeding point is unknown pre-operatively the main problem at laparotomy is to find the source of the bleeding. Even though the diverticula are situated on the left side of the colon the bleeding *is more often from the right side.*

A right paramedian incision is made and the whole of the colon inspected. If the source of bleeding is obscure there are then two alternatives: (*1*) to carry out a right-sided transverse colostomy; during the next 24 hr it will transpire whether the bleeding is coming from the left or right side of the colon; (*2*) to perform a total colectomy; either an ileorectal anastomosis can be made if the condition of the patient allows or the ileum should be brought out as an ileostomy and the distal end of the bowel as a mucous fistula. Continuity of the bowel can be restored later.

Of these two operations the latter is preferred, though the mortality can be in the region of 10–20 per cent.

[The illustrations for this Chapter on Operations for Diffuse Diverticular Disease of the Colon were drawn by Mr. G. Lyth from drawings by Mr. P. Drury.]

Ileocolic Anastomosis

W. W. Slack, M.Ch., F.R.C.S.
Consultant Surgeon, The Middlesex Hospital, London

PRE - OPERATIVE

Indications

An anastomosis of the ileum to any part of the colon, without any resection of a pathological lesion in the colon or terminal ileum, has a limited place in modern surgery. The exceptions are in some cases of obstructive Crohn's disease or in the presence of an irremovable tumour of the caecum or colon proximal to the sigmoid. Whenever possible, a primary growth in the colon should be removed and continuity restored, even though there may be secondary deposits in the liver. If the tumour is left *in situ*, haemorrhage from the ulcerated surface will continue and pericolic abscesses around the tumour may occur. An ileocolic anastomosis, therefore, in the presence of malignant disease is only palliative.

Preparation of patient

This operation is usually performed as an emergency for obstruction without any adequate bowel preparation. If time allows, an accepted antibiotic regime should be instituted pre-operatively, together with washouts of the distal colon.

THE OPERATIONS

1

Obstructing lesions of the terminal ileum and ileo-caecal region. The easiest operation is a side-to-side anastomosis between the ileum above the obstruction and the transverse colon.

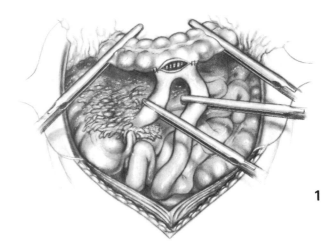

1

2

Obstructing lesions between the hepatic flexure and the descending colon. Similarly a side-to-side anastomosis is performed but between the ileum and the sigmoid colon.

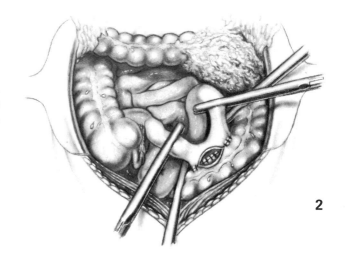

2

In both operations the technique is the same. A loop of ileum about 10 cm proximal to the obstruction is placed adjacent to either the transverse or the sigmoid colon and a series of interrupted seromuscular thread sutures (size 20) inserted between the two for a length of about 6–7 cm. Non-crushing clamps are then applied to the small intestine above and below the site of the anastomosis and if possible the colon as well, though the latter will probably be empty. The small and large intestine are then opened over a length of 4–5 cm and an all-layer suture of continuous 0/0 chromic catgut inserted to anastomose the opposing edges. The clamps are then removed and the anterior layer of seromuscular interrupted thread sutures is inserted.

It is advisable to leave a drain down to the site of all ileocolic anastomoses.

[*The illustrations for this Chapter on Ileocolic Anastomosis were drawn by Mr. G. Lyth from drawings by Mr. P. Drury.*]

Operations for Volvulus of the Colon

Murray T. Pheils, M.Chir., F.R.C.S., F.R.A.C.S.
Professor of Surgery, University of Sydney;
Surgeon, Repatriation General Hospital, Concord,
New South Wales

INTRODUCTION

Volvulus of the large bowel most frequently affects the sigmoid colon and is estimated to account for about 2 per cent of acute colonic obstructions in Western Communities. The condition occurs more frequently in Eastern Europe, in Asia amongst Indians, and in Africa amongst Bantu Communities. Volvulus of the caecum is a much rarer emergency and occasional cases have been reported of volvulus of the splenic flexure.

Volvulus of the sigmoid colon can only occur when there is an abnormally long pelvic mesocolon. This can be due to congenital factors, but in Western Communities it is usually acquired as a result of chronic constipation. The condition is consequently seen more frequently in the elderly and in patients with mental disorders. The increased incidence in other parts of the world is believed to be due to a diet with a high cereal content.

PRE - OPERATIVE

1

Clinical features

The patient presents with complete large bowel obstruction. There is gross abdominal distension with pain and tenderness in the left iliac fossa. The abdominal x-ray is diagnostic showing an enormously dilated sigmoid colon with a characteristic 'birds beak' or reversed U-sign appearance. This may be extended over the mid-line and up into the left hypochondrium. Non-operative reduction may be attempted by the method described by Bruusgaard.

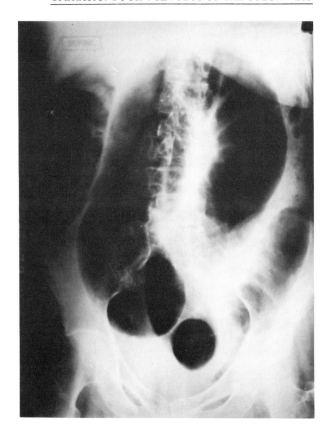

1

2

Non-operative reduction

The patient is placed in the knee—elbow position. A sigmoidoscope is inserted up to the site of the torsion and a lubricated rubber tube 60 cm in length is gently inserted. It may help to untwist the volvulus if a little air or water is instilled gently into the tube when it cannot be inserted further. If decompression is successful, the rectal tube is kept in place by suture to the peri-anal skin.

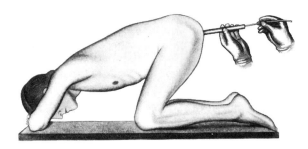

2

Indications for operation

Immediate laparotomy is indicated if non-operative reduction is unsuccessful, or if there is clinical, or sigmoidoscopic evidence of bowel strangulation. Elective resection is indicated after successful non-operative reduction in the majority of patients because of the risk of recurrence.

Preparation for laparotomy

The stomach should be emptied by means of naso-gastric suction. Blood should be available for transfusion in case strangulated bowel has to be resected. Intravenous infusion is commenced before induction of anaesthesia. Cephaloridine is administered at the start of the operation and for 48 hr postoperatively.

THE OPERATION

The incision

A lower (L) paramedian, or rectus-splitting incision provides the best exposure. The enormously distended sigmoid loop is delivered and examined for viability, especially at its base.

3

Untwisting

The torsion is usually in an anticlockwise direction and the bowel is gently untwisted. If the bowel is gangrenous, it should not be untwisted and immediate resection should be undertaken.

Resection

There are several alternative techniques. The traditional method is by the Paul Mikulicz exteriorization technique. Unfortunately this is unsatisfactory because the site of torsion is at the rectosigmoid junction and is too distal to be exteriorized. There have been several instances reported of ischaemia occurring in the distal segment after a Paul Mikulicz-type resection.

4

Preparation for resection

Vessels in the mesocolon are divided and doubly ligated. The affected segment of bowel is mobilized in preparation for resection. The distal end may be deep in the pelvis and require some mobilization posteriorly from the sacrum. If necessary the superior rectal vessels can be divided, but this is not mandatory as in cancer resection. Crushing clamps are placed on the segment of bowel to be resected, a non-crushing clamp is used to occlude the proximal bowel.

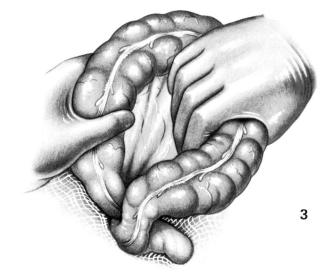

3

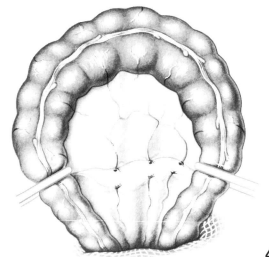

4

End-to-end anastomosis

Indications

Elective resection and end-to-end anastomosis is undertaken at least 7 days after successful non-operative reduction. Routine mechanical and antimicrobial bowel preparation is administered for 4 days pre-operatively. End-to-end anastomosis can also be undertaken as an emergency procedure in selected cases, such as in fit patients in whom the proximal bowel is empty and in whom non-operative reduction has been unsuccessful.

Preparation for anastomosis

The distal bowel is not clamped, but stay sutures are placed to demonstrate its lumen and facilitate anastomosis.

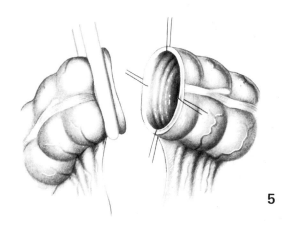

5

Anastomosis: posterior layer

The anastomosis is technically easy as there is an adequate length of bowel with a sizeable lumen. A posterior layer of 3/0 Ethiflex vertical mattress sutures is inserted through all layers.

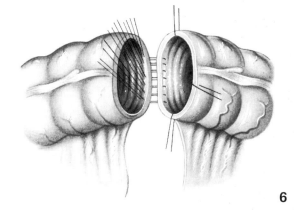

6

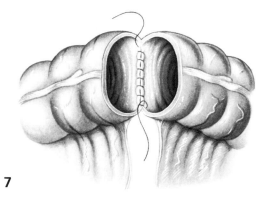

7

Anastomosis: inner layer

A continuous inner layer of 3/0 chromic catgut is inserted with some re-inforcing Ethiflex sutures at intervals.

8

Completion of anastomosis

The anterior layer 3/0 Ethiflex Lembert sutures completes the anastomosis. If the presacral space has been opened, it is drained with low-pressure suction for 2–3 days postoperatively. The mesentery is closed with interrupted stitches.

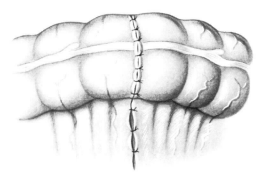

8

9

Excision without anastomosis

This is indicated in poor-risk patients, patients with a loaded proximal bowel and patients with a gangrenous loop. The proximal bowel can be brought out as an end colostomy through a muscle-splitting incision in the left iliac fossa. The distal end is either brought out through the lower end of the wound, or if there is insufficient length to bring it up to the abdominal wall, it can be closed in two layers and left in the pelvic peritoneal cavity.

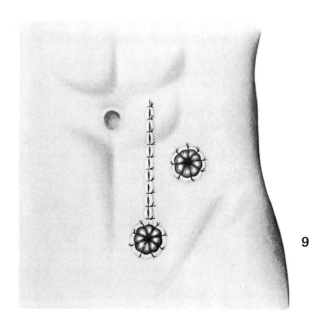

9

Closure of abdomen

The abdominal wound is closed with great care due to the risk of dehiscence. Non-absorbable sutures are used for the fascial layers and 2/0 nylon tension sutures are inserted through all layers except the peritoneum.

Formation of colostomies

Interrupted mucocutaneous sutures with 2/0 chromic catgut on an atraumatic needle are inserted around both proximal and distal colostomies. A plastic bag is fitted to the proximal colostomy in the operating theatre.

Closure of colostomy

This requires formal re-opening of the abdominal wound and mobilization of the proximal and distal ends. The anastomosis is carried out by the same technique as has been described for one-stage resection. The operation should be delayed until the patient is completely fit and all signs of local sepsis has subsided. This is usually at least 6 weeks after the resection, but can be deferred indefinitely in poor-risk patients.

Special risks

Anastomotic leak with consequent intraperitoneal sepsis is an especial risk following one-stage anastomosis and resection. The surgeon should not hesitate to carry out a temporary transverse colostomy should this occur. Careful attention to bowel habit is necessary during rehabilitation, as many of these patients have poor colonic tone resulting from chronic constipation.

Volvulus of the caecum

This is dependent on the caecum being intraperitoneal and having a mesentery. The straight x-ray is diagnostic, the distended caecum being situated in the left hypochondrium. The operation of choice is a standard right hemicolectomy with anastomosis of the ileum to the transverse colon. In poor-risk patients a simpler procedure is to untwist the volvulus and to fix the caecum in the right iliac fossa by means of a formal caecostomy with a skin-to-mucosa suture.

Reference

Bruusgaard, C. (1947). 'Volvulus of the sigmoid colon and its treatment.' *Surgery* **22**, 466

[*The illustrations for this Chapter on Operations for Volvulus of the Colon were drawn by Mr. M. Courtney.*]

Intractable Constipation and Adult Megacolon

Ian P. Todd, M.S., M.D.(Tor.), F.R.C.S., D.C.H.
Consultant Surgeon, St. Bartholomew's Hospital, St. Mark's Hospital
and King Edward VII Hospital for Officers, London

INTRODUCTION

A certain number of adults who have intractable constipation, require operation as the laxative life becomes intolerable, as each medicine in turn seems to become less and less effective as the large intestine becomes decompensated and unable to contract. Some of these patients have megacolon. Some have adult Hirschsprung's disease (aganglionosis). The author has one patient who had no bowel action for more than 1 year. As far as possible a diagnosis should be reached. In the author's opinion, a full thickness rectal biopsy should be taken, under anaesthesia, in all cases of adult megacolon, to prove or exclude Hirschsprung's disease. It is easy to mis-diagnose, and x-rays, internal sphincter function tests and special staining techniques of mucosal biopsies are less dependable in most people's hands.

If medical treatments have failed and surgery has been decided upon, the surgeon may be left in doubt as to what to do. The operation of choice in adult Hirschsprung's disease is Duhamel's operation with or without Martin's modification. Clamps will probably have to be used instead of stapling of the spur; most of the mega segment will need resection and a caecostomy may be wise, but otherwise the technique is much the same as in the infant (*see* pages 271–282).

Most authors agree that sigmoid colectomy is an unsatisfactory operation for idiopathic megacolon and even if there seems to be a redundant sigmoid colon improvement is seldom maintained for more than a few months. It is important to note the state of the colonic and rectal muscle when the abdomen is open. If the bowel is dilated and thin-walled, it is wiser to carry out a subtotal colectomy with caecorectal (or ascending colorectal) anastomosis (*see* pages 19–25). An ileorectal anastomosis is best avoided as incontinence, urgency or excessive frequency of actions often result (Lane and Todd). If the intestine is hypertrophic throughout but maximally in the rectum, this is probably due to a disorder of the rectosphincteric inhibitory reflexes: a resection is probably contra-indicated and a colostomy may be fashioned. Sphincterectomy procedures would seem logical but have seldom helped. This latter condition is, however, excessively rare.

FULL THICKNESS RECTAL BIOPSY

Pre-operative

As these patients may be very constipated, it may be necessary to spend many days cleaning out the intestine. It is, however, essential that the bowel should be clear before this diagnostic procedure is carried out if dangerous extrarectal sepsis is to be avoided.

THE OPERATION

A general anaesthetic is necessary. The patient is placed in the lithotomy position and an Eisenhammer or Parks speculum passed. The biopsy is best taken from the left posterior quadrant. It must be from above the upper limit of the internal sphincter muscle which is an aganglionic area. Stay sutures of 2/0 catgut should be placed through the full thickness of the rectal wall in this area, having palpated the anorectal ring, the upper limit of the sphincteric complex, with the finger. These should be 2–3 cm apart and each should be tied.

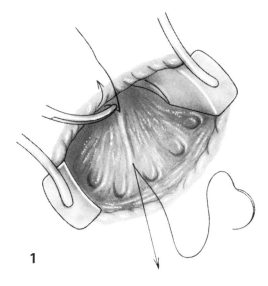

1

One end of the upper stitch is left long. An artery forcep is placed on to the other short end and this is pushed forwards and upwards by an assistant. One end of the lower stitch is pulled downwards and backwards by the operator. The other with the atraumatic needle still attached is left to oversew, in one full thickness layer, the defect when the piece of tissue has been removed. It is then tied to the remaining long end of the upper stitch. The purpose of the two stay stitches is, however, to raise and control a full thickness ridge of rectal wall to facilitate removal of the tissue. A sucker to remove blood is advisable.

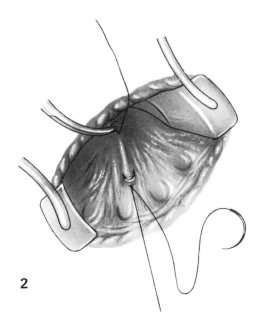

2

A 3 mm transverse incision is made with scissors directly backwards through the full thickness of the bowel wall, immediately above the lower stay stitch. As soon as the muscle coat is seen, it should be grasped with forceps and it should not be let go of, as it tends to contract excessively and a mucosal biopsy can easily result.

3 & 4

Parallel cuts 3 mm apart are then made vertically up (longitudinally) the rectum to the upper stay suture, when the biopsy is removed. The defect is then closed with the running continuous sutures of 2/0 catgut of the lower stay stitch and tied to the upper stay. The retractor is closed slightly to see if bleeding is controlled. A further full thickness stitch may be inserted if necessary and a piece of haemostatic gauze placed on to the area (Oxycel).

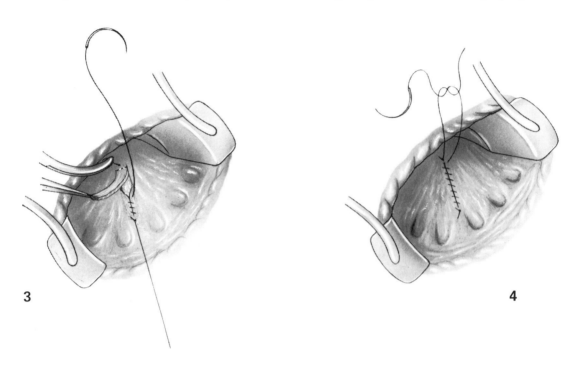

3   4

POSTOPERATIVE CARE AND COMPLICATIONS

No special care is needed postoperatively but hydrophilic bulk stool softeners are to be preferred to paraffin to initiate bowel actions. No postrectal abscesses or fistulae have resulted from this procedure in the author's series. Nor has a secondary haemorrhage occurred.

[*The illustrations for this Chapter on Intractable Constipation and Adult Megacolon were drawn by Mr. F. Price.*]

Hirschsprung's Disease

H. Homewood Nixon, M.A., M.B., B.Chir., F.R.C.S.(Eng.), Hon. F.A.A.P.
Consultant Paediatric Surgeon, The Hospital for Sick Children,
Great Ormond Street, Paddington Green Children's Hospital,
and St. Mary's Hospital Group, London

PRE - OPERATIVE

Most patients now present in the first weeks or months of life when a colostomy is the usual primary treatment. Should the baby have a complicating enterocolitis this treatment may be a matter of great urgency.

Right transverse colostomy is preferred in the usual case. Ileostomy may be necessary if a long aganglionic segment is present. Should unrelieved obstruction necessitate colostomy in the first days of life the author prefers Swenson's plan of colostomy immediately above the transition to ganglionic bowel so that all the normal bowel continues to function, develop and lengthen its mesenteric vessels. This facilitates the later pull-through procedure.

Cases, diagnosed when older, may sometimes be maintained in good health by daily rectal irrigations for primary definitive operation—at which time the author now always performs a covering colostomy, although some believe this to be unnecessary. Colostomy cover does not reduce the incidence of anastomotic complications but virtually eliminates serious consequences.

Four main operations are extant (*see Illustrations 1–3*). Duhamel's operation modified by the use of the mechanical stapler is found more convenient in infancy but there is little to choose between it and the Swenson operation except for long-segment cases. In these the extra 'reservoir' of the Duhamel neorectum seems to make convalescence easier. When total colectomy is necessary a period of several months with an ileostomy to allow 'colonization' of the ileum appears more useful than the construction of a longer neorectum in avoiding later fluid balance problems. Both the Swenson and Duhamel operations have been found satisfactory over a long period of follow-up.

Whilst the results of Soave's operation have been good the need for postoperative dilatations can be troublesome. The 'sutured Soave' (Denda operation) avoids this need but requires great care in suturing to avoid retraction of the colon within the muscular cuff.

On theoretical grounds the author has not used Rehbein's operation but good results in large carefully followed series are reported.

For secondary treatment after an inadequate resection, Duhamel's operation is usually preferred since a second eversion of the anal canal may jeopardize its blood supply. The colon is brought down to one side of the mid-line to avoid crushing the marginal vessels to the bowel brought down at the previous operation.

For those cases requiring a secondary operation for rectovaginal or recto-urethral fistula following unsatisfactory earlier surgery the Soave procedure is preferred. It avoids a difficult dissection which may damage the nerve supply to the bladder neck.

Definitive surgery has been carried out from 6 weeks old onwards. If colostomy has been carried out, delay for 6–9 months is usual. 'Toddlers' are more likely to be upset by operation and may be difficult to train afterwards.

Pre-operative preparation

If a neonatal colostomy has been made a weekly rectal digital examination and distal loop irrigation should be carried out. This minimizes disuse contracture of the anus and avoids inspissation of mucus and retention of any overflow faeces in the bowel.

Those without a colostomy have daily rectal irrigations of normal saline (using up to 11·5 litres in small quantities in older children) until thoroughly clear. This may take 1 or even 2 weeks.

Five days' bowel preparation with an insoluble sulphonamide is given but more reliance is placed on thorough mechanical cleansing.

TYPES OF OPERATION

1a-d

Swenson's operation

Resection of the aganglionic segment and pull-through abdomino-anal anastomosis. Dissection *on* muscle coat to avoid pelvic splanchnic damage.

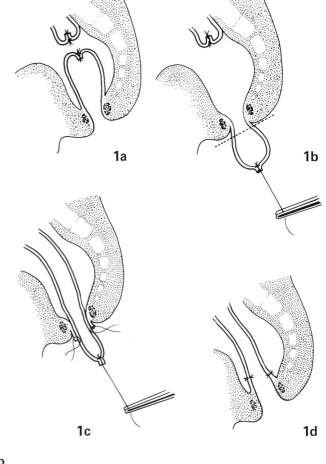

1a

1b

1c

1d

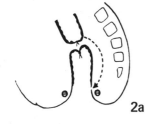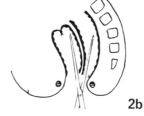

2a

2b

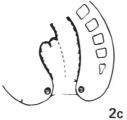

2c

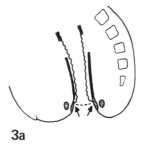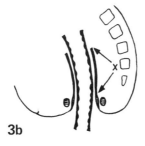

3a

3b

2a, b & c

Duhamel's operation

Rectorectal transanal pull-through.

3a & b

Soave's operation

Submucous endorectal pull-through.

Rehbein's operation (not illustrated)

Anterior resection with forcible divulsion of the sphincter.

THE OPERATIONS

SWENSON'S OPERATION

4a&b

Position of patient

Semilithotomy position on a baby table (made by the hospital carpenter) to strap on to the main table allows the use of the main tilt and elevation controls.

The sacrum is extended over the table end, falling back to allow a direct view down the pelvis, since all dissection is from the abdomen. The catheter in the bladder is left open to drain during the operation.

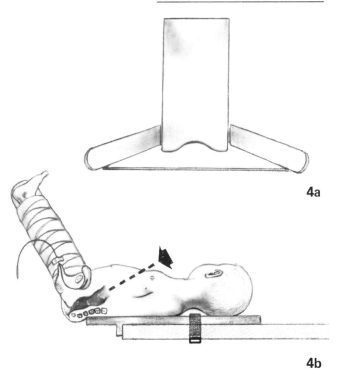

4a

4b

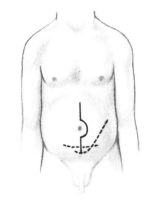

5

5

The incision

The author prefers a mid-line incision. If there is a left iliac fossa colostomy a hockey stick incision may be preferred to include this.

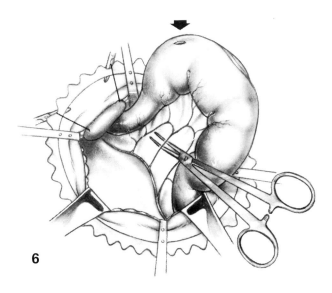

6

6

Placing of Denis Browne retractor

The bladder is drawn forward out of the pelvis by stay sutures. The retractor is positioned. A biopsy for frozen section confirms the safe level for resection (arrowed). Disposition of sigmoid vessels is demonstrated by transmitted light after division of the lateral 'congenital adhesion' to the sigmoid mesentery.

7

Mobilization of the sigmoid

The sigmoid vessels are divided individually retaining the marginal vessels. The superior rectal artery is ligated in continuity to reduce bleeding during pelvic dissection. A marker stitch is placed at the level of good blood supply.

The peritoneal incision is carried around the bowel high *above* the pelvic reflection and deepened to expose the longitudinal muscle layer of the upper part of the rectum.

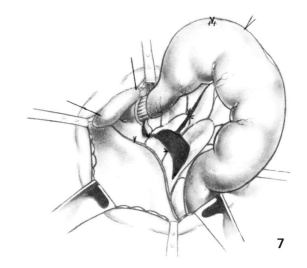

8

Dissection on muscle coat of rectum down to upper end of anal canal

Individual terminal branches of vessels are tied or diathermied as the assistant demonstrates them by traction on the rectum upwards and away from each quadrant in turn. The muscular plane is *crucial* to preservation of the pelvic splanchnics.

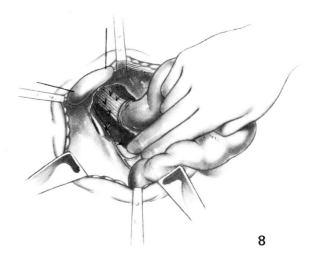

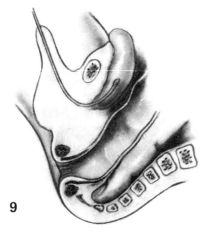

9

A finger tip rocking the coccyx indicates that the correct level is reached. It can be confirmed if necessary by putting a second glove over that on the left hand and bimanual palpation with a finger in the anus.

10

Resection of segment of bowel

The segment of bowel between the rectum and the site confirmed by biopsy and blood supply as suitable for pull-through is resected and the ends oversewn.

At this point time is saved if the team divides with an anal and an abdominal operator.

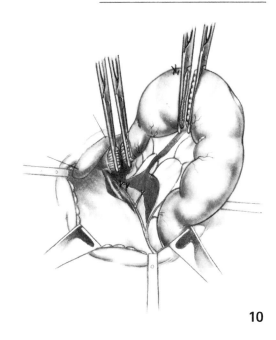

10

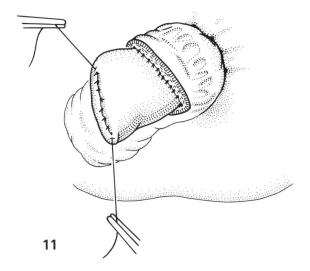

11

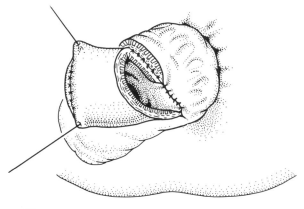

12

Anal phase

Prolapse of rectum and pull-through anastomosis

The mobilized rectum is prolapsed outside the anus by passing a forceps from the anus up its lumen, seizing the upper end and withdrawing it, and its mucosal surface cleansed with antiseptic. (If freeing is found to be incomplete it can be returned to the abdomen for further mobilization.) Ideally the mobilization should allow complete eversion of the anal canal when traction is exerted on the rectum but with spontaneous re-inversion of the anal canal when traction is released.

11 & 12

One half of the rectum is transected from a level 1–2 cm above the dentate line anteriorly (depending on the size of the patient) and extending obliquely down to the dentate line posteriorly (this should, therefore, include an upper partial internal sphincterectomy). The colon is drawn down to this incision and an outer layer of 3/0 silk sutures is placed. The same side of the end of the pulled-through colon is then opened and an inner layer of 3/0 chromic catgut sutures is placed.

The other half of the anastomosis is then made similarly and is allowed to retract within the anus.

Further abdominal phase

The pulled-through colon is attached to the posterior abdominal wall by a few sutures to close the potential gap behind the mesenteric vessels. No attempt is made to close the pelvic peritoneum.

A soft drain is laid in the pelvis and the upper end brought out through a stab wound in the left iliac fossa. Low pressure suction-drainage is preferred for 48 hr.

A proximal covering colostomy is made if not already present.

The wound is closed in layers.

POSTOPERATIVE CARE

The urethral catheter is removed after 24 hr. The abdomen should remain flat and the colostomy usually acts within 48 hr. No routine rectal examination is carried out for 7 days. A radiographic 'distal loopogram' is performed 10 days after operation. If satisfactory the colostomy is closed 14 days after operation. If a leak is revealed this is delayed.

VARIATIONS IN PARTICULAR CIRCUMSTANCES

Denis Browne modification

The object is to avoid any division of bowel within the abdomen. It is applicable when the megacolon is not too gross.

13

Introduction of sigmoidoscope

A sigmoidoscope is passed up to present its distal end above the pubes. A needle longer than the sigmoidoscope is threaded with a 1·5-m loop of thick 'plaited silk' passed around the mobilized bowel. The needle is then inserted through the bowel wall just proximal to the sigmoidoscope, withdrawn outside the anus and the silk snugged down at the distal end of the instrument. Traction on the silk and sigmoidoscope together prolapse the bowel.

Incision of outer layer

The outer layer is incised down to just above the anal canal anteriorly—from 1 cm above the anal columns in a small infant to 2 cm in an adolescent.

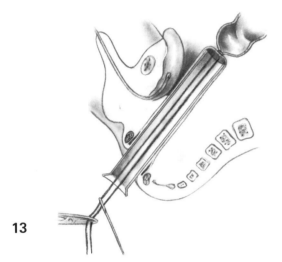

13

14, 15a & b

Completion of bowel division

The inner layer is withdrawn until the marker stitch and is opened in turn. A 'suture plug' of suitable size is inserted and circumferential division of the bowel completed in quadrants, attaching each in turn to the plug for control during the anastomosis. The anastomosis is made obliquely reaching down almost to the dentate line posteriorly. Denis Browne mattress sutures are used and should be tied fairly loosely.

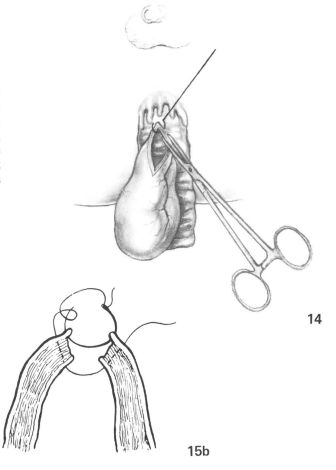

14

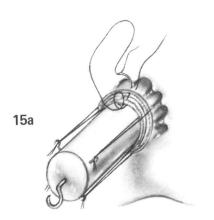

15a

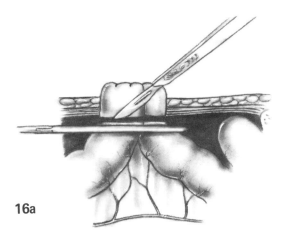

15b

16a & b

Presence of preliminary colostomy

If a preliminary colostomy has been made just above the cone this is taken down and both ends of the bowel closed by suture. The bowel distal to the colostomy is then mobilized in the usual way for resection and that proximal to it is mobilized for the 'pull-through' to the anal canal.

If a right transverse colostomy has been made for a usual length segment it is left as a covering colostomy and closed 2 weeks later when the anastomosis is soundly healed.

Long segment cases

If a long segment involves pull-through of right colon this is completely mobilized and rotated 180° down around the axis of the ileocolic vessels. If only a part of the ascending colon is ganglionic it is preferable to resect this and perform an ileorectal Duhamel procedure after at least 3 months with an ileostomy.

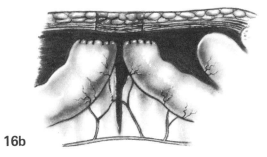

16a

16b

DUHAMEL OPERATION WITH STAPLER

Mobilization of the sigmoid

Exposure is obtained as in the Swenson operation, the sigmoid colon is mobilized in the same way but the superior rectal artery is preserved because the rectum is retained in this operation.

Division of the colon

The bowel is divided at a suitable point for pull-through as confirmed by frozen section biopsy.

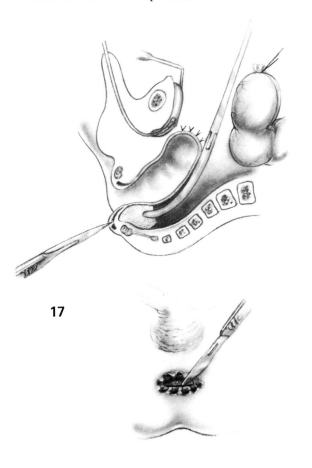

17

17

Retrorectal, transanal pull-through

The colon is drawn forward over the pubes and the retrorectal space is easily opened by blunt dissection with the index finger.

A small swab held in a long curved forceps is then thrust down this space to evert the posterior wall of the anal canal. An incision is made across the posterior wall of the anal canal just above the dentate line exposing the swab. (This leaves the lower half of the internal sphincter intact.)

The swab is seized from below with another forceps and this forceps is guided up into the abdomen by traction on the upper forceps. The swab is released and the sutures on the colon are grasped in the forceps. The colon is then drawn down to the incision in the anal canal, sutured to this incision and its end opened.

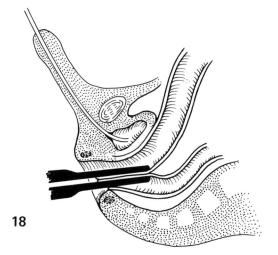

18

18

Application of the stapler

The GIA stapler is then inserted, one limb in the rectum and the other in the pulled-down colon. Activation of the stapler then divides the septum between colon and rectum over 5 cm leaving two overlapping layers of staples on each side of the cut.

Note: The bowel wall in Hirschsprung's disease is commonly so thickened that the 'adult' sized staples may be needed for all but young infants, rather than the 'paediatric' size.

19

Division of the rectum

The distal colon is drawn upwards and forward demonstrating the upper end of the stapled 'lateral anastomosis'. The rectum is divided at this level, cutting obliquely forwards and downwards. The open end is closed with a running 3/0 catgut suture and a second layer of interrupted 3/0 silks.

The author completes the operation with a proximal colostomy although many believe it unnecessary. A drain is placed from the left iliac fossa before the abdomen is closed in layers.

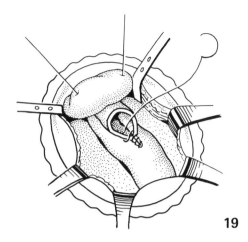

19

The Duhamel operation in older children

In older children the 5 cm division by the stapler does not reach the level of the peritoneal reflection which is preferred for division of the rectum. In such cases the stapler is first applied from within the

abdomen. A stab wound is made in the rectum at the level of the peritoneal reflection and another in the adjacent anterior wall of the colon. The stapler is then placed with one limb in each and its action then forms the upper part of the neorectum. The instrument is then re-inserted from below to complete the division of the septum.

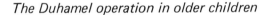

DUHAMEL OPERATION WITHOUT THE STAPLER

20a & b

Martin's modification

The upper end of the rectum is left open and sutured to an incision in the anterior surface of the colon at the same level. The modified Lloyd-Davies' or similar crushing clamp is then placed with one blade in the rectum and the other in the pulled-down colon as illustrated, under direct vision before the anastomosis of the upper end of the rectum to the opening in the colon is completed. The clamps are tightened in the usual way and separate in 4–5 days. (This avoids any risk of a blind anterior pouch which sometimes followed the original Duhamel technique if the spur was not crushed right to the apex. Such a pouch could be the site of faecal impaction.)

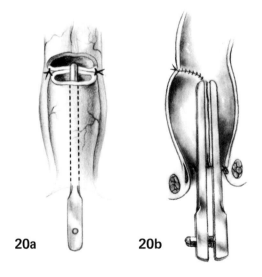

20a   **20b**

SOAVE'S OPERATION

21

In this procedure also care is taken to retain the superior rectal artery because the muscle coat of the rectum is to be retained.

Saline injections help to find the submucous plane in which blunt pledget dissection is carried down to the anal canal. A few scissor snips may be required. Gauze pressure is sufficient to stop bleeding from the small vessels divided. The rectal muscle tube is slightly dilated.

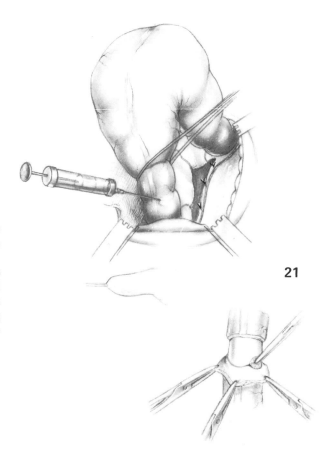

21

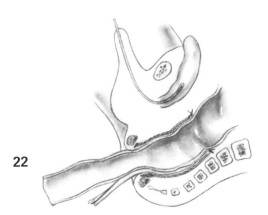

22

22

The anastomosis

The anus is dilated and the mucosa divided at the upper end of the anal canal. The colon is pulled through to the desired level and fixed with sutures to the upper end of the rectal muscle tube. A few loosely tied sutures also hold the bowel to the skin at the anal verge and a Penrose drain lies in the space between the colon and the rectal muscle tube.

A few inches of colon are left protruding; 21 days later, when the colon is adherent to the rectal muscle, the external excess is cut off with diathermy at the anal orifice.

Dilatations of the 'non-suture anastomosis' will be necessary daily for several weeks. At first the anastomosis feels very thickened (like a cervix) but this settles down surprisingly well.

23

Denda's technique

A similar procedure has been described by Scott Boley. The colon is divided at the anus and sutured to the free edge of the mucosa at the upper end of the anal canal. It is *essential* also to place a few deep sutures through the full thickness of the lower rectal wall to avoid retraction within the rectal cuff. These sutures are placed by everting each quadrant of the anal canal in turn with Allis' forceps.

A covering colostomy is constructed before wound closure.

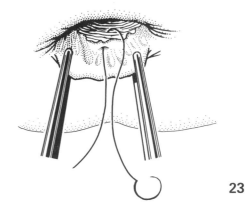

23

Anorectal myectomy for ultrashort segment Hirschsprung's disease

A group of patients with milder symptoms of constipation has been recognized in recent years and called ultrashort segment disease. Barium enema may not demonstrate an unexpanded distal segment but anorectal manometry and/or biopsy may be typical of aganglionosis. Anorectal myectomy to weaken the internal sphincter may be adequate treatment for these.

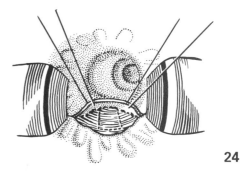

24

24

The anus is held open with a child-sized Goligher retractor and a transverse incision is made across the posterior wall of the anal canal just above the dentate line. The mucosa is elevated from the underlying muscle largely by blunt dissection and held forward by stay sutures.

A strip of internal sphincter is excised from 5 to 10 mm wide depending on the size of the child and the excision is extended as far proximally as can conveniently be reached—usually 5–8 cm.

The wound is then closed with a running suture of catgut without drainage.

Note: although these are called ultrashort segment cases, sometimes the entire resected strip is aganglionic even though the operation is clinically successful. It would be more precise to say that they are an uncommon mild variant presenting as chronic constipation without obstructive symptoms and usually having a very short segment. The variation in histological picture of aganglionic segments described by Garrett and Howard (1969) would explain this presentation.

References

Boley, S. J., Lafer, D. J., Kleinhaus, S., Cohn, B. D., Mestel, A. L. and Kottmeier, P. K. (1968). 'Endorectal pull-through procedure for Hirschsprung's disease with and without primary anastomosis.' *J. pediat. Surg.* **3**, 258

Denda, T. (1966). 'Soave-Denda operation.' *J. Jap. Ass. ped. Surg.* **2**, 37

Duhamel, B. (1960). 'A new operation for the treatment of Hirschsprung's disease.' *Archs Dis. Childh.* **35**, 38

Ehrenpreis, Th. (1970). *Hirschsprung's Disease.* Chicago: Year Book Medical Publishers

Garrett, J. R., Howard, E. R. and Nixon, H. H. (1969). 'Autonomic nerves in rectum and colon in Hirschsprung's Disease.' *Archs Dis. Childh.* **44**, 406

Lynn, H. B. (1968). 'Personal experience with rectal myectomy in the treatment of selected cases of aganglionic megacolon.' *Z. Kinderchirurg.* **5**, suppl. 98

Martin, L. W. and Caudill, D. R. (1967). 'A method for elimination of the blind rectal pouch in the Duhamel operation for Hirschsprung's disease.' *Surgery* **62**, 951

Rehbein, F. and von Zimmermann, H. (1960). 'Results with abdominal resection is Hirschsprung's disease.' *Archs Dis. Childh.* **35**, 29

Soave, F. (1964). 'Hirschsprung's disease: A new surgical technique.' *Archs Dis. Childh.* **39**, 116

Steichen, F. M., Talbert, J. L. and Ravitch, M. M. (1968). 'Primary side to side colorectal anastomosis in the Duhamel operation for Hirschsprung's disease.' *Surgery* **64**, 475

Swenson, O. (1964). Sphincterotomy in the treatment of Hirschsprung's disease.' *Ann. Surg.* **160**, 540

[*The illustrations for this Chapter on Hirschsprung's Disease were drawn by Mr. G. Lyth and Mr. P. Jack.*]

Imperforate Anus with Low Opening

Alexander H. Bill, Jr., M.D., F.A.C.S.
Chief of Surgical Services, The Children's Orthopedic Hospital and
Medical Center, Seattle, Washington and Clinical Professor of Surgery,
University of Washington School of Medicine

PRE-OPERATIVE

Indications

In about half of the infants born with imperforate anus
the lower end of the rectum and its opening lie below
the pubococcygeal line. In these cases the rectum is
within the grasp of the puborectalis muscle, which
provides much of the rectal control.

1

Low abnormal rectal openings of male

In males, the openings will be on the perineum
anterior to the position of the normal anus. Sometimes there will be a small tract extending to the
scrotum.

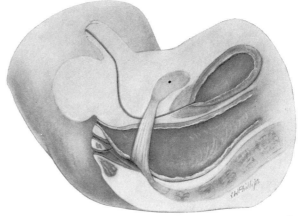

1

283

2

Usual low abnormal rectal openings in female

In the females, the opening will be into the lower vagina, the fossa navicularis, or anteriorly placed on the perineum.

In these infants, both male and female, the surgical aim is to bring the rectal opening back within the external sphincter muscles, and to make the opening large enough.

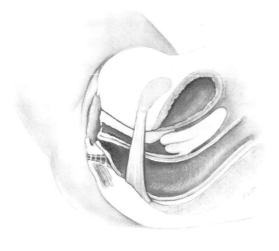

2

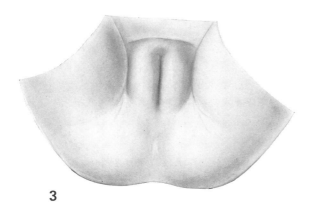

3

3

Appearance of female with rectofourchette fistula

The female infant who is born with no opening on the perineum will usually have a fistula into the fourchette. These may be predicted by the presence of a normal appearing hymen. The fistula is always distal to the hymen. These infants may be treated by means of a single operation without a preliminary colostomy.

4

Dilatation of rectofourchette fistula

When such an infant is first seen, the tip of a haemostat is pushed gently against the area of the fourchette. If it enters a fistula just distal to the hymen, the fistula is dilated. If the fistula is found to be just beneath the cervix, the rectum is above the levators. Then a preliminary colostomy must be done, followed later by an abdominoperineal procedure (*see* Chapter on 'Conservative Excision of the Rectum', pages 26–29).

The low fistula is kept dilated to allow passage of faeces until the child is established. At about 8–10 lb (4–5 kg), the definitive repair is done. Before operation, the rectum must be cleansed thoroughly by antibiotics and enemas.

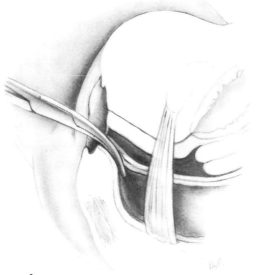

4

THE OPERATION

5

Position on table

The infant is positioned on the operating table with the lower legs folded over the abdomen and the thighs drawn up. The legs are secured in place by adhesive tape. An intravenous cannula is inserted into an arm or hand vein.

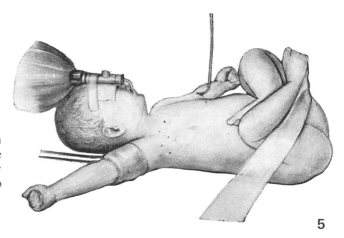

5

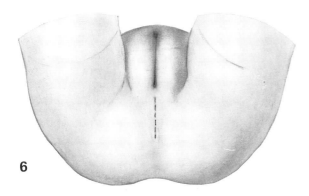

6

6

The incision

The incision is made from just behind the fourchette to a point just behind the position for the external sphincter muscles. These are beneath a flat area of skin which is somewhat shinier than the skin of the rest of the perineum.

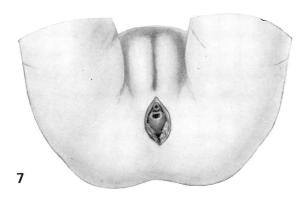

7

7

Division of fistula and dissection

The dissection is carried carefully to the lower surface of the rectum and its fistula into the vagina. Posteriorly, the sphincter muscles are divided in the mid-line. The sides of the rectum and the fistula are freed. The fistula to the fourchette is then divided.

8

Dissection of rectum from vagina

After the fistula is divided, the anterior rectal wall is meticulously separated from the posterior vagina. The tissues are very thin! The rectum is then dissected from its lateral attachments to allow it to swing downward and posteriorly.

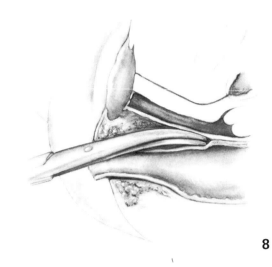

8

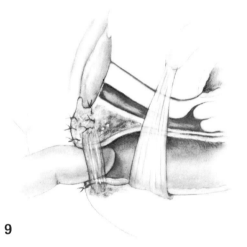

9

9

Retropositioning of tip of rectum

The rectum is moved posteriorly so that the rectal opening lies between the divided external sphincter muscles. The opening is made large enough to accept the operator's little finger. Care is taken that it will remain in the normal position without tension.

10

Final suture lines

The perineal body is then reconstructed with a few fine sutures. The rectal opening is sutured full thickness to the skin within the grasp of the external sphincter muscles. The perineal skin is closed.

Postoperatively the infant's legs are suspended by skin traction and the area is left exposed during healing.

The new anus should be dilated every day by the mother's finger for several months, starting 10 days after surgery.

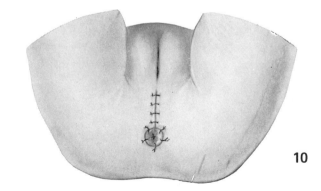

10

RECTOPERINEAL FISTULAE

Infants with the rectal opening anteriorly placed comprise about one-half of those with anorectal anomalies. These lesions are frequently unrecognized at birth, and are only diagnosed after the infant has become intractably constipated. The constipation is caused by the fact that the passage from the rectum is smaller than the normal anus, and is not distensible.

This condition is known by a variety of terms, including 'anteriorly placed rectal opening', 'covered anus', 'imperforate anus with rectoperineal fistula', and 'ectopic anus'. These lesions should be repaired at whatever age they are recognized. They may be repaired on the first day of life.

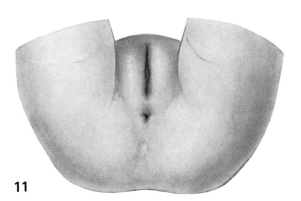

11

11

Rectoperineal fistula in female

In the female, the opening may be anywhere from the fourchette back to a position where it lies partly within the grasp of the external sphincter muscles. In all cases, the sphincter muscles should be in their normal position. The position of the sphincter can be recognized by the shiny, flat area of skin which overlies it.

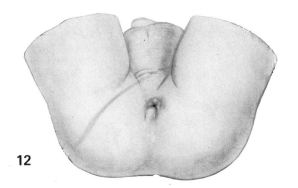

12

12

Rectoperineal fistula in male

In the male the small anterior opening may be anywhere from the posterior scrotum to the anterior part of the sphincter area. Sometimes there is a tiny meconium-filled tract along the median raphé of the scrotum.

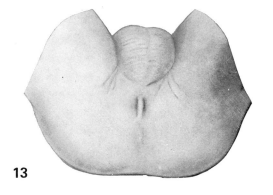

13

13

'Congenital median band' in male

In some male infants, the abnormal opening is covered by a longitudinal band of tissue covered with skin. This is known as a 'congenital median band'. The opening beneath it may be tiny. While it may appear to be normally placed, it is always anterior to the sphincters.

14

Skin incision for repair

The aim of the repair is to enlarge the opening and to bring most of it within the grasp of the external sphincter muscles. To do this, a triangular flap of skin and subcutaneous tissue is raised. Its base is over the posterior end of the sphincters. Its apex is at the posterior margin of the abnormal opening.

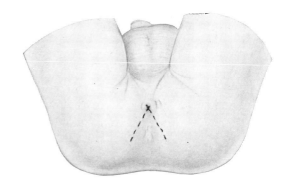

14

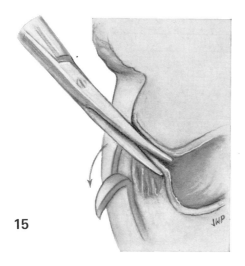

15

15

Division of lower wall of tract

When the skin flap is raised, the sphincter fibres will be found beneath and posteriorly; these are separated. Beneath these the wall of the lower rectum and the abnormal tract are dissected free. A mid-line incision is made through this.

16

Appearance of sphincters and incised tract

The posterior part of the enlarged opening will have sphincter fibres beside it along its posterior position. These provide control together with the puborectalis muscles.

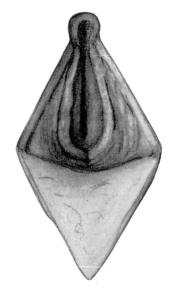

16

17

Placement of flap

The skin flap is brought inwards to lie in the posterior part of the incision in the bowel wall. It is sutured in place with 4/0 catgut sutures. The more anterior part of the incised tract is then sutured to the skin with similar through-and-through sutures of 4/0 catgut.

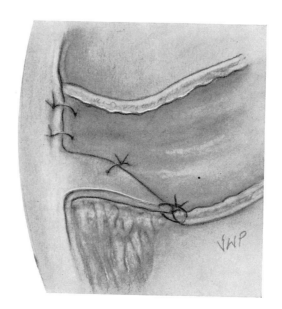

17

18

Final appearance

The new opening is lined by skin posteriorly. This prevents contracture. The skin on the sides tends to pull inwards with time, giving an adequate skin lining all around.

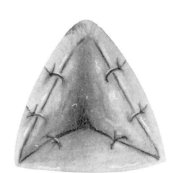

18

POSTOPERATIVE CARE

There is very little postoperative care necessary for this operation, other than ordinary cleanliness. After 12 days, dilatations with the mother's finger are started. These are continued for 2–3 months.

The following section on The 'Cutback' for 'Ectopic Anus' has been contributed by Mr. H. H. Nixon, F.R.C.S., Consultant Paediatric Surgeon, The Hospital for Sick Children, Great Ormond Street, London.

The 'cutback' for 'ectopic anus'

Forms 4, 15, 16, 17 and 18 of the International Classification of Anorectal Anomalies (Santulli *et al.*, 1970) consist of an anteriorly placed anus which has been called either a fistula or an ectopic anus. The point of practical importance is that the opening is below the levator ani sling and is proven capable of normal continence, retaining all the functional components of an anal canal except the unimportant subcutaneous external sphincter.

In Great Britain and some other regions a simple technique to enlarge this orifice in the first days of life is commonly the preferred primary treatment. It does not prevent anal transplantation (described on page 286) as a secondary procedure for that minority who require it for hygienic reasons. This can be done when the child is older, co-operative and continent.

The opening is, however, commonly too small. Dilatation alone is insufficient for more than a minor anterior displacement in the perineum because straining tends to force the stool down behind the opening ('defaecation block'). Hence there is a tendency to constipation which may lead eventually to overflow soiling. A simple mid-line episiotomy ('cutback') reduces this tendency.

19

One blade of the scissors is inserted into the orifice as far back as it will go under the skin. It is *not* allowed to go deeper lest the all important puborectalis sling be damaged. The other blade remains outside and closure of the scissors produces the episiotomy. The opening in the newborn will then be dilated to take a size 12 or 13 Hegar or the fifth finger. A few sutures may be placed for haemostasis but healing is probably better without careful complete mucocutaneous closure which may retain infection and encourage fibrosis.

Aftercare

The fifth finger or a similar sized dilator should be inserted daily for the next *3 months* until the anal canal is supple to avoid a tendency to develop rectal inertia and constipation. The mother can almost always be taught to do this from a few days after the operation. So the aftercare is completed before the baby reaches a psychologically vulnerable age (dilatations after about the fourth or fifth month of life can be very disturbing, hence delay in managing these conditions never benefits the patient).

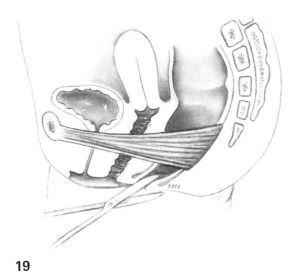

19

20

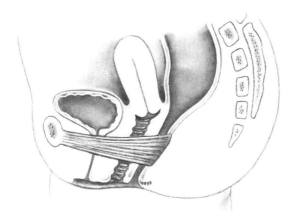

20

NOTE: A less common variant (Rectovestibular fistula, No. 20 in the International Classification) has a narrow segment running up parallel with the vagina before opening into a rectal ampulla. It can be recognized from the common type by probing. It is not suitable for cutback. Colostomy is usually the safest primary treatment.

References

Bill, A. H., Jr., Johnson, R. J. and Foster, R. A. (1958). 'Anteriorly placed rectal opening in the perineum; "Ectopic anus".' *Ann. Surg.* **147**, 173

Bill, A. H., Hall, D. G. and Johnson, R. J. (1975). 'Position of rectal fistula in relation to the hymen in 46 girls with imperforate anus.' *J. pediat. Surg.* **10**, 361

Browne, D. (1951). 'Some congenital deformities of the rectum, anus, vagina and urethra.' *Ann. R. Coll. Surg. Engl.* **8**, 173

Gross, R. E. (1953). *The Surgery of Infancy and Childhood.* Philadelphia: Saunders

Louw, J. H. (1965). 'Congenital abnormalities of the rectum and anus.' In *Current Problems in Surgery.* Chicago: Year Book Medical Publishers

Santulli, T. V., Kiesewetter, W. B. and Bill, A. H., Jr. (1970). 'Anorectal anomalies: a suggested international classification.' *J. pediat. Surg.* **5**, 281

Stephens, F.. D. (1963). *Congenital Malformations of the Rectum, Anus and Genito-Urinary Tracts.* Edinburgh and London: Livingstone

Stone, H. B. (1936). 'Imperforate anus with recto-vaginal cloaca.' *Ann. Surg.* **104**, 651

[The illustrations for this Chapter on Imperforate Anus with Low Opening were drawn by Mrs. J. W. Phillips and Mr. G. Lyth.]

Imperforate Anus with High Fistula

Alexander H. Bill, Jr., M.D., F.A.C.S.
Chief of Surgical Services, The Children's Orthopedic Hospital and
Medical Center, Seattle, Washington and Clinical Professor of Surgery,
University of Washington School of Medicine

PRE-OPERATIVE

Indications

Almost all babies with imperforate anus can be
expected to have a small fistulous connection from
the tip of the rectum to some other structure. Very
few will have a blind rectum.

Rectal continence will depend on the proper
placement of the rectum within the levator sling
muscles, as well as reconstruction of the external
sphincter muscles. The innervation of these muscles
must also be intact for function. When the fistula
is above the pubococcygeal line, the rectum will
not have descended to lie within the grasp of the
puborectalis muscles of the levator group.

Meticulous technique within the pelvis is necessary
in the reconstruction of the puborectalis muscular
sling. This is best done, following an initial colostomy,
when the infant is larger.

Pre-operative preparation for colostomy in the newborn

The colostomy should be carried out within the first
24 hr of life in order to prevent over-distension
and possible rupture of the thin bowel wall. During
the pre-operative period a suction tube should be
placed in the infant's stomach to remove as much
swallowed air as possible.

Anaesthesia and special aids

General anaesthesia administered through an intra-
tracheal tube is most satisfactory. A small plastic
cannula should be inserted in an ankle vein in the
operating room. Fluids may be given through this
during both the operative and the postoperative
periods, until the colostomy begins to function.

1

Positions of fistulae in male

In the male, the fistula will be to the lower bladder or to the urethra, usually through the prostate. If the rectum has 'descended' further, the opening will be on the perineum anterior to the normally placed external sphincter muscles.

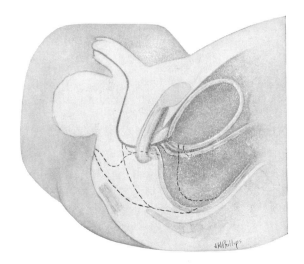

1

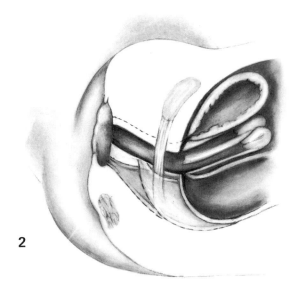

2

2

Positions of fistulae in female

In the female, the fistula will be to the posterior wall of a cloacal remnant, the fourchette or the perineum. Most frequently it is to the fourchette. In this chapter, however, we shall consider the treatment of the rectum lying high in the pelvis.

3

External appearance of male with fistula

The external sphincter muscles will usually be present in their usual position. Overlying them, the perineum is flat, and the skin is of slightly different texture from that of the surrounding area. If the innervation is intact, the underlying sphincter muscles can be made to pucker by pricking the adjacent skin with a pin. A colostomy is the first step preliminary to the repair.

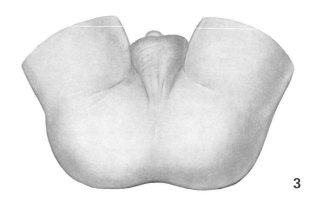

3

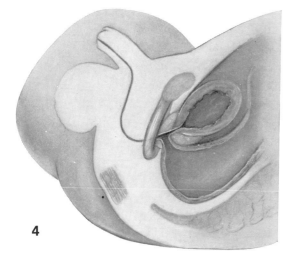

4

4

Sagittal section of male

The infant male with no opening on the perineum will almost always have a fistula from the rectum to the bladder or the urethra. This may be very tiny, and is sometimes impossible to demonstrate by urethrogram or the passage of meconium. The so-called upside-down x-ray view of the pelvis will very frequently *not* show the end of the rectum. This is likely to be full of meconium, which will not allow air beyond it.

THE OPERATION

5

Division of sigmoid

A subumbilical transverse incision is made, dividing
the rectus muscles. The enlarged sigmoid colon is
brought out through the incision. This bowel
is divided at its apex. The mesentery is divided and
dissected back from each end of the bowel for a
distance of 1·5 cm.

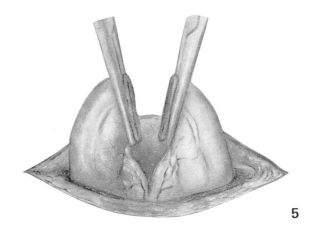

5

6

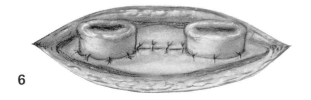

6

Peritoneal closure around bowel

The proximal end of the sigmoid is brought out at
the left extremity of the incision, and the distal end
at the right. The peritoneum is carefully sutured to
the serosa of the bowel with interrupted stitches of
5/0 silk on atraumatic needles. The openings through
the peritoneum are left large. The peritoneum between
the two pieces of bowel is closed.

7

Superficial closure and postoperative care

The fascia is closed between the bowel ends, and the
skin closed with subcuticular sutures of 5/0 or 6/0
silk.

When the colostomy site is healed, it is essential
that the stomas be dilated once daily by the parents.
A suitable sized Hegar dilator is excellent. The
dilatations must be continued as long as the colostomy
is maintained.

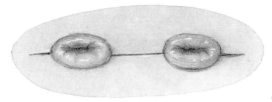

7

PULL-THROUGH OPERATION

Indications

The infant with the colostomy is then allowed to grow to a weight of 15 lb (6·8 kg). During the interval an intravenous urogram is performed to search for renal anomalies, which are not infrequently present. A film of the sacrum is also inspected. In the presence of important anomalies of the sacrum, the nerve supply to the perineum and to the pelvic structures may be absent, precluding successful control of the bladder or of a reconstructed rectum. In such a case, the child will need a permanent colostomy.

When his size and condition are adequate for repair, the proximal and distal sigmoid are cleansed by enemas and antibiotics.

8

Position on table

In the operating room the entire lower trunk, perineum, and thighs are prepared and draped. The infant is placed on sterile drapes so that he may be turned over without redraping. An intravenous cannula is inserted in an arm vein. A small metal sound is inserted into the urethra.

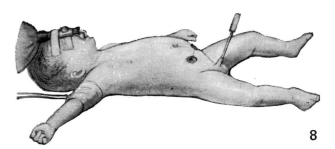

8

9

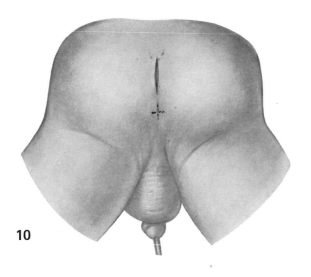

9

Position with buttocks elevated

The infant is then turned over with the tip of the sound in the bladder. The buttocks are elevated by means of a rolled sterile drape under the abdomen and hips.

10

Skin incision

A mid-line posterior perineal incision is made from the coccyx to a point 1·5 cm, posterior to the smooth area of skin which overlies the external sphincter muscles.

10

11

Exposure of urethra and puborectalis muscle

The incision is deepened carefully in the mid-line until the urethra is identified by feeling the sound. Surrounding the postero-inferior aspect of the urethra will be found the puborectalis muscle sling. The puborectalis muscle is *carefully* dissected from the urethra and then stretched *very gently* by means of a curved clamp to receive the bowel which will be brought down from above.

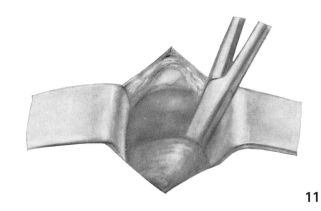

11

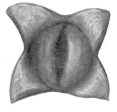

12

12

Incision over anal sphincters

A cruciate incision is made over the external sphincter muscles. The four small triangular flaps of skin and subcutaneous fat are turned back. The underlying sphincter muscles are identified and carefully dissected in the mid-line.

13

Haemostat placed in pelvis

A light curved haemostat is passed through the external sphincter muscles and up through the puborectalis sling. It is sutured firmly in place at the skin of the new anus, so that it will not slip out when the infant is turned over.

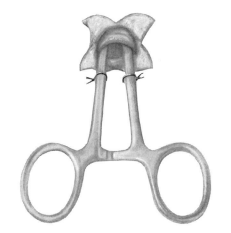

13

14

Closure of perineal incision

With the tip of the instrument 2 cm above the pubo-rectalis muscle, and with the handle sutured to the skin, the posterior perineal incision is closed in layers.

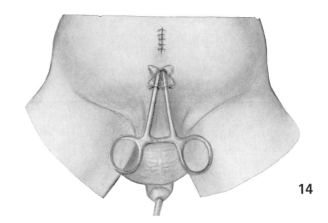

14

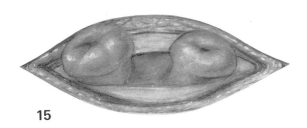

15

15

Re-opening of colostomy incision

The infant is then turned face upwards without redraping. The urethral sound is removed. The original transverse abdominal incision is re-opened, and the two ends of the sigmoid are dissected from the layers of the abdominal wall and from the peritoneum.

16

Shortening of distal bowel

The distal sigmoid is divided at the level of the bladder. The proximal sigmoid is temporarily closed with sutures which are left long. The inferior mesenteric vessels may require division to ensure that the end of the proximal bowel will reach the new anus.

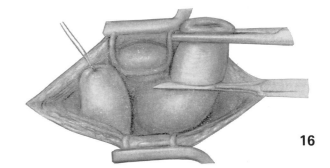

16

17

Dissection of mucosa of rectum

The mucosa of the distal sigmoid and rectum is dissected gently from the inside of the muscularis. This dissection is carried down to the fistula. Bleeding is controlled with the cautery.

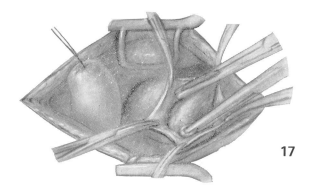

17

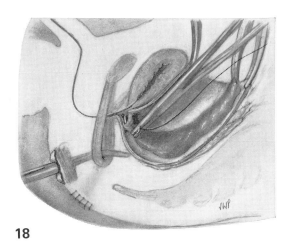

18

18

Closure of fistula

At this point, the mucosa is transfixed and tied off as it enters the fistula in the bladder or urethra. The mucosa is then divided proximal to the closed fistula and removed.

19

Incision of base of rectum

The serosa and muscularis of the rectum have been shortened to a level just above the pelvic peritoneal floor. The temporary sutures holding the clamp to the perineal skin are cut. The clamp is now thrust against the under-side of the original rectal stump. An incision is made through this from above, and the tip of the clamp pushed through it. The incision is widened adequately to accept the proximal bowel.

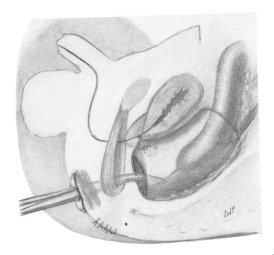

19

20

Proximal colon pulled through pelvis

The proximal bowel, which was once the colostomy stoma, is now pulled down by the sutures used to close it. It will traverse the serosa and muscularis of the original rectum, and it will be surrounded by the levators and the external sphincters.

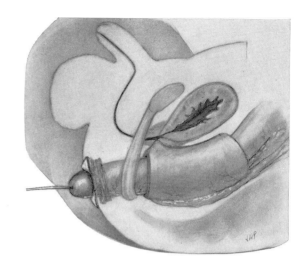

20

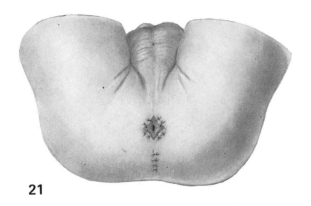

21

21

Construction of new anal opening

The end of the bowel is trimmed so that it will lie without tension at the level of the new anal skin. Four small notches are cut out, and the four triangular skin flaps are sutured into them with 4/0 chromic sutures.

22

Postoperative position

Postoperatively the patient is placed in balanced skin traction to the legs for 1 week with the incisions exposed. The incisions are cleansed frequently.

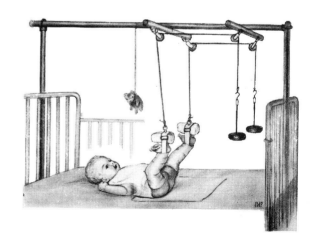

22

POSTOPERATIVE CARE

Starting on the tenth day after surgery, the new rectum is dilated daily for 2 months. The mother's finger, covered by a rubber finger cot, makes an excellent dilator. The dilatations must extend up through the levator muscle sling.

23

Female with high rectofourchette fistula

Although most female infants with imperforate anus will have a *low* rectofourchette fistula which can be treated without a colostomy (*see* Chapter on 'Imperforate Anus with Low Opening', pages 283–291), a few females will have a high fistula entering a cloacal remnant above the puborectalis muscle. Usually the urethra enters the cloacal remnant high on its anterior surface. These infants must have a colostomy and a later definitive operation, as in the preceding description for the males. In some, the rectum is so high that it is well to excise it entirely. The upper bowel is brought down without bringing it through the remnant of the rectum.

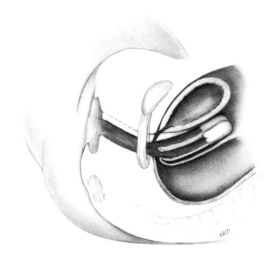

23

References

Bill, A. H., Jr. and Johnson, R. J. (1958). 'Failure of migration of the rectal opening as the cause for most cases of imperforate anus.' *Surgery Gynec. Obstet.* **106**, 643

Johnson, R. J., Palken, M., Derrick, W. and Bill, A. H. (1972). 'The embryology of high anorectal and associated genitourinary anomalies in the female.' *Surgery Gynec. Obstet.* **135**, 759

Kiesewetter, W. B. (1966). 'Imperforate anus: The role and results of the sacro-abdominoperineal operation.' *Ann. Surg.* **164**, 655

Kieswetter, W. B. and Nixon, H. H. (1967). 'Imperforate anus. 1. Its surgical anatomy.' *J. pediat. Surg.* **2**, 60

Louw, J. H. (1965). 'Congenital abnormalities of the rectum and anus.' In *Current Problems in Surgery*. Chicago: Year Book Publishers

Palken, M., Johnson, R. J., Derrick, W. and Bill, A. H. (1972). 'Clinical aspects of female patients with high anorectal agenesis.' *Surgery, Gynec. Obstet.* **135**, 411

Soave, F. (1964). 'Hirschsprung's disease: A new surgical technique.' *Archs Dis. Childh.* **39**, 116

Stephens, F. D. (1963). *Congenital Malformations of the Rectum, Anus, and Genito-Urinary Tracts.* Edinburgh: Livingstone

[*The illustrations for this Chapter on Imperforate Anus with High Fistula were drawn by Mrs. J. W. Phillips.*]

Coccygeal Teratoma (Sacrococcygeal Tumour) and other Postrectal Masses

John F. R. Bentley, F.R.C.S., F.R.C.S. (Ed.), F.R.C.S. (Glas.)
Consultant Surgeon, Royal Hospital for Sick Children,
Glasgow

PRE-OPERATIVE

This teratoma originates from totipotent cells derived from the primitive knot of the embryo. It is attached to the coccyx, and most often evident at birth as a large or gigantic mass taking one of three forms: (*1*) pedunculated; (*2*) sessile; or (*3*) dumb-bell, with an extension into the pelvis between the rectum and the sacrum, when the external protrusion is occasionally insignificant. The overlying skin is often normal, but it is infiltrated by angiomatous tissue on occasion. Sometimes large veins are visible through the skin. Ulceration can occur spontaneously, and this can be followed by dangerous haemorrhage. The tumour is partly cystic and partly solid and it is usually well defined. It contains glial elements and various other tissues such as nerve cells and fibres, dermal elements, pancreas, hamartomatous connective tissue, muscle and bone. Calcification is present in one third of the lesions, and three out of four occur in girls. Additional anomalies are present in nearly one fifth of the patients, these mostly affect the musculoskeletal system including the spine, but pre-operative neural deficit is rare. The differential diagnosis includes a low meningocele, which may be anterior to the spine, chordoma, neuroblastoma, hamartoma (lipoma or angioma), a cystic duplication of the rectum or a postrectal abscess. All these lesions are exceedingly rare, but the operative management for coccygeal teratoma can be adapted for their treatment.

Indications

The bulk of the tumour is often disfiguring and incapacitating but, more significantly, there is malignant change in half of the tumours excised after the first month of life. The benign tumours are often cystic with some calcification. The need for removal is particularly urgent with solid and dumb-bell tumours but seldom essential within a few days of birth. A further indication for early excision is the danger of bleeding from an ulcer. The overall mortality rate is about 25 per cent and pedunculated tumours have the best prognosis.

Contra-indications

Operation is contra-indicated where there is evidence of metastatic spread or other irremediable conditions such as other gross anomalies or generalized disease.

Pre-operative preparation

General preparation

Certain metabolic disorders of the newborn are rectified if they are present. They include:

(1) Hypoprothrombinaemia, which is remedied by the routine subcutaneous injection of 1 mg Konakion (phytomenadione) Hepatic biosynthesis of the vitamin K dependent clotting factors can be deficient so a 'thrombotest' is performed. If this is under 20 per cent, give 10 ml/kg body weight of fresh frozen plasma by intravenous infusion. Thereafter monitor the need for a repeated infusion by repeating the thrombotest after an interval of 10–12 hr.

(2) Hypoglycaemia, which is most common in premature, postmature and 'small for dates' infants and in those suffering neonatal asphyxia or with diabetic mothers. The condition is detected by frequent screening tests (with Dextrostix) and it seldom persists for more than 48 hr after birth. Treatment by the addition of glucose to the feeds is sufficient when the blood sugar is in the range 20–40 mg per cent but when the level is lower intravenous glucose is required (the initial dose of glucose 50 per cent solution is 2 ml/kg body weight; it is followed by divided doses of 10 per cent glucose, 50–100 ml/kg body weight per day).

(3) Hypocalcaemia may occur during the first 3 days of life in infants who have had exchange transfusions or in the second week of life in bottle-fed babies who are intolerant of the heavy phosphate load in cow's milk. It is often sufficient to sedate these hyperexcitable infants with 60 mg of chloral hydrate in syrup given 4-hourly but the addition of 1 g calcium lactate in each 45 ml of the feed will assist in restoring a biochemical balance.

Special preparation

Where impediment to the vesical outflow could be a result of pressure from a bulky tumour, an expressed mid-stream sample of urine is examined for evidence of infection so that appropriate medication can be given. In these circumstances it is wise to estimate the blood urea or serum creatinine and to perform excretory urography as hydronephrosis may be present. The bladder is emptied immediately before operation by a balloon catheter which is left in place. An opaque enema examination will seldom yield more information about the extent of the pelvic mass than can be deduced from the excretory urogram, abdominal palpation and digital rectal examination. Radiography of the lungs and skeleton is undertaken to exclude evidence of metastatic spread which is evident in 5 per cent of patients at the primary examination. Sonar scan may identify cystic lesions with their better prognosis. Radiotherapy may reduce the size of massive presacral lesions to facilitate excision. It is prudent to correct possible anaemia and to cross-match two units (each of 500 ml nominal) of donor blood of appropriate group to compensate for loss during and after operation.

Special equipment

The body temperature of a small infant is prone to fall during a major operation. When the operating room temperature is adjusted to allow the surgical team to work in comfort, special apparatus is needed to keep the infant warm. This can be done with a simple and effective device that is placed on the operating table; it consists of a small porous air mattress. A draught of warm air is impelled into the side by a tube from an electric blower (Climator, Type W. H., Howorth, Surgicair, Farnworth, England). The blood to be transfused is also warmed to body heat and warm, moist gases are used in inhalation anaesthesia. Temperature is monitored by a thermocouple probe in the oesophagus.

Anaesthesia

General endotracheal inhalation anaesthesia is preferred but for a major operation on an infant this requires special apparatus and skill. If excision of the tumour must be attempted when adverse circumstances preclude the use of general anaesthesia it is feasible to operate with local or spinal anaesthesia.

Sedation is then essential; it is obtained by subcutaneous injection of pethidine hydrochloride 1 mg/kg body weight. The use of local anaesthesia is restricted to pedunculated lesions; 0·5 per cent procaine with 1:250,000 adrenaline is infiltrated around the coccyx and into the pedicle in a dose not exceeding 5 mg (5 ml)/kg body weight. Spinal anaesthesia can be used for sessile or dumb-bell lesions. The infant is held with the back erect and cinchocaine (Nupercaine, Ciba 0·5 per cent solution, diluted with 7·5 parts of sterile 5 per cent dextrose injection B.P.), 1:1500 solution at 41°C is injected into the spinal theca through the interspace between the *fourth* and *fifth* lumbar vertebrae. Both the volume of anaesthetic used and the length of time the infant is held erect after the onset of the injection determine the upper level of the spinal block. The volume and time for obtaining blockade to thoracic 5 in infants is computed as follows.

Measure the distance (H) from the inter-nipple level (thoracic 4) to the inter-cristal level (lumbar 4) and where H occupies the range 7·5–17·5 cm or 3·5–7 inches the following formulae apply:

$$\text{Dose in ml} \quad \frac{H \text{ cm}}{50} \quad \text{or} \quad \frac{H \text{ inches}}{2}$$

$$\text{Time erect in sec} \quad \frac{H \text{ cm}}{5} \quad \text{or} \quad 5\,H \text{ inches}$$

(Four-fifths of these times will give mid-spinal anaesthesia).

Supportive treatment during operation

This is directed towards avoiding hypoxia, maintaining body temperature and combating oligaemic shock. The 'guesstimated' blood loss is replaced by transfusion as it occurs and *in addition* blood amounting to 22 ml/kg body weight is given slowly to occupy the expansion in the vascular compartment that occurs in response to bodily trauma. The rate and volume of transfusion may be monitored by measurement of the central venous pressure. The blood is infused through a nylon cannula 0·75 mm internal diameter inserted through the median cubital vein and arranged to communicate with a simple manometer. The transfusion is adjusted to restore the pre-operative level of central venous pressure (5–9 cm). To counter the chelating action of acid–citrate–dextrose donor blood, the cannula is flushed

with isotonic saline and 5 ml (50 mg) of 1 per cent calcium gluconate solution is injected after each 50 ml of blood is infused. The cannula is flushed again with isotonic saline before transfusion is resumed.

Positioning and draping

For opening the abdomen at the beginning and at the end of the operation the patient is supine, but for excising the tumour itself the patient is prone. For this perineopelvic phase of the operation a rolled towel supports the shoulders and a sandbag supports the pubes so that there is a free ventilatory excursion and the hips and knees can be flexed. Sterile drapes are placed to surround the operative field; they are renewed after each change of position.

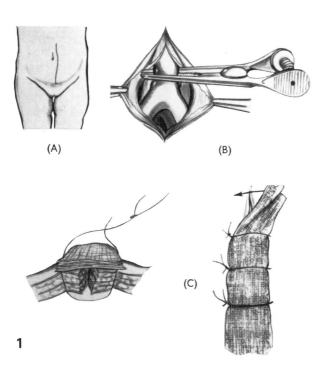

(A)

(B)

(C)

1

THE OPERATION

1

Preliminary exploratory laparotomy

A left lower paramedian incision (*A*) is made in patients with dumb-bell tumours (*1*) to determine the extent of the lesion within the pelvis, (*2*) to exclude gross metastatic spread within the abdomen, and (*3*) to define the distal aorta or common iliac arteries to which Potts' spring clamps (*B*) are applied to curtail haemorrhage during dissection of the tumour. The abdominal incision is then closed temporarily with transfixing 2/0 sutures tied over a gauze dressing (*C*) so that the patient can be repositioned for the perineopelvic dissection. Thereafter the patient is again placed supine and the abdominal wound is re-opened to remove the vascular clamps and to rectify any damage sustained by the pelvic peritoneum. Formal suture of the abdominal wall is then completed.

Perineopelvic excision of tumour

The coccyx is always excised together with the tumour but the muscles of the pelvic floor and the rectum and anal canal are preserved. The details that follow refer to the excision of a dumb-bell tumour.

2

Preliminary suture of anus

The rectum is packed with gauze impregnated with liquid paraffin (mineral oil) so that it can be felt more easily during dissection in the pelvis. The anus is then sutured temporarily with 2/0 silk. The suture and pack are removed at the conclusion of the operation.

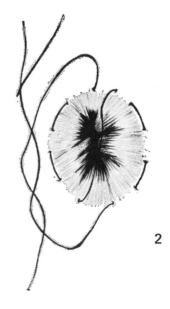

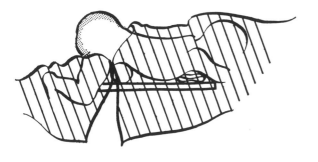

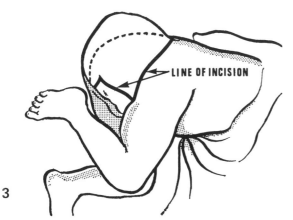

3

The incision

An inverted chevron incision is made extending behind the anus. From the lateral ends of this incision a second inverted chevron incision is made to pass behind the basal parts of the tumour. The apex of this incision extends posteriorly into the natal cleft to reach just proximal to the base of the coccyx.

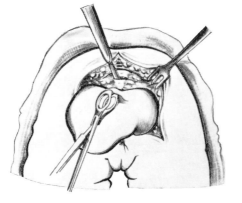

4

Posterior dissection

Define the base of the coccyx and divide the sacrococcygeal junction with a scalpel. Apply traction to the coccyx with Lane's tissue forceps and enlarge the sacrococcygeal cleft to admit the index finger.

5

Lateral dissection

Pass the tip of an index finger forwards and laterally deep to the mobilized coccyx and separate the muscles of the pelvic floor on each side from the surface of the tumour. Divide the muscles only at their medial margins around the tumour end and at their attachment to the coccyx.

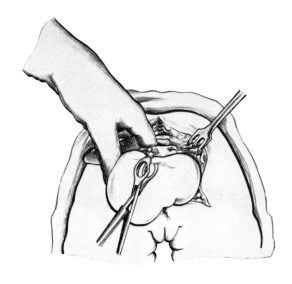

5

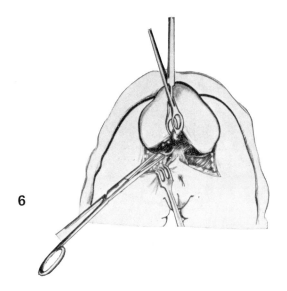

6

6

Anterior dissection

Displace the anal canal and rectum forwards and define the anterior surface of the tumour by finger dissection.

7

Enucleation of the pelvic extension

Enucleate the mass from the presacral space by a combination of traction and finger dissection. Secure haemostasis of the tumour bed with coagulating diathermy (blood flow through the vertebral anastomosis is sufficient to permit the bleeding points to be defined).

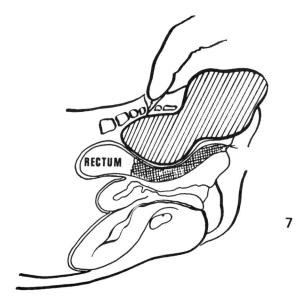

RECTUM

7

8

Closure of perineal wound

The muscles of the pelvic floor are stitched together in the mid-line with a continuous 3/0 chromic catgut suture. The presacral space is drained by a strip of corrugated rubber ensheathed in Paul's tubing or a Ragnall drain placed to emerge posteriorly at the apex of the wound. The skin is sutured with interrupted stitches of 3/0 silk. The anal suture and rectal pack are removed. Finally a pressure dressing is applied to the perineum with a crêpe bandage. Thereafter, the vascular clamps are recovered from the abdomen.

Very occasionally a two-stage operation may be indicated to resect residual or locally recurrent tumour, or to perform urinary or faecal deviation.

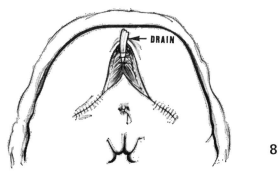

8

POSTOPERATIVE CARE

Small infants are nursed in an incubator to curtail the risk of cross-infection. Regulation of the controlled temperature within the incubator allows rapid restoration of normothermia, and enriching the atmosphere with oxygen helps to compensate for the increased alveolar dead space that accompanies oligaemic shock. Wrapping the infant in insulating aluminium foil is helpful in a convected heat incubator but it impairs the efficiency of a radiant heat incubator.

Management of oligaemic shock

Oligaemic shock follows extensive excisional surgery within the pelvis despite replenishment of the circulating volume during operation. Augmentation is therefore continued after operation on the same scale as that for a 30 per cent deep cutaneous burn, but blood is given in preference to plasma or dextran as oozing from the wound is probable. The volume to be transfused in the first 8 hr after operation will be approximately the equivalent in millilitres to 30 times the postoperative body weight in kilograms. The efficacy of this treatment can be monitored by the output of urine and the central venous pressure but the placement of a suitable cannula can present problems. For this reason it is often more practical to relate cardiac output and tissue perfusion to the pulse rate as determined electronically.

Acid-base balance

Metabolic acidosis is anticipated with oligaemic shock. It can be monitored with the Astrup apparatus on samples of arterial or capillary blood. Acidosis beyond a 'base excess' of −4 mEq/l of bicarbonate is reduced by the intravenous injection of 8·4 per cent sodium bicarbonate (dose in millilitres = one-third of the excessive base deficit multiplied by the body weight in kilograms). No attempt is made to neutralize the metabolic acidosis completely as a delayed metabolic alkalosis is probable when the citrate that accompanies the donor blood is metabolized to bicarbonate. This alkalosis is gradually rectified by the kidneys.

Postoperative sedation

Pethidine hydrochloride 1 mg/kg body weight is given by subcutaneous injection 4-hourly, if required.

Urinary drainage

Pelvic dissection is prone to disturb the reflex of micturition so balloon-catheter drainage of the bladder is continued for at least 3 days; it is resumed if there is a persisting liability to urinary retention. During this period prophylactic co-trimoxazole 62·5 mg is given 8-hourly by intramuscular injection, and the effect is observed by repeated culture of the urine.

Nutrition, including salt and water balance

Feeding is resumed gradually as soon as it is feasible but as the restoration of alimentation may be delayed by paralytic ileus 20 per cent laevulose is given intravenously in the interim to supply both water and calories. The water loss to be replenished daily can vary greatly; it is increased by pyrexia and a hot dry atmosphere, and conversely the trauma of birth or operation is followed by retention of water and sodium. Thus a *healthy* new-born infant in a temperate atmosphere needs only 40 ml of water per kilogram of body weight per day but this requirement increases fourfold at the age of 6 days. In the postnatal week the trauma of operation does not aggravate water and sodium retention very much but thereafter it will halve the renal loss for about 2 days. If the infant develops gaseous distension of the abdomen or bilious vomiting a nasogastric tube is inserted. It is kept unspigoted and aspirated to keep the stomach empty. To compensate for the consequent loss of secretions a comparable volume of half isotonic saline is added to daily intravenous intake. In view of the potassium load conferred by blood transfusion arbitrary intravenous replacement of potassium is contra-indicated.

Care of the wound

The pressure dressing and drain are removed as soon as the serous exudate ceases. The perineum is cleaned with 0·5 per cent aqueous chlorhexadine as soon as faecal soiling occurs and the wound is dried and dusted with compounded neomycin powder. The skin stitches are removed when the wound is healed, on about the tenth postoperative day.

Follow-up examinations

The patient is examined at regular intervals of a few months for 5 years to elicit signs of recurrence or metastasis. Radiotherapy or chemotherapy may be useful for residual or recurrent malignant tumours, specially if histology indicates a predominantly endodermal type of malignant component. Unhappily, there is no evidence that such treatment is effective for metastases. When complications in the urinary tract have included infection, hydronephrosis or a neuropathic bladder their progress is reviewed periodically and appropriate treatment is arranged.

References

Altman, R. P., Randolph, J. G. and Lilly, J. R. (1974). 'Sacrococcygeal teratoma: American Academy of Paediatrics, Surgical Section Survey, 1973.' *J. pediat. Surg.* 9, 389

Izant, R. J. (1962). 'Sacrococcygeal teratoma', In *Paediatric Surgery*, Vol. 2, p. 849. Chicago: Year Book Publishers

[The illustrations for this Chapter on Coccygeal Teratoma (Sacrococcygeal Tumour) and other Postrectal Masses were drawn by Miss J. McDonald.]

Excision of Peri-anal Haematoma

C. V. Mann, M.Ch., F.R.C.S.
Consultant Surgeon, St. Mark's Hospital, London
and The London Hospital

PRE-OPERATIVE

Indications

The lesion usually develops suddenly as a result of rupture of one of the subcutaneous external veins alongside the anal verge. The natural history of the condition is of an acutely painful swelling for several days, after which the lesion slowly subsides as the clot is re-absorbed. Occasionally, the haematoma causes pressure necrosis of the overlying skin and is extruded spontaneously: sometimes this process is incomplete.

As the usual course of the condition is to proceed to spontaneous cure, there is no absolute indication for surgical intervention. The later the patient is seen, the stronger is the case for conservative management unless complications have developed.

However, if the patient is seen early on, and especially if the pain is exceptionally severe, operative treatment can be advised. Surgery is indicated if the clot remains partially evacuated, or if an abscess develops. If an abscess is not operated upon, a subcutaneous fistula may result: this must also be treated surgically.

Contra-indications

As the operation can be performed satisfactorily under local anaesthesia, there are no general contra-indica-

tions. The patient's circumstances should be taken into consideration before advising surgery, as strenuous activity or prolonged sitting are best avoided for a few days afterwards.

Pre-operative preparation

No preparation is needed.

Anaesthesia

The operation can be performed under infiltration of the overlying skin by 1 per cent lignocaine solution plus adrenaline 1:200,000.

As the insertion of the local anaesthetic solution can be painful at the beginning, if the patient is exceptionally young or very nervous, a light general anaesthetic is to be preferred.

Position of patient

For the operation to be performed under local anaesthesia, the Sims position with the pelvis raised on a sandbag as described in the Chapter on 'Sigmoidoscopy' (*see* page 5) is ideal. The upper buttock should be strapped or held back by an assistant.

Under general anaesthesia, the lithotomy position can also be used.

THE OPERATION

1

Injection of local anaesthetic

The skin around the lesion is carefully cleaned with Hibitane 1:2000 solution. The finest needle should be used for the injection as the skin is very sensitive. The infiltration should include the area around the swelling, as indicated.

The best technique is to start the infiltration of the subcutaneous tissues around the haematoma before putting any of the solution beneath the skin directly over the lesion, where the increase in tension can cause considerable pain.

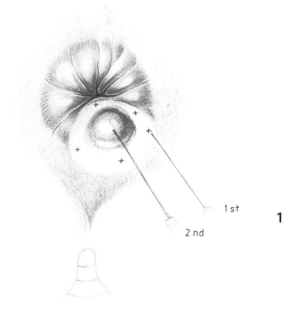

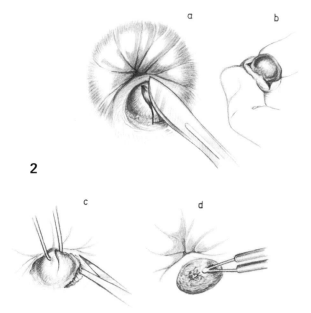

2

Evacuation of the haematoma

A short radial incision 1–2 cm long is made directly over the haematoma. The clot can then be squeezed out by gentle pressure with the thumbs and forefinger. Sometimes the haematoma is adherent, in which case it may have to be removed by sharp dissection with fine pointed scissors (iridectomy scissors are ideal for this purpose).

After the lesion has been removed, the cavity should be 'curetted' gently to ensure that no fragments are left behind. The wound is left open to drain.

3

Excision of haematoma

If the haematoma is very large, or multiple contiguous lesions are present, simple evacuation of the haematoma will leave a large cavity surrounded by folds of skin, in which infection can take place, or a fistula or large skin tag result later on. Under these circumstances, it is better to remove the haematoma plus any redundant skin around to produce a flat shallow cavity. The wound edges can be approximated at the end of the excision by several stitches of fine 00 chromic catgut or left open.

Postoperative care is carried out in the same way as after simple evacuation of the haematoma.

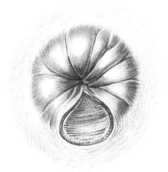

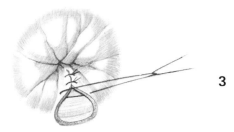

3

POSTOPERATIVE CARE AND COMPLICATIONS

For the first 24 hr a gauze dressing lightly soaked in 1:2000 Hibitane solution is applied and held in place by a 'T' bandage. A stool softener or gentle aperient is administered every evening for a few days to ensure easy, complete defaecation the following morning.

After the first day, the patient is advised to take frequent hot baths, which soothe and cleanse the operation site. It is particularly necessary to bathe the area thoroughly after each defaecation. After the first 24 hr, a soft dry dressing (paper gauze or a cotton-wool pad) is all that is required.

When the wound is healed, which may take 5—7 days, all dressings are discarded, but Vasogen cream may be applied daily for 2 weeks to prevent chaffing.

While the wound is healing, strenuous activity or prolonged sitting should be avoided.

Infection and abscess formation

If the clot is incompletely evacuated either by partial failure of spontaneous expulsion or by faulty surgical technique, the wound can become infected. If this happens, the wound should be inspected to ensure that adequate drainage is present, and any trimming of wound edges or evacuation of retained products

carried out under general anaesthesia. Antibiotics are not usually required.

If an abscess develops, this should be incised and deroofed under a general anaesthetic.

Skin tag

This should not happen after surgery if excision as opposed to evacuation is carried out when indicated, and no redundant skin folds remain.

However, conservative management of a large peri-anal haematoma may leave behind a skin tag after the clot has been re-absorbed. This does not usually require treatment, but can be excised if it gives rise to symptoms, e.g. pruritis.

Fistula

If large loose folds of skin are left after evacuation of the haematoma, superficial cross-healing of the wound edges can occur, leaving a subcutaneous track or fistula beneath.

Under these circumstances, the wound must be laid open again to obtain proper healing by secondary intention from below upwards.

References

Goligher, J. C. (1975). *Surgery of the Anus, Rectum and Colon*, 3rd Edition, page 163. London: Balliere Tindall
Bailey and Love (1975). *Short Practice of Surgery*, 16th Edition, page 1023. London: H. K. Lewis

[The illustrations for this Chapter on Excision of Peri-anal Haematoma were drawn by Mr. R. N. Lane.]

Injection of Haemorrhoids

C. V. Mann, M.Ch., F.R.C.S.
Consultant Surgeon to St. Mark's Hospital, London
and The London Hospital

PRE-OPERATIVE

Indications

Injection treatment can give excellent results in *first-degree* haemorrhoids (bleeding is the only symptom), although the treatment may have to be repeated at intervals. In *second-degree* haemorrhoids the results are less predictable, although some cases may obtain substantial relief of symptoms: results can be improved if the injection is combined with elastic band ligation of some of the larger haemorrhoids. In *third-degree* haemorrhoids the results are poor, and can cause an acute thrombosed prolapse to occur: it is rare that a patient cannot have treatment by banding or surgery under caudal anaesthesia even in extreme old age or infirmity, and during pregnancy manual dilatation of the anus (*see* pages 319–323) is an alternative to injection treatment.

Contra-indications

An injection treatment within 3 weeks of a previous treatment may cause the complication of injection ulcer with severe haemorrhage: it is usually recommended that injection treatments should be spaced at 4–6 week intervals for this reason.

Injections are contra-indicated during or soon after an attack of thrombosis/prolapse.

The presence of a chronic fissure or fistula is an indication for surgical treatment, although injection treatment can be used as a temporary expedient to stop bleeding from associated haemorrhoids. However, injection treatment makes subsequent surgical procedures more difficult, and should not be used without due consideration of any future proposed surgical procedures.

The presence of proctocolitis, Crohn's disease, tropical infestations (e.g. amoebiasis, schistosomiasis) and rectal neoplasms must be excluded by careful examination and sigmoidoscopy before starting a course of injections for haemorrhoids.

A general and abdominal examination should also be carried out to exclude heart failure or portal hypertension as a cause of the piles, for which other treatment is needed.

Pre-operative preparation

No special preparation is needed providing the rectum is not loaded with faeces. If a loaded rectum is discovered, prior to injection an immediate evacuation by disposable enema (sodium di-hydrogen phosphate) solution should be carried out.

Anaesthesia

If properly given, the injection is painless, and should lead only to a slight feeling of rectal distension which soon passes off. No anaesthetic, local or general, is needed.

Position of patient

The Sims position with the pelvis raised on a sandbag as described under Sigmoidoscopy (*see* page 5) is comfortable for the patient and convenient for the surgeon.

THE OPERATION

1

Instruments

A good light is essential. A tubular illuminated procto-scope as already illustrated on page 2 is the one preferred. A 10 ml syringe with three-finger grip, fitted with a long needle attaching by a bayonet lock, is used for the injection (Gabriel pattern). The solution used is 5 per cent phenol in vegetable (arachis) oil, with 0·5 per cent menthol added. Total dose of any one treatment should not exceed 10–15 ml, and it is wise not to put in more than 5 ml to the base of any individual haemorrhoidal mass. Forceps and sponges should be available to wipe away faecal waste, and to apply pressure to the injection site if bleeding occurs.

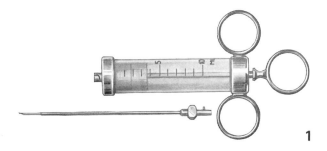

2

Place to inject

All three main haemorrhoidal masses may be injected at one time if necessary. The proctoscope is moved and tilted until the proposed site of each injection is clearly seen. The patient should not strain while an injection is being performed. The site for each injection is at the base of the haemorrhoidal mass just above the level of the mid-anal point, as identified by the dentate line. If pain is experienced as the needle is inserted, the needle should be removed and re-inserted at a higher level.

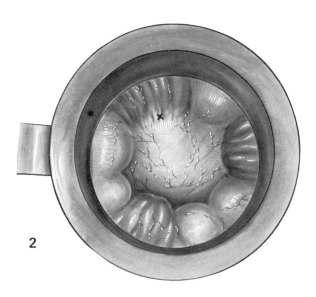

3

The injection

The solution is injected in the submucosal zone and should flow with light pressure. At the site of injection the mucosa should be seen to expand and resemble a blister as the injection proceeds. If a dead white patch appears, the injection is too superficial and must be stopped immediately. Once 3–5 ml have been injected into each haemorrhoid pedicle, the site of injection should be changed until not more than 9–15 ml have been given *in toto*. A few seconds delay before removing the needle at the completion of each injection lessens escape of solution or bleeding at the site of the injection.

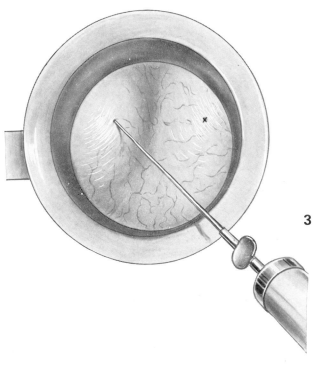

4

As shown in the diagram, the injection is given above the mid-anal point, and should cause no pain to the patient but only a sensation of mild discomfort or distension.

Should bleeding occur when the needle is withdrawn, it is usually easily arrested by a few minutes pressure with a cotton-wool swab. If bleeding persists, the site of the injection can be encircled with an elastic band (*see* page 317).

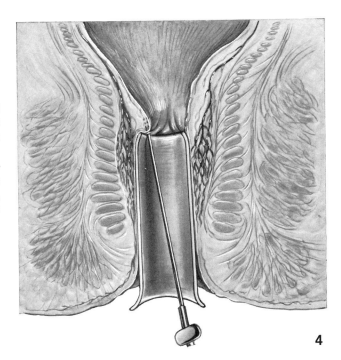

4

POSTOPERATIVE CARE AND COMPLICATIONS

The patient is advised to avoid physical exertion or prolonged standing for 24 hr after the injection. The next bowel movement should if possible be postponed until the day after the injection. If the rectum was loaded prior to the injection treatment, or if the patient has a history of chronic straining to defaecate, a laxative may be given for a few days after the injection to promote easy defaecation.

It is usual for the patient to notice a sense of fullness and heaviness in the rectum for 24 hr after an injection: analgesics that are known to cause or aggravate constipation should be avoided.

Injection ulcer

This should not occur if the proper solution is used and the injection given in the correct (submucosal) plane. However, if an intramucosal injection is administered, or too big a dose is given, mucosal sloughing may occur. This is usually accompanied by haemorrhage, which can be severe if a large artery is eroded. Treatment is by packing, as described under secondary haemorrhage after haemorrhoidectomy (*see* pages 331–337).

Other complications

Severe pain can occur if the injection is placed too low in the anal canal. Prolapse/thrombosis may be precipitated if *third-degree* haemorrhoids are injected. Intraprostatic injection can cause haematuria or a sterile prostatic abscess. Submucous abscess formation is occasionally seen. Stricture of the anus, and oleogranuloma formation do not occur if a 5 per cent phenol solution in vegetable oil is used, and is put into the proper site of election.

Reference

Gabriel, W. B. (1963). *The Principles and Practice of Rectal Surgery*, 5th Edition, p. 132. London: Lewis

[*The illustrations for this Chapter on Injection of Haemorrhoids were drawn by Mr. R. N. Lane.*]

Barron Band Ligation of Haemorrhoids

C. V. Mann, M.Ch., F.R.C.S.
Consultant Surgeon, St. Mark's Hospital, London
and The London Hospital

PRE-OPERATIVE

Indications

Many internal haemorrhoids are too large to respond satisfactorily to injections, but do not give rise to such severe symptoms that the patient is willing to have an operation. In some cases, haemorrhoids recur after excision and the patient is reluctant to have further surgical treatment.

When other treatments have failed, or do not seem to have reasonable prospect of success, banding ligation of the haemorrhoids can be tried, although surgical removal is still the best treatment for third-degree haemorrhoids.

The ideal case for treatment by this method is a patient with one or two large second-degree haemorrhoids, i.e. those which prolapse but return spontaneously after defaecation. Early small haemorrhoids are best treated by injections.

Contra-indications

As with all other operations in the anal region, this procedure should not be done in the presence of any dysenteric infection, Crohn's disease or colitis (*see* Chapter on 'Haemorrhoidectomy', page 331). Preliminary diagnostic sigmoidoscopy is required to exclude a rectal neoplasm or proctocolitis.

A general and abdominal examination should be carried out beforehand to exclude conditions such as heart failure or portal hypertension requiring other treatment.

Banding treatment should not be attempted if an anal fissure or fistula is present.

Preparation

No special preparation is necessary. The rectum should not be loaded, and habitual constipation should be corrected by suitable treatment before banding is carried out. A normal defaecation on the day of the procedure is the best preparation, but if necessary the rectum can be evacuated by a disposable (sodium di-hydrogen phosphate) enema immediately beforehand.

An assistant is required.

Anaesthesia

If properly performed, the banding is painless, although it may cause mild aching discomfort. No anaesthetic, local or general, is required, but if the patient is particularly nervous a general anaesthetic can be given.

Position of patient

The left lateral (Sims) position with the pelvis raised on a sandbag (as described on page 5) is a good position for the procedure to be performed. It can also be carried out in the knee-elbow or jack-knife positions.

The lithotomy position is not a good posture in which to carry out banding, as anteriorly situated haemorrhoids are difficult to visualize.

THE OPERATION

1

Instruments

Banding is carried out through an ordinary tubular proximally illuminated proctoscope as illustrated on page 2. The proctoscope is passed and then held in position by the assistant. The banding instrument consists of a double drum carrying elastic bands $\frac{1}{16}$ inch in diameter when unexpanded. This double drum is mounted on a long shaft, at the base of which is a trigger mechanism which can release the rings as required. The elastic bands are loaded by a separate conical device which slots into the end of the barrel and enables the bands to be slipped over from the loader onto the drum. The third essential piece of equipment is a special pair of grasping forceps, which are passed through the hollow core of the drum to grasp each haemorrhoid in turn.

The drum is loaded with two bands before each application.

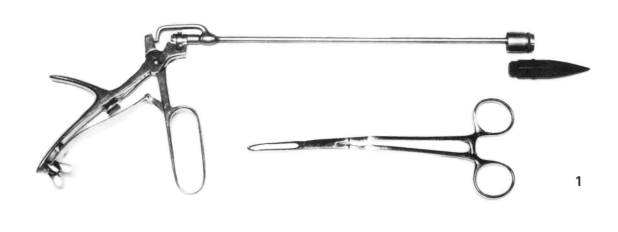

1

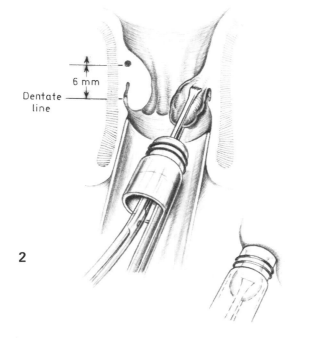

2

2

The banding procedure

Each haemorrhoid is grasped at its base by the grasping forceps. It is important that the point selected for application of the forceps is at least 6 mm above the dentate line, and that the patient does not experience *any* pain when they are applied.

Gentle traction is then applied to the forceps, and at the same time the banding instrument is pressed firmly forwards: this combination of traction and pulsion draws the pile into the drum, the distal edge of which comes opposite the base of the haemorrhoid.

3

The bands are now released by 'firing' the trigger mechanism, which allows the bands to snap around the pedicle of the haemorrhoid.

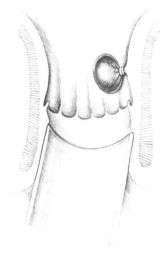

3

The end-point

When the bands are in position, and the banding instruments have been released and withdrawn, a small ball of tissue the size of a cherry is seen, with its base constricted by the bands.

It is not wise to 'band' more than two individual haemorrhoids at each treatment, as severe pain can result from too many rings being applied.

Editorial comment

The editor sometimes injects a little saline or 1:200,000 lignocaine through the finest needle into the 'cherry' to make it more tense and thus encourage sloughing. He has the impression that this also eases the discomfort which sometimes occurs.

At least 3 weeks should elapse between treatments.

POSTOPERATIVE CARE AND COMPLICATIONS

Providing the bands have been put on correctly, the patient should not experience more than a mild aching discomfort, which usually goes after 48 hr. If the patient is very tense, extra analgesia may be required (Pethidine 50–75 mg every 8 hr for 24–48 hr) but normally a few Paracetamol or Distalgesic tablets are all that is required.

Constipation should be prevented by administering the appropriate laxative: Milpar 15 ml every evening is usually enough, and the patient should be told to avoid straining to pass stool.

The haemorrhoid necroses and sloughs away between the fourth and tenth postoperative days, at which time the patient may notice slight bleeding on defaecation: the bands may also be observed by the patient after they have separated who should be warned to expect both these possibilities.

Severe pain

If too many haemorrhoids have been banded at one treatment, or if the bands have been applied too low in the anal canal (thereby including sensitive squamous cell epithelium in the banded area), severe pain can result. Unless the pain can be relieved by strong analgesics (Pethidine 100 mg every 6 hr), the bands may have to be removed. This is a difficult business, and should be carried out under a general anaesthetic, the rubber rings being divided by a small knife.

Oedema and thrombosed external haemorrhoids

Occasionally after a banding treatment the tissues at the anal verge become slightly swollen. This subsides after a few days and does not require treatment, but hot baths are soothing and may hasten resolution of the tissue oedema.

Very rarely, thrombosis of an external haemorrhoid may happen. This should be treated with frequent baths, and the application of hygroscopic ointments (Ung. magnesium sulphate).

Prolapse

Providing constipation is prevented, this complication can be avoided. However, if the patient strains at defaecation within a few days of a banding, prolapse and thrombosis of internal haemorrhoids can occur. This complication is handled conservatively, but the patient may require admission to hospital for a few days.

'Ulcer' and secondary haemorrhage

After an internal haemorrhoid has sloughed away, a small ulcer is left on the mucosa, surrounded by an area of oedema. The ulcer heals rapidly, and a normal appearance returns after 2–3 weeks.

In 1–2 per cent of cases, separation of the dead pile is accompanied by moderate haemorrhage from the bed of the ulcer, and more rarely the bleeding can be severe. If serious blood loss occurs, the patient should be admitted to hospital and the same measures instituted as for secondary haemorrhage after haemorrhoidectomy (*see* page 337).

References

Barron, J. (1963). 'Office ligation of internal haemorrhoids.' *Am. J. Surg.* **105**, 563
Goligher, J. C. (1975). *Surgery of the Anus, Rectum and Colon*, 3rd Edition, page 137. London: Balliere Tindall

[*The illustrations for this Chapter on Barron Band Ligation of Haemorrhoids were drawn by Mr. R. N. Lane.*]

Maximal Anal Dilatation

Peter H. Lord, M.Chir., F.R.C.S.
Consultant Surgeon, Wycombe General Hospital,
High Wycombe and The Chalfonts and Gerrards Cross
Hospital

INTRODUCTION

Haemorrhoids consist of normal tissue which is present in the form of vascular cushions or pads, situated in the submucosa at the lower extremity of the rectum and upper anus. These pads are in the well recognized positions — left lateral, right posterior and right anterior. The vascular pads are present at birth, become larger at puberty and persist throughout life (Thompson, 1975). They can give rise to symptoms if they become over-filled with blood. We then call them haemorrhoids which may bleed, or thrombose, or prolapse. This over-filling is always associated with defaecation and is presumably due to obstruction of venous return by increased intrarectal pressure. This in turn is believed to be caused, certainly in the vast majority of sufferers, by a constricted outlet which will not dilate sufficiently to allow the faecal bolus to pass easily. The congested haemorrhoids further restrict the outlet, and it is the aim of the dilatation procedure and regime to break this vicious circle.

PRE-OPERATIVE

Pre-operative preparation

Little pre-operative preparation is required. An enema is not necessary. Premedication is not essential for such a brief procedure, but is useful if the patient is apprehensive, and even the routine pre-operative sigmoidoscopy can be deferred if the patient has a tender anus. It is easily and quickly achieved under anaesthesia, though it should be repeated afterwards if the view at operation is obstructed by faeces in a loaded rectum. A sort of 'retention with overflow' is common in patients with anal problems.

Anaesthetic

The procedure is usually carried out in the anaesthetic room. The patient is asked to lie on the left side; intravenous Epontol (Propanidid) is used for induction; this is supplemented by halothane inhalation anaesthetic if necessary. Normally the procedure takes only a few minutes, including the sigmoidoscopy.

THE OPERATION

1

Identifying the constriction

The surgeon's first move is to identify the constrictions involving the lower end of the rectum and the anal canal. These are not apparent in the unanaesthetized patient, nor can they be felt with the fingers of one hand. The surgeon stands at the patient's back. He inserts two fingers of the left hand and pulls upwards. Then the index finger of the right hand is inserted, pressing downwards, and the constriction can be felt (*see Illustration*). This is often at the level of the pecten, and in most patients consists of the lowermost fibres of the internal sphincter, which have undergone a change and which are no longer able to relax. The nature of this change is not known, it is not apparent on histological examination, but it is probably much the same as the change seen at the rectosigmoid junction in diverticular disease. These constricting fibres must be stretched, or sometimes even torn, in order to achieve the dilatation.

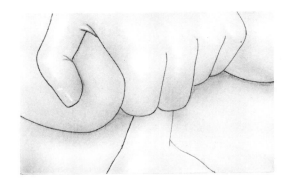

1

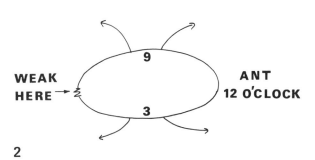

2

2

The dilatation

The dilatation procedure should be gentle and controlled. It starts using the index finger of each hand; the surgeon gradually inserting more fingers as the constriction is overcome. By careful manipulation it is possible to throw the strain of the dilatation on to the constricting bands in the left lateral and right lateral positions, i.e. at 3 and 9 o'clock, and to avoid damaging the sphincter at 12 o'clock, and particularly at 6 o'clock where it is relatively weak. The degree of dilatation varies, and it is clearly better to do too little than to risk damage to the sphincter; usually six to eight fingers can be inserted, and often constrictions can be felt in the lower rectum as high as the fingers can reach. These also should be made to give way laterally.

The sponge

At the end of the dilatation procedure it should be clear that there is no constriction between the upper rectum and the exterior, and that defaecation is able to take place without any significant rise in intra-rectal pressure.

3a, b & c

At this point, without removing his fingers, the surgeon stands to the side, and the theatre nurse inserts the sponge, using a sponge-holding forceps. This is easier if the specially designed forceps are employed, though these are not essential. The sponge should be inserted gently and goes in more easily if it is well soaked in a soapy solution such as Hibitane, 1:200,000. The surgeon's fingers guide the sponge into position, and if the special introducer is used, the nurse can then spring open the sponge holding forceps and remove the blades one at a time. With an ordinary forceps there is a tendency for the sponge to be pulled down again as the forceps are removed. The sponge exerts gentle pressure on the walls of the lower rectum and anal canal where the dilatation has been carried out, thereby reducing the risk of haematoma formation.

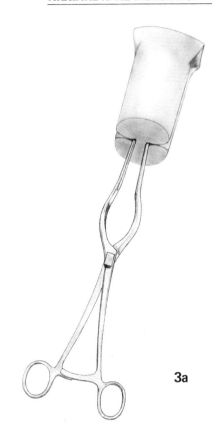

3a

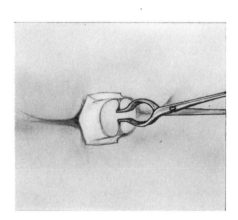

3b

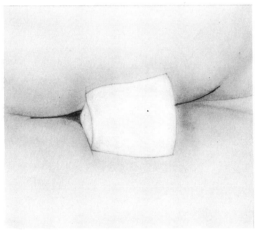

3c

It is important to stress that all these manoeuvres are carried out with great gentleness and that the surgeon must feel what he is doing — there should be no tearing of mucosa or damage to the delicate anorectal sphincter mechanism. It is worth repeating that it is far better to do too little than to do too much and thus cause damage.

The sponge stays in place for at least 1 hr. It can then be removed. This part of the procedure may cause pain to the patient, so Pethidine 100 mg can be given intramuscularly half an hour before removing the sponge.

POSTOPERATIVE REGIME

4

It is important that the anorectal region should not narrow down again during the healing period. It is the aim of the postoperative regime to prevent this possibility. A special dilator (illustrated) has been designed for this purpose, and the patient is trained to insert this when well relaxed after a hot bath in the evening before retiring. If the dilator goes in easily, then it can be used less often, but once a day for 2 weeks, then twice a week, once a week, etc., has usually been the pattern among the author's patients.

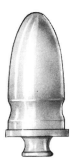

4

A bulk evacuant, Normacol, is used as a routine postoperatively so that the patient passes a soft bulky stool. Once a good bowel habit is established, it is usually a wise precaution for the patient to supplement the normal diet with natural bran.

The patient is seen 2 weeks after the procedure to make sure that all is well, and 2 months afterwards for a final check and discharge.

Discussion

Although the author carries out the procedure and regime in much the same way as originally described (Lord, 1969) the method has been modified by others who claim satisfactory results. Some surgeons have stopped using the sponge and say it has made no difference to their haematoma rate.

It is difficult to know if the dilator is vital to the success of the method. Some surgeons claim that they get good results without its use. On the other hand, many of the author's patients have volunteered that they find the dilator very helpful in the early postoperative phase, and that they feel more comfortable after using it.

The dilator

The dilator is left with the patient who is instructed that if at any future date any anal symptom occurs, the dilator should be used a few times to make quite sure that the constriction has not recurred.

Complications

Incontinence is the complication most feared by the patient and by the surgeon not familiar with the method. It is a fair statement that this complication

does not occur, and that if it did, the method would be unacceptable, but this statement needs to be qualified as follows:

(*1*) Incontinence of flatus for a few days after dilatation is usual, and this may persist for a few weeks.

(*2*) If the patient previously had a particularly tight outlet, things are very different after dilatation from the situation before, and the patient may take a little time to get used to the new condition. There may be a feeling of unsureness of the sphincter mechanism and encouragement and sphincter exercises are needed for a few weeks.

(*3*) A number of cases have now been reported where the sphincter mechanism has been damaged at 6 o'clock, producing the so-called key-hole deformity of the anus. Faecal-stained mucus can escape down the groove leading to soiling and soreness. This complication is avoided by good technique, and particularly by ensuring that the strain of the dilatation is thrown on to the lateral aspect of the anus.

Bruising. Modest peri-anal bruising is normal after this procedure and is of no significance. A large amount of bruising can lead to pain and may require several days' treatment with analgesics, but fortunately this does not adversely affect the end result.

Note

Excessive haematoma formation may occur in a patient with a bleeding diathesis, e.g. haemophilia. The method is not contra-indicated in these patients, but should be carried out with great gentleness — in stages if necessary — and with full haematological cover.

Mucosal prolapse. Some degree of postoperative prolapse is commonly seen after the dilatation in those patients who had appreciable haemorrhoidal prolapse pre-operatively. This will gradually improve with the postoperative regime and sphincter exercises and the majority resolve, but if still persistent at 2 months, a further procedure is necessary.

A prolapse is abolished either by: (*1*) Barron band ligation; (*2*) cryo-destruction, or (*3*) clamp excision using the author's peri-anal clamp.

Acute thrombosis of the haemorrhoidal tissue. This complication is fortunately rare — it is not clear why it occurs to these few patients, nor what can be done to prevent it. It is an embarrassment since the patient gets a considerable swelling with some soreness, though usually not severe pain. This settles gradually and usually leads to an excellent end result, but the patient requires much reassurance.

Complications not seen

Urinary retention; faecal impaction; deep vein thrombosis; pulmonary embolus.

5a, b & c

Use of the clamp

Persistent mucosal prolapse if present is usually in the right anterior position (*Illustration 5a*). Under general anaesthetic, as already described, this is grasped in Duval forceps, pulled down, the Lord pattern peri-anal clamp (*Illustration 5b*) is applied across the base, and the excess mucosa removed. The clamp is curved to the buttocks, it is strapped in position and left on for 1 hr (*Illustration 5c*). The jaws are of a crushing haemostatic design so that when the clamp is removed, there should be no bleeding and the patient is allowed home when recovered from the brief anaesthetic. This clamp can also be used for skin tags and anal polyps.

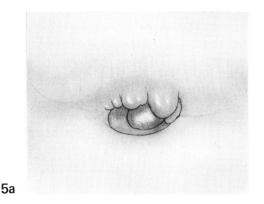

5a

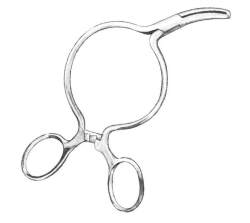

5b

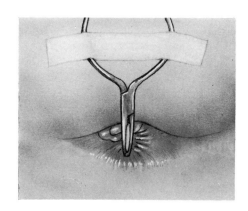

5c

References

Lord, P. H. (1969). 'A day-case procedure for the cure of third-degree haemorrhoids.' *Br. J. Surg.* **56,** 747
Lord, P. H. (1972). 'A new approach to haemorrhoids.' *Prog. Surg.* **10,** 109
Thomson, W. H. F. (1975). *Br. J. Surg.* **62,** 542

[*The illustrations for this Chapter on Maximal Anal Dilatation were drawn by Mr. F. Price.*]

Cryosurgery of Haemorrhoids

K. Lloyd Williams, M.D., M.Chir., F.R.C.S.
Consultant Surgeon, Royal United Hospital, Bath

INTRODUCTION

Cryosurgery is the technique of freezing living human tissue. Tissue once frozen, becomes white and solid. To achieve freezing, tissue temperatures around $-20°C$ are needed. Frozen tissue undergoes a sequence of changes. The white solid mass rewarms at a variable rate depending upon the heat flow and vascularity of the surrounding area, but usually takes 2 or 3 min.

Immediately after rewarming the frozen tissue looks exactly the same as unfrozen tissue, a point of some importance which will be referred to later. Within the first 15 min after rewarming, swelling of the frozen area occurs, with oedema and increase in vascularity. Within 6 hr, microscopically there is demarcation between the frozen and unfrozen cells. By 24 hr thrombosis and infarction of the frozen area occurs, and over the next 24 hr the tissue becomes black and necrotic. During this time there is a profuse serous discharge. Sloughing takes from 10 to 14 days. Haemorrhage and infection are rare. Healing on a mucous surface occurs with no detectable scar formation.

1,2&3

There are three commonly used methods of freezing living human tissue.

(*a*) Applying a spray of liquid nitrogen producing local temperatures of $-180°C$.

(*b*) Applying a closed probe in which either liquid nitrogen or liquid nitrous oxide is allowed to boil off. Liquid nitrogen boils at $-196°C$: Liquid N_2O boils at $-90°C$ (*Illustration 1*).

(*c*) Applying a closed probe in which pressurized gas is allowed to expand rapidly after passing through a narrow orifice. The expanding gas takes up heat from its surroundings (Joule–Thompson effect) (*Illustration 2*). The commonest gas used is nitrous oxide at a pressure of 650–750 lb/in^2 which will produce a tip temperature of $-75°C$.

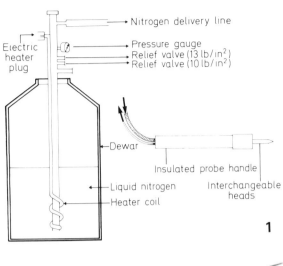

1

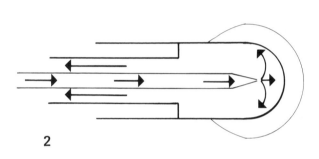

2

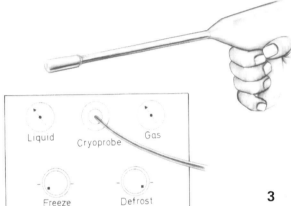

3

Spray techniques are unsatisfactory for haemorrhoids but either of the closed probes can be used. Because of the greater cooling power both liquid nitrous oxide and liquid nitrogen freeze tissue faster and produce a larger ice ball than Joule–Thompson cooling.

A nitrous oxide probe when applied to moist tissue becomes firmly attached and cannot be removed without rewarming. This has some advantages in manipulating the tissue, as for example exerting traction to prolapse a pile or diminish the blood supply to it.

A cooled liquid nitrogen probe when applied to moist tissue does not stick, and can be easily removed without rewarming.

Cooling tissues numbs sensation. Freezing produces anaesthesia of the frozen area, thus accounting for the relative painlessness of cryosurgical procedures.

SELECTION OF CASES

Though cryosurgery will effectively destroy all haemorrhoidal tissue, it is useful to separate patients with symptoms of bleeding, prolapse, anal discomfort, discharge, or tenesmus into two functional groups:

(*1*) Those with a normally relaxing or lax anus.

(*2*) Those with tight, unrelaxing, or spastic anal musculature—with pain on dilatation.

Into the first category fall the elderly patients with lax musculature, where bleeding, discharge and prolapse are prominent symptoms, and younger patients with a lax mucous membrane, who often have arteriovenous anomalies and a family history. Into group 2 fall patients with a history of loose bowel movement, accentuated gastrocolic reflex, anal fissure, peri-anal haematoma and duodenal ulcer, often tense people with a tense anus.

In practice the two groups can be readily separated into those whose anus will comfortably dilate to accommodate two well lubricated fingers (3 cm dilatation), and those in whom two fingers cannot be passed because of spasm, rigidity or pain.

The former group can be treated by cryosurgery as out-patients; the latter will require a general anaesthetic and manual dilatation of the anus to six fingers (7 cm), before proceeding to freezing of their haemorrhoids.

GROUP 1. NORMALLY RELAXING OR LAX ANUS

No pre-operative preparation is required. No anaesthesia is normally required but, in an anxious patient, 5–10 mg of diazepam may be injected intravenously. The patient lies on a couch in the left lateral position with the knees well drawn up to the stomach.

The right buttock should be raised, preferably by the curled fingers of the patient's right hand. The anus should then be gently dilated with a well lubricated gloved finger. K-Y jelly is used as lubricant, as this produces good thermal contact with the probe. The largest proctoscope which will pass with ease is used to examine the haemorrhoidal area.

4

A diagram of the anal area is made showing the site and size of the haemorrhoids, to assist in planning treatment and form an operative record.

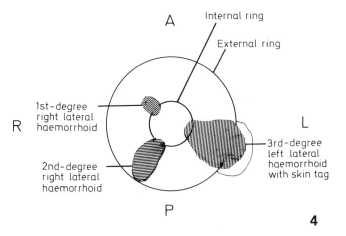

4

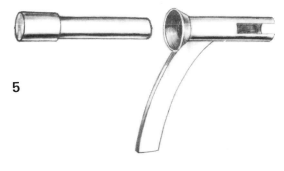

5

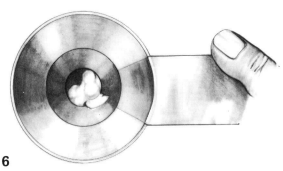

6

5 & 6

For treatment, a plastic proctoscope is preferable as it acts as a thermal insulator. It should be modified as illustrated. The 1·5 cm slit allows the haemorrhoid to prolapse into the lumen of the proctoscope.

The cryoprobe is applied with its tip at the apex of the pile, at the anorectal ring. If a nitrous oxide probe is used, the 'trigger' should be pressed or the foot switch depressed and freezing begun.

7&8

After a few seconds, the probe will stick to the mucosa and gentle traction can be exerted. The tissue in contact with the probe becomes white and hard. Freezing is continued until all of the pile tissue becomes white and solid. This will take 2 or 3 min with a nitrous oxide probe. It is important that only the haemorrhoid is frozen and the probe should be moved to ensure that the frozen haemorrhoid is free on the underlying muscle.

When the freezing is complete, the probe should be turned off, allowed to rewarm and detached. A nitrous oxide probe should not be broken off the tissue, otherwise the mucosa will be torn and bleeding result. After freezing the haemorrhoid, the proctoscope should be withdrawn, the still solid tissue sliding along the slit of the proctoscope. The obturator should then be replaced in the proctoscope which is re-introduced into the anus, and rotated so that the slit coincides with the next haemorrhoidal area to be treated.

Treatment is concluded when all haemorrhoidal areas have been treated.

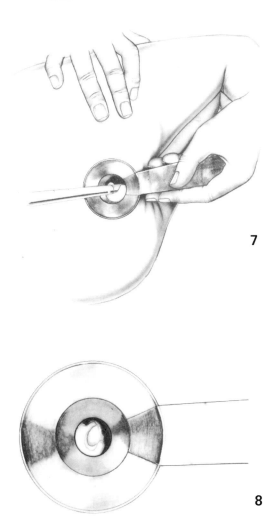

7

8

POSTOPERATIVE CARE

Pain is rarely severe and mild analgesics will usually suffice to control it.

Patients should be warned of the swelling which occurs in the first 24 hr and the discharge, which will require the wearing of a pad or sanitary towel. Saline baths will be found comforting, but no local application should be necessary. Discharge is worst with prolapsed or third-degree haemorrhoids, and both discharge and discomfort worse when skin areas are frozen. In patients with first- or second-degree haemorrhoids and a competent anus, discharge may be retained in the rectum and voided with the motion, and hence not noticed by the patient.

The bowels should be kept loose and regular with bran or Isogel.

Healing should be complete within 3 weeks.

GROUP 2. PATIENTS WITH AN UNRELAXING, SPASTIC, OR TIGHT ANUS

General anaesthesia is necessary.

9

The patient may be positioned in the left lateral or Trendelenburg position, according to preference. If in the left lateral, a nurse should be positioned on the opposite side of the table facing the patient, to retract the right buttock upwards.

The anus is well lubricated. The index finger of the right hand is inserted pointing pulp forwards, the index finger of the left hand is then inserted with the pulp facing backwards. The tips of the fingers are forced apart and the fingers gradually withdrawn, ironing out and stretching any bands or rings felt in the muscle. Further fingers of both hands are inserted until the index, middle and ring fingers of both hands can be inserted together. Stretching should be done gently, should take approximately 5 min to perform and the aim should be to achieve dilatation without mucosal tearing.

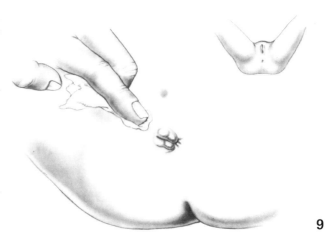

9

10

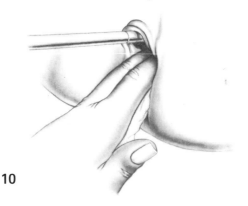

10

After dilatation, the haemorrhoidal area should be examined with a speculum. Prolapsing or redundant haemorrhoids should be frozen with a liquid nitrogen probe. The probe is applied at the internal ring at the apex of the pile, the pile and redundant skin are moulded around the probe with the gloved finger; pressure will diminish the blood supply and increase the freezing effect.

11 & 12

When the skin and haemorrhoidal area, which would normally be excised in a classical haemorrhoidectomy, have been rendered hard and white by the freezing, the probe should be detached by twisting it. Usually the probe will be easily detached. On occasion, if the probe temperature is not low enough ($<-70°C$) it cannot be detached. When this occurs, the nitrogen supply should be turned off and the probe tip warmed by pouring warmed water over it. After removal of the probe, the junction of normal and frozen skin should be marked with indelible ink. This is a wise precaution, as it is important to preserve intact skin bridges between the frozen areas in order to prevent anal stenosis, as on rewarming the demarcation between the frozen and unfrozen area disappears.

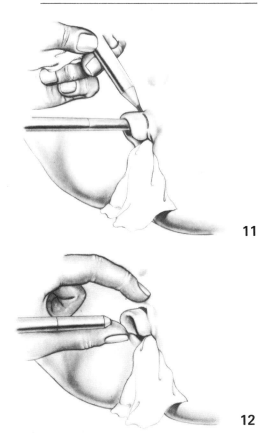

11

12

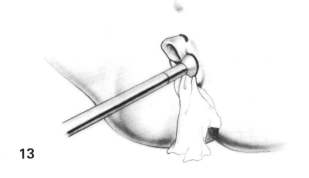

13

13, 14 & 15

The cryoprobe is then applied to the next haemorrhoidal area and the procedure continued as before. When all the haemorrhoidal areas have been frozen in turn the operation is completed by introducing a small gauze swab into the anus to act as a wick, and a pad and a T bandage are applied.

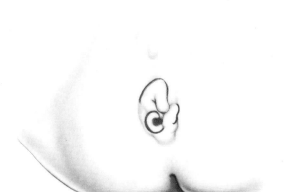

14

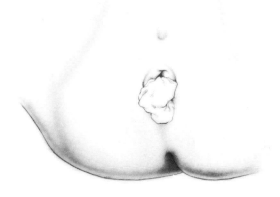

15

POSTOPERATIVE CARE

Pain

One-third of patients will require strong analgesics such as morphia or pethidine postoperatively for 24 hr. Two-thirds will require either no analgesic or mild analgesic such as (Veganin or Disprin) compound aspirin tablets.

The anus should be examined with a well lubricated finger the day after operation. This has the dual advantage that it proves to the patient that opening the bowels will not be too painful, and to the surgeon that there is no spasm of the anal musculature. If spasm exists a St. Mark's dilator lubricated with 2 per cent lignocaine jelly should be passed daily for a week.

The motion should be kept soft with Isogel or bran. The patient may leave hospital once the bowels have been opened. They must be warned of the swelling, and unpleasant appearance of the anus, and the profuse discharge which will occur up to 10 days after cryosurgery. During this time frequent changes of an absorbant dressing such as a sanitary towel, and frequent saline sitz baths will be required. The aim should be to keep the anal area as dry as possible as otherwise excoriation may occur. Healing should be complete in 3 weeks.

Complications

Urinary retention, haemorrhage and sepsis are very rare. Anal stenosis has not occurred.

Residual anal skin tags are not uncommon. If these give rise to symptoms they may require a further freeze or local excision. The skin tag may be frozen without an anaesthetic and on rewarming the tag may be clamped across and the redundant tissue excised. The clamp should be left on for 1·5 hr, and then removed. Note that the clamp must be applied within the area frozen, otherwise it will be painful. Excising the tags in this manner does not diminish the recovery period, but it does cut down the amount of discharge.

[The illustrations for this Chapter on Cryosurgery of Haemorrhoids were drawn by Mr. G. Lyth.]

Haemorrhoidectomy (St. Mark's Ligation/Excision Method)

C. V. Mann, M.Ch., F.R.C.S.
Consultant Surgeon to St. Mark's Hospital, London
and The London Hospital

and

H. E. Lockhart-Mummery, M.D., M.Chir., F.R.C.S.
Consultant Surgeon, St. Thomas's and St. Mark's Hospitals,
and King Edward VII Hospital for Officers, London

PRE-OPERATIVE

Indications

Surgical removal offers the best chance of permanent cure of haemorrhoids. If the haemorrhoids are very large and prolapse occurs to more than a moderate extent, other treatments are likely to fail. Associated anal pathology (e.g. chronic fissure, large skin tags or a fistula) are additional strong reasons for surgical removal. Rarely, severe anaemia can be caused by persistent bleeding from large haemorrhoids.

Failure of other methods of treatment is probably the commonest reason for surgical removal.

The method of ligation/excision combines adequate removal of the haemorrhoidal masses with excellent drainage of what is theoretically a septic wound; the complication rate of this operation is, therefore, very low, and the success rate very high.

Contra-indications

All operations on the anal region are best avoided in the presence of any dysenteric infection, Crohn's disease or proctocolitis; not only are the wounds likely to be slow to heal and indolent, but the colitis may be aggravated by the operation. Operation should be postponed on patients with active pulmonary or intestinal tuberculosis, as tuberculous infection of the anal wounds can result.

Severe constipation should be relieved before haemorrhoidectomy. Similarly, chronic diarrhoea from laxative addiction should be corrected before surgery.

Prolapsed thrombosed haemorrhoids should not be operated upon unless the patient presents within 24–48 hr; after this, the potential risk of portal pyaemia contra-indicates surgery until the thrombosis has completely subsided.

During pregnancy, palliative treatment is best for the condition which will improve soon after delivery.

Providing a safe anaesthetic can be given, old age is not a contra-indication to surgical treatment, but the establishment of a regular bowel habit is advisable before the operation is performed, in order to avoid anal stenosis afterwards.

Sigmoidoscopy to above the rectosigmoid is essential in every patient prior to haemorrhoidectomy, to ensure that no rectal disease is present, and in particular to exclude a neoplasm. When indicated, a barium enema may have to be performed for the same purpose. If a rectal polyp is present, this should be removed prior to haemorrhoidectomy in case malignant change has occurred.

331

Preparation

The patient should be admitted to hospital the day before operation.

A simple soap and water enema should be given soon after admission.

The peri-anal skin should be carefully shaved, and the patient should bath.

A laxative should be given if the patient is constipated, and a normal evacuation encouraged on the morning of the operation.

One hour before the operation, and prior to any premedication, a rectal washout is given with a tube and funnel and *all* the fluid carefully siphoned back.

Anaesthesia

General anaesthesia supplemented by local anaesthesia is best; the local anaesthetic enables a much lighter plane of general anaesthetic to be used because stimulation from the anal area is markedly reduced; in particular, the risk of laryngeal spasm or cardiac arrhythmias is much less by the use of this combined technique. Lignocaine 1 per cent with adrenaline 1:200,000 is a very satisfactory solution to use for the local infiltration.

In elderly or unfit patients, a caudal block can be used.

Some surgeons employ epidural anaesthesia to supplement the general anaesthetic, as this produces excellent relaxation of the anal sphincters and reduces oozing from the wounds during the operation. Epidural anaesthesia can be used instead of a caudal to provide local anaesthesia of the anal area.

Position of patient

The patient is placed in the full lithotomy position, with the buttocks lifted well down over the edge of the table, the lower flap of which should be removed.

This is an embarrassing and uncomfortable position if the operation is being carried out under local anaesthesia. In this situation, the Sims position with the buttocks raised on a sandbag (*see* page 5) offers reasonable exposure, especially if the upper buttock is retracted by strapping; if the patient is a cardiac 'cripple', this position is safer than the lithotomy position.

THE OPERATION

1

Injection of local anaesthetic

With the patient anaesthetized and in the lithotomy position, the peri-anal skin is carefully cleaned with Cetrimide solution. The anal canal is carefully swabbed out with cotton-wool soaked in Cetrimide until all faecal particles have been removed.

With a finger in the anal canal as a guide, a No. 20 2-inch (5 cm) needle on a syringe is passed from a central puncture into each ischiorectal fossa in turn, and the lignocaine–adrenaline solution injected (5–7 ml each side) alongside the medial aspect of each ischial tuberosity. Further smaller amounts (2–3 ml each) are then injected subcutaneously opposite to each haemorrhoid site at the muco-cutaneous junction.

It is advisable to wait 3–5 min after the local infiltration to allow the full effect of the solution to occur.

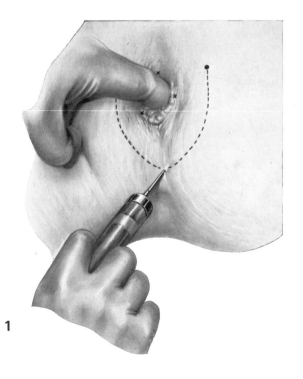

1

2

Eversion of the anal canal

A gentle two-finger dilatation of the anal canal is performed.

Dunhill forceps are placed on the peri-anal skin just outside the mucocutaneous junction, opposite to the primary haemorrhoidal positions (left lateral, right anterior and right posterior). Skin tags should be included in the area of peri-anal skin removed. Gentle traction on the forceps brings the internal haemorrhoids into view.

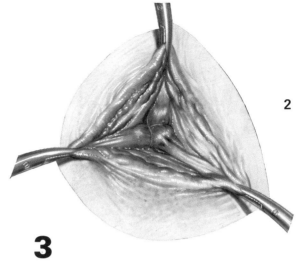

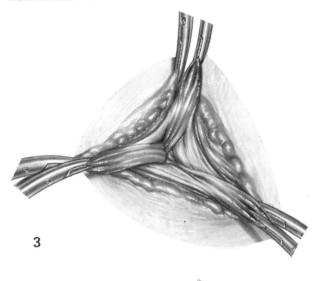

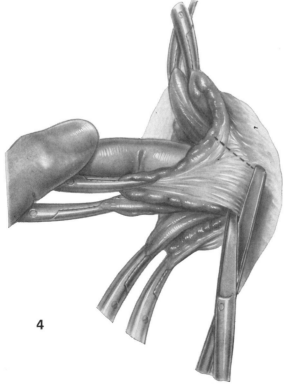

3

Triangle of exposure

As the internal haemorrhoids are pulled down, a second Dunhill forceps can be applied to the main bulk of each haemorrhoidal mass; further traction exposes the pedicles of the haemorrhoids, and produces the so-called 'triangle of exposure' which is caused by the triangular stretching of pink columnar cell mucosa at the apex of the wound between the pedicles of the haemorrhoids. When the second Dunhill forceps are clipped on the haemorrhoid, care must be taken not to include the internal sphincter muscle by a too deep bite. Intervening secondary haemorrhoids are taken with separate forceps, and approximated to the nearest primary forceps, so as to be included with the main haemorrhoid in the subsequent dissection.

Once the triangle of exposure has been achieved, the haemorrhoids are ready for removal by dissection and ligation/excision. It is a mistake to carry the dissection higher than this point.

4

Start of the dissection

The haemorrhoids are dissected in turn. For a right-handed surgeon, it is convenient to start with the left lateral, with the others held out of the way under slight traction by an assistant. The two forceps are held in the palm of the left hand with the left forefinger in the anal canal on the base of the haemorrhoid and pressing outwards. The blades of a pair of blunt-nosed scissors are placed alternately at each edge of the base as seen from its cutaneous aspect, and the tissues divided towards the median plane. This opens the subcutaneous space superficial to the lowest whitish fibres of the internal sphincter muscle.

5

Further dissection

Dissection is continued in a coronal plane superficial to the internal sphincter muscle towards the tip of the left forefinger. The haemorrhoids should not be dissected beyond the base of each pedicle as previously defined by the 'triangle of exposure'. As the dissection proceeds, the tissues on either side of the haemorrhoidal mass are snipped through, narrowing the line of dissection towards the apical point of the pedicle.

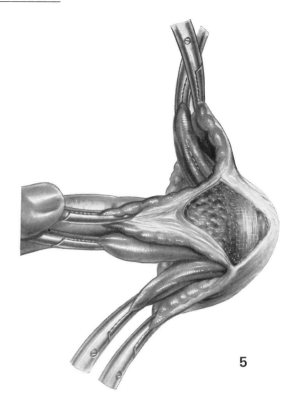

5

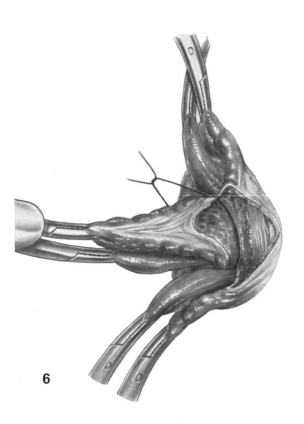

6

6

Ligation of pedicle

As the pedicle is defined by the dissection, traction on the haemorrhoid should be eased. Once defined, the pedicle is transfixed and ligated with strong silk or catgut, with the knot tied on the lumen side. If the pedicle is large, a second ligature can be applied. The pile can then be cut away allowing a good cuff of tissue distal to the ligature. The ligatures are cut long.

7

Procedure for remaining haemorrhoids

The other haemorrhoids are dealt with in turn by an identical method. Intact 'bridges' of skin and mucosa (which should not be less than 1 cm in width) are preserved between each dissection site. If large external veins are seen beneath the residual bridges, these can be removed by dissection from each side beneath the margin of each strip of skin ('filletting').

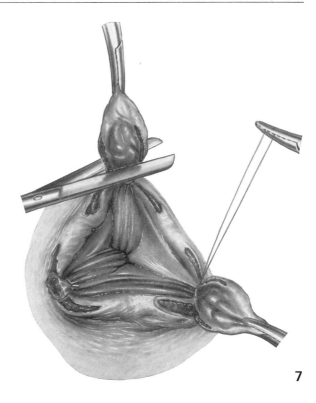

7

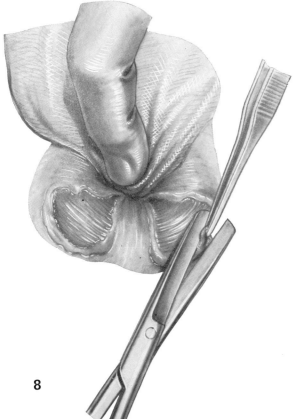

8

8

Trimming of wounds

The pedicles are returned to their normal situation in the upper part of the anal canal. The external wounds are then inspected, and redundant skin tags trimmed away to produce flat firm edges with no puckering or pocketing. This process may lead to brisk capillary bleeding from the divided edges, which can be stopped by application of a swab soaked in 1:1000 adrenaline solution. Other minor bleeding points may be cauterized.

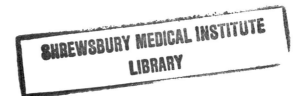

Final appearance; dressing

The final appearance of the operated area should resemble a three-leafed clover, and the wounds should be absolutely dry before a dressing is applied.

Dressings are a matter of choice, except that oily substances and materials should be avoided as they interfere with proper drainage and cleansing of the wounds.

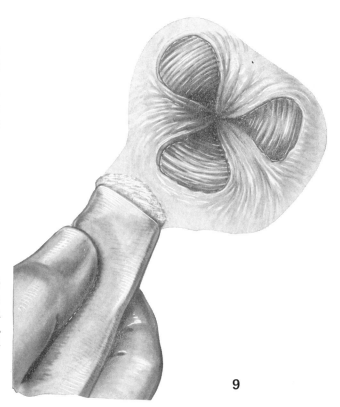

9

A good dressing is gauze lightly soaked in 1:2000 Hibitane solution. The gauze should be applied so that it lies flat and does not wrinkle. After each wound has been separately dressed with the gauze, a pad of cotton wool or Gamgee is applied and held in place by gentle pressure by a 'T' bandage.

9

POSTOPERATIVE CARE AND COMPLICATIONS

The dressings are left undisturbed for 24 hr, but after this they are changed twice daily. At each dressing, the patient should have a warm bath, and on return to bed the wound is thoroughly irrigated with hydrogen peroxide followed by Hibitane 1:2000. A gauze dressing moistened either in the same solution or 1:40 Milton solution (1 per cent sodium hypochlorite) is placed over the wounds and cotton wool is applied beneath a 'T' bandage, as previously.

In order to make the first evacuation easier, an aperient is administered each evening after the day of operation. A small dose of magnesium sulphate solution (10 ml) is sufficient for this purpose in most patients. If defaecation has not occurred by the third day after the operation, a disposable (sodium dihydrogen phosphate) enema should be administered. Once the first action has taken place, the aperients should be stopped and a bulk-forming laxative substituted; any hydrophilic colloid (Cologel, Isogel, Normacol, etc.) is suitable and the patient's preference can be indulged. After each defaecation, the usual bath followed by irrigation and dressing should be carried out.

A finger should be passed on the fifth postoperative day. If there is any stenosis (there should not be, if the operation has been correctly performed), or if there is any undue spasm or pain, it is wise to ask the patient to use a dilator (St. Mark's pattern – size No. 2) twice daily for several weeks after the operation. If there is difficulty in establishing a regular daily bowel action of reasonable bulk, it is also necessary to recommend the use of a dilator.

Final healing takes several weeks, although the patient can leave hospital between the sixth and tenth postoperative days.

The patient should return for examination 3 weeks after the operation. A finger should be passed to check that stenosis has not occurred, but a proctoscope should not be used, as it is liable to precipitate an acute fissure by breaking open the healing wounds.

Retention of urine

This can occur unexpectedly in stoical patients, but is more common in nervous subjects or patients with a lot of pain. The incidence can be reduced by pre- and postoperative use of suitable sedatives, tranquillizing agents and analgesics. The condition usually responds to simple measures, but catheterization is occasionally necessary.

Reactionary haemorrhage

Haemorrhage from a pedicle is very rare. Bleeding may occur from a small vessel in the external wound but can be stopped nearly always by local application of pressure with a gauze swab soaked in 1:1000 adrenaline solution. If this fails, the vessel must be clipped and ligated or diathermied.

If a ligature slips on a main pedicle, the patient must be re-anaesthetized for the rectum to be packed, or the bleeding point identified and religated. The latter is the better procedure.

Secondary haemorrhage

This occurs in 1–2 per cent of cases between the sixth and twentieth postoperative days. The haemorrhage is often severe, requiring blood transfusion as well as local measures to stop the bleeding.

Occasionally a single bleeding point can be identified after washing blood and clots out of the rectum, in which case diathermy coagulation or an under-running suture may be used to stop the bleeding. More frequently, the haemorrhage must be stopped by applying pressure. This is done by passing a large protoscope, after which a large piece of rubber tubing wrapped around by dry gauze is passed through the 'scope into the rectum. Sufficient gauze wrapping should be used to exert firm pressure on the wall of the anal canal and lower rectum. The patient should be given enough sedation to prevent straining, which can cause the tube to be expelled before the bleeding has been controlled. A little traction on the tube to assist the haemostasis can be achieved by wrapping more gauze between the anus and a safety-pin passed through the tube 2 inches (5 cm) from the anal verge. The tube and gauze are left for 48 hr and are then gently removed. A Foley catheter blown up in the rectum can be used as an alternative to a gauze-wrapped tube; after the balloon is distended, traction is applied to the stem of the catheter, which is then fixed firmly to the thigh — after which normal after-care is continued. As a general rule, sepsis is a necessary accompaniment to all cases of secondary haemorrhage and broad-spectrum antibiotic cover should be given (ampicillin 250 mg every 6 hr for 5 days).

Fistula

Occasionally, the superficial margins of the wound fall together and heal, leaving a track or pocket beneath the surface; a fistula then results.

If this happens, the wound must be laid open to allow secondary healing to occur from the depths of the wound towards the surface.

Anal stenosis and cross-healing

If the anus is not regularly expanded during the postoperative period (by a formed stool, or a dilator), the anal orifice can over-contract, leading to stenosis. If this occurs, the anal orifice must be dilated manually under a general anaesthetic. For the same reason, cross healing can occasionally take place between two separate wounds, which then requires breaking down under a general anaesthetic.

A dilator should be used for several weeks after these complications.

References

Goligher, J. C., Leacock, A. G. and Brossy, J. J. (1955). *Br. J. Surg.* **43,** 57
Milligan, E. T. C. and Morgan, C. N. (1934). *Lancet* **2,** 1151, 1213
Milligan, E. T. C., Jones, L. E. and Officer, R. (1937). *Lancet* **2,** 1119

[*The illustrations for this Chapter on Haemorrhoidectomy (St. Mark's Ligation/Excision Method) were drawn by Mr. R. N. Lane.*]

Closed Haemorrhoidectomy

Stanley M. Goldberg, M.D.
Clinical Professor of Surgery and Director, Division of
Colon and Rectal Surgery, University of Minnesota
Medical School, Minneapolis, Minnesota

INTRODUCTION

Over 200 years ago the French anatomist Petit first attempted to eradicate haemorrhoids without denuding the lower anal canal of its mucosa. The technique, modified by many surgeons and popularized in the United States by Ferguson and Fansler, involves saving the anoderm, removal of haemorrhoidal tissue and replacement of the anoderm into its normal position. The advantages over open haemorrhoidectomy are that the anal canal is covered with its own anoderm, no postoperative dilatations are required and primary healing is secured, resulting in much less discomfort for the patient. Frykman modified the partially closed technique of Fansler to the completely closed technique. Fansler advocated closing the wound only to the dentate line; however Frykman extended closure to include the undercut and mobilized peri-anal skin. The same technique, used by us for 30 years, is described in this chapter.

PRE - OPERATIVE

Indications

Since the advent of the rubber band ligature technique for bleeding internal haemorrhoids, our indications for closed haemorrhoidectomy have been limited to: (*1*) prolapse; (*2*) pain; (*3*) bleeding not controlled by rubber band ligature or injection; (*4*) association with other surgical conditions of the anal canal, e.g. fissure, fistula.

The most frequent indication for haemorrhoid-ectomy, in our practice today, is rectal mucosal prolapse associated with prolapsing mixed haemor-rhoids. Pain associated with haemorrhoids is always associated with thrombosis. When thrombosis is extensive, haemorrhoidectomy is indicated although the majority of painful thrombosed haemorrhoids can be handled with simple excision of the entire haemorrhoidal complex, under local anaesthesia. When surgery is required for fissures or fistulae associated with haemorrhoids, haemorrhoidectomy may be added at that time.

Pre-operative evaluation

All patients undergoing haemorrhoidectomy have pre-operative sigmoidoscopy at the time of their first examination; if they are beyond the age of 40 years and their symptoms suggest additional pathology, a barium enema examination is indicated. Special care is always taken with any patient who has a history of soft stools or diarrhoea to rule out the possibility of undiagnosed inflammatory bowel disease, which is a specific contra-indication for haemorrhoidectomy. The usual laboratory tests to rule out a bleeding diathesis are obtained.

The patient is informed that he will be in the hospital for 4–5 days and that he should refrain from any heavy lifting for a period of 2 weeks follow-ing surgery. He is told complete healing will not occur for a period of approximately 3–4 weeks and that his chance of returning to the operating room for a complication, related to surgery, is usually about 1 in 100.

Pre-operative preparation

No oral pre-operative preparation is indicated for our technique. One disposable packaged enema is given the evening before surgery and another approximately 1 hr before surgery. Neither laxatives nor antibiotics are used pre-operatively or during the procedure.

1

Position of patient

Traditionally anorectal procedures have been done in the lithotomy position or the left lateral position as favoured in certain parts of North America. However, we use the semiprone or jack-knife position with soft rolls under the hips and ankles of the patient ensuring that the patient is comfortable on the table. The advantages of this position are that any bleeding that occurs will fall away from the operative field, it affords comfort for the operating surgeon, and access to the operative field is superior.

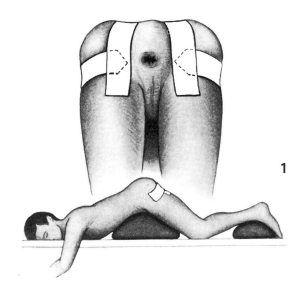

1

Preparation of skin

No attempt is made to sterilize the skin other than using Zephiran (tincture of benzalkonium chloride). The operative area is not shaved and adhesive tapes are applied to the buttocks to provide lateral traction.

Anaesthesia

The prone position lends itself well to a combination of general and local anaesthesia. We use Pentothal (thiopentone sodium) intravenously as a sedative and inducing agent combined with 0·5 per cent Xylocaine and 1:200,000 adrenaline solution locally. Regional anaesthesia, either spinal or caudal, can be used in this position; however, local anaesthesia is preferred since there is an inherent fear on the part of the patient for regional types of anaesthesia. With certain patients it is necessary to use an endotracheal tube in the prone position; however, in all cases local infiltration with Xylocaine and adrenaline is employed.

2

If local anaesthesia is used alone it is most important that infiltration be carried out correctly. Forty to fifty millilitres of a 0·5 Xylocaine and 1:200,000 adrenaline solution is injected through a No. 22 needle into the skin picking up the cutaneous nerves. Following this a direct injection into the muscle, as pictured, is carried out in order to pick up the branches of the inferior haemorrhoidal nerve resulting in immediate relaxation of the sphincter muscle; no manual dilatations or stretching of the sphincter muscle are carried out. No specific attempt is made to inject the anoderm directly in the area of the haemorrhoids or to 'balloon up' the mucosa. The anaesthetic usually lasts for 40–60 min, more than sufficient for the operative procedure, and it also provides considerable relief in the immediate postoperative period. Elderly patients with hypertension or cardiovascular problems present no difficulty with the low concentration of adrenaline.

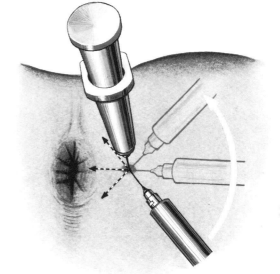

2

Another important point regarding anaesthesia is the use of minimal volumes (less than 50 ml) of intravenous solutions during surgery, a principle which has helped keep our catheterization incidence under 3 per cent. We believe that by keeping the patients dehydrated in the postoperative period their bladders are not distended, resulting in spontaneous voiding within the first 20 hr.

PROCEDURE

Following the introduction of local anaesthesia which relaxes the sphincter, the anal canal is examined digitally and then by a Pratt bivalve speculum introduced into the anal canal, examining carefully the specific haemorrhoidal areas; the operation is planned in greater detail at this moment. No dilatations are carried out with the bivalve speculum. The largest haemorrhoidal complex is removed first; the quadrants usually involved are the left lateral, right posterior and right anterior. No suction is necessary during the procedure. Small 7·5 cm² gauze sponges which fit through the operative scope are used as an alternative to suction. Having examined the area with the Pratt bivalve speculum, we then employ the Fansler operating anoscope.

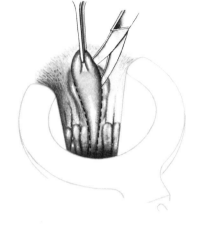

3

3&4

Dissection is started on the peri-anal skin. No attempt is made to remove all the tissue in one motion. An elliptical incision is made with fine dissecting scissors removing skin and haemorrhoidal tissue down to the underlying internal sphincter.

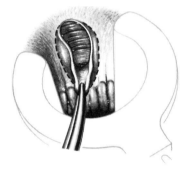

4

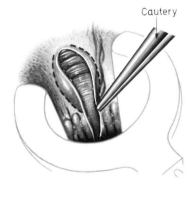

Cautery

5

5

Redundant rectal mucosa is excised high up to and sometimes even beyond the first valve of Houston in order to correct the rectal mucosal prolapse. No crown suture is placed on the pedicle. Most of the bleeding occurs from edges of the mucosa; individual bleeders in the mucosa are coagulated using a Medtronic forceps.

6

At this point the mucosa is elevated, haemorrhoidal tissue is dissected from beneath the mucosal flaps, other bleeding points are electrocoagulated and the anodermal flaps are undercut adequately so that they can be closed without tension.

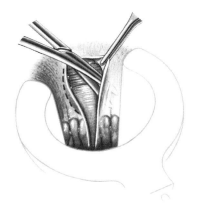

6

7

After dissecting the secondary haemorrhoidal vessels from beneath the anodermal skin flaps and controlling the bleeding, the wound is closed starting at the apex utilizing a running suture of 3/0 chromic catgut. The mucous membrane is sutured down to the underlying sphincter mechanism in an attempt to create a longitudinal scar which will prevent further prolapse. Trimming of excess skin is carried out, but *it is essential that the wounds be closed without tension.* A loose knot is tied at the completion of the procedure. Rarely is any clamping of vessels necessary and no pile clamps are used.

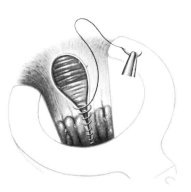

7

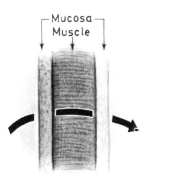

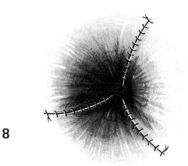

8

8

The procedure is carried out in three major areas and in as many additional areas as necessary; in certain cases of prolapsed thrombosed haemorrhoids, as many as six areas may be excised and primarily closed.

When the anal canal does not accept the operating anoscope easily, a partial internal sphincterotomy is carried out in the base of a wound, usually in the right posterior or left lateral quadrant. At the completion of the procedure all quadrants are examined carefully, and blood clots are removed. No packing or dressing is placed in the anal canal or peri-anal area. The average operating time is 35 min.

POSTOPERATIVE CARE

Postoperatively our patients are encouraged to have only sips of water until such time as they void spontaneously. Since we have instituted this programme of dehydration, catheterization rate on all patients has been under 3 per cent. Having voided postoperatively the patients are allowed fluids and food as desired. One of the advantages of the operative technique as described is that little pain is experienced. However, our patients receive meperidine (pethidine) on demand for the first 3–4 days and are also given an oral pain medication consisting of aspirin and meprobamate four times daily during their hospital stay.

Early activity is encouraged. Warm packs are applied to the perineum during the immediate postoperative period. After 24 hr, patients are encouraged to take as many sitz baths as required for cleanliness and comfort. A small cotton dressing is put in the peri-anal area to collect whatever discharge or drainage may be present. No other local treatment is carried out. The patients are started immediately on Metamucil (psyllium hydrophilic mucilloid), one package twice daily and Kondremul (55 per cent liquid paraffin in Irish Moss emulsion) twice daily, the latter being stopped immediately after the first bowel movement. Because the patients receive only a small (100 ml) packaged enema the evening before surgery and the morning of surgery, they usually have their first bowel movement the second or third postoperative day. If they do not, a tapwater enema is given on the third postoperative day using a soft rubber catheter.

No dilatations are carried out in the hospital. Patients are usually discharged from the hospital between the fourth and fifth postoperative day, our average being 4·1 days. Patients are instructed not to do any lifting or straining, and to report back to the clinic in 10–14 days for examination. They are discharged with Metamucil, one package per day and some oral analgesics consisting of aspirin and meprobamate to use as necessary.

Follow-up

Patients return to the clinic, 10–14 days following surgery, and are examined very carefully with a digital and anoscopic examination. It is apparent at this time that a percentage of the wounds have failed to remain closed; however, the majority have healed primarily. Secondary haemorrhage has occurred in 0·3 per cent of our cases. Less than 1 per cent of our patients return to the operating room for a second operative procedure resulting from an unhealed wound or a persistent sinus tract. Postoperative infection has not been a problem but in two isolated cases an attempt was made, on the part of the surgeon, to reduce postoperative pain by re-injecting the peri-anal tissue with local anaesthetic at the completion of the procedure, resulting in two ischiorectal abscesses. No further infections have occurred since discontinuing the re-injection technique.

Skin tags

Skin tags may result from any operative procedure on the peri-anal area, however no greater incidence of skin tag formation occurs with the closed technique. A large skin tag can be removed under local anaesthesia in the clinic, however, we do like to have a 'pleat' so that the patient does not split the peri-anal skin when the anal canal opens at the time of defaecation.

Anal stenosis and anal stricture have been reported following the closed technique, and usually result from the removal of too much normal skin in the peri-anal area. With attention to detail, however, these complications have not been a problem.

SUMMARY

Closed haemorrhoidectomy is an effective and safe alternative to open haemorrhoidectomy, resulting in rapid healing and minimal postoperative discomfort for the patient. The use of the prone position and infiltration of local anaesthetic facilitates the procedure.

References

Fansler, W. A. (1934). 'Surgical treatment of hemorrhoids.' *Minn. Med.* **17**
Ferguson, J. A., Mazier, W. P., Ganchrow, M. I. and Friend, W. G. (1971). 'The closed technique of haemorrhoidectomy.' *Surgery* **70,** 480
Parks, A. G. (1971). 'Haemorrhoidectomy.' *Adv. Surg.* **5**
Petit, J. L. (1774). *Traite des maladies chirurgicales et des operations qui leur convenient, Paris,* **2,** 137

[*The illustrations for this Chapter on Closed Haemorrhoidectomy were drawn by Mr. M. J. Courtney.*]

Haemorrhoidectomy

A. G. Parks, M.Ch., F.R.C.S., F.R.C.P.
Consultant Surgeon, St. Mark's Hospital, London
and The London Hospital

INTRODUCTION

There are at least three entities which may occur separately or together and which are generally regarded as being encompassed by the term, haemorrhoids. The most widely recognized is dilatation of the veins of the submucosa of the upper anal canal (internal haemorrhoids), in some cases coupled with similar change in the lower anal canal (intero-external haemorrhoids). The reason for this change is not known but it may be due to two factors acting simultaneously. Even in normal people there is, during defaecation, some eversion of the anal canal with prolapse of the upper anal mucosa. This allows the veins of the upper anal submucosa to be exposed to atmospheric pressure. If defaecation straining is excessive, pressure in the superior haemorrhoidal veins is high (up to 500 cm of water). This pressure, when communicated to the exteriorized veins of the upper anal submucosa, causes their sudden distension which, if repeated over a long period of time, may produce permanent varicosities. Vascular haemorrhoids of this type are commoner in men. In women simple protrusion of the upper anal mucosa, without varicose change, is commoner but this too is called haemorrhoids. It is particularly prone to occur in those who have lax perineal musculature; during defaecation straining the pelvic floor drops, the anal canal is shortened by eversion and prolapse occurs.

1

In either situation, once the stage of conservative treatment is passed there is almost always descent of the whole anal lining. Mucosa of the lower rectum enters the anal canal, forcing the columnar mucosa of the upper anal canal down beyond its usual termination in the mid-anal region. In its turn the lower squamous mucosa is driven out of the canal. There are several important consequences of these changes. During embryonic development the migration of skin and squamous mucosa into the last 2 cm of the gut replaces insensitive, mucus-secreting epithelium with dry epithelium. As a result, the normal person does not experience any mucous leakage. In addition the squamous mucosa is rich in nerve endings (Duthie and Gairns, 1960), is very sensitive and forms an important part of the mechanism of continence. Once this state of affairs is changed by the drop of the whole anal lining, several unfortunate events are apt to ensue. Firstly, columnar epithelium secretes mucus with consequent soreness and pruritus. Secondly, the sensitive squamous mucosa is no longer so effective a part of the continence mechanism because it is now situated outside the anal canal (the columnar epithelium itself has virtually no sensory receptors). Thirdly, the exteriorized squamous mucosa protrudes as a so-called 'tag'. Its delicate epithelium is liable to be the site of irritation and soreness.

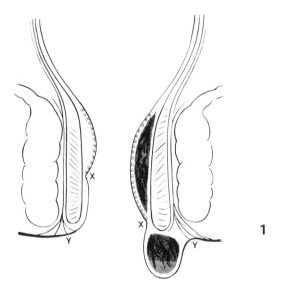

1

Some of the symptoms associated with haemorrhoids are therefore due to mucous secretion by columnar epithelium which is intermittently exteriorized and also to the total exteriorization of the squamous mucosa which forms an irritable tag. Further symptoms can be caused by impairment of anal sensation with resultant soiling and, if the mucosal prolapse of the upper and lower rectum is marked, by obstruction during defaecation as the mucosa descends into the anal canal. In most standard operations the exteriorized squamous mucosa (the anoderm) is usually excised as a worthless tag. Part of the prolapsing columnar mucosa is also removed but not a great deal. The canal becomes partially lined by columnar epithelium and partially by regenerating squamous mucosa from the skin edges. Most of the sensitive anal mucosa is lost and there is still columnar mucosa at a relatively low level which secretes mucus. In most cases the latter undergoes partial squamous metaplasia but only after some time has passed. In summary, the tissue which should be removed (that is the upper columnar type mucosa) has been retained and the anoderm, which should be conserved, is excised. The aim of the procedure to be described is to reverse this situation. The anoderm is carefully preserved but upper anal and lower rectal mucosa is

excised in an amount appropriate to the prolapse. In addition the vascular submucosa in each haemorrhoidal area is completely excised.

Salmon (quoted by Allingham) in the early part of the last century carefully dissected haemorrhoidal tissue from the internal sphincter and then performed a high ligation of the pedicle. Following this operation patients had little pain and did well initially but the risk of subsequent stenosis was as high as 10 per cent. To avoid the latter complication, a low ligature operation was introduced by Milligan and Morgan (1937), whereby the pile pedicle was sutured to the lower anal muscle wall, thus avoiding a large wound with consequent stenosis. However, Watts *et al.* (1964) have shown that the pedicle retracts, leaving a considerable area of denuded muscle. Haemorrhoidal change may affect a large part of the circumference of the anal canal and, if a radical procedure is performed, much of the normal mucosa may be removed. The principle of the present method is to excise all the vascular submucosa in each haemorrhoidal area, together with an appropriate amount of prolapsing columnar-type epithelium. The vascular plexus in the submucosa is carefully freed from the underlying internal sphincter; the exposed muscle is not left as an open wound but is covered by squamous mucosa conserved during the dissection and advanced into the anal canal as a plastic procedure. The theoretical objection that the space between the mucosa and muscle is an undrained cavity in which infection will occur, does not hold in practice; in fact one of the main advantages of the procedure is that the wounds heal more quickly, with less induration and scarring than with other methods. In this way it combines the benefits of the high ligation operation without having its disadvantages. This principle of conservation of mucosa was first enunciated in 1774 by Jean-Louis Petit and has been practised by others intermittently since then.

2

There is one anatomical point of importance if this technique is adopted. At the mucocutaneous junction, approximately half way within the anal canal, the epithelium is tethered to the underlying internal sphincter; above and below this point it is readily separated from underlying structures. Here then care must be taken in the dissection lest the mucosa fragments and becomes non-viable. The anal crypts occur at this level and they too are a hazard in dissection, as they are easily 'button-holed'. The haemorrhoidal plexus itself is adherent to the internal sphincter by smooth muscle and connective tissue strands for a variable distance above the mucocutaneous junction. If these strands are not divided, the muscle bundles of the sphincter are drawn down and incorporated into the ligature; this may be a major factor in the cause of post-haemorrhoidectomy pain (*see Illustration 10b*).

Normal anal mucosa is thin and easily lacerated; the submucosal plexus is tenuous and is also difficult to manipulate without fragmentation. When haemorrhoidal change is advanced, the mucosa becomes tougher and fibrous tissue is deposited in the submucosa; both these changes make the performance of the operation relatively easy.

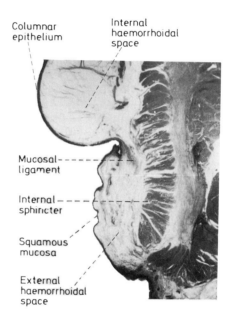

Columnar epithelium

Internal haemorrhoidal space

Mucosal ligament

Internal sphincter

Squamous mucosa

External haemorrhoidal space

2

PRE-OPERATIVE

Pre-operative preparation

Preparation for operation is minimal; it is not necessary to administer antibiotics. A mild laxative, such as paraffin emulsion is given 24 hr before, and then 4 hr prior to operation two glycerine suppositories are administered.

Position of patient

The operation is usually performed in the lithotomy position, but the jack-knife position is equally suitable. It is important that the external sphincter be completely relaxed to allow the introduction of the anal retractor without tearing anal mucosa. This may either be obtained by using relaxant drugs or by local infiltration with analgesic agents, such as lignocaine.

THE OPERATION

3

The speculum

The operation is performed through a speculum which enables the operator to see the mucosa *in situ*, undistorted by traction. The speculum is self-retaining and has winged blades which hold the rectal wall away from the field of operation.

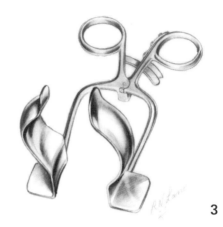

3

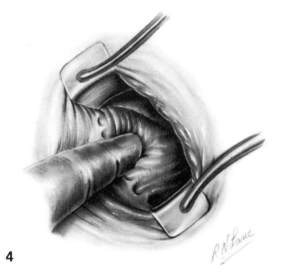

4

4

Insertion of anal retractor

After the anal canal has been inspected to find out the situation and extent of haemorrhoidal change, the skin distal to the right posterior haemorrhoid is grasped with a haemostatic forcep. The anal retractor is inserted and as the blades are opened the mucosa is gently 'milked' into the aperture between the blades.

5

Exposure of haemorrhoid

The haemorrhoid is seen as a wedge-shaped structure whose apex lies at the mucocutaneous junction. The pedicle depicted in many texts is largely an artefact created by traction.

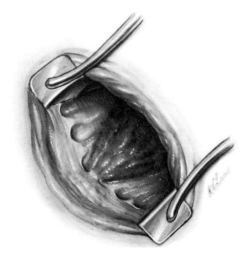

5

6

Injection of adrenaline

A weak solution of adrenaline in isotonic saline solution (1 part adrenaline in 300,000 parts of saline solution) is then injected just under the surface of the mucosa of the haemorrhoid. The needle is first introduced at the mucocutaneous junction where the mucosa is attached to the muscle. If it is not placed here at the start, the tissue on either side of the mucocutaneous junction distends and leaves the junction as a deep furrow which is difficult to dissect free.

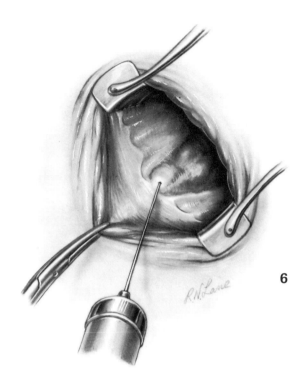

6

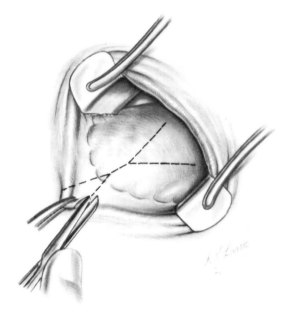

7

7

Skin incision

After this region has been infiltrated, about 20 ml of fluid is injected under the mucosa of the internal haemorrhoid and a few millilitres are put into the peri-anal space. This manoeuvre creates a plane between the mucosa and the vascular plexus in which dissection can be performed. The skin incision starts at the outer edge of the anus and is carried around both sides of the forceps holding the anal skin, keeping close to them to avoid removing more anoderm than is absolutely necessary.

8

The incision

The skin and squamous mucosa of the lower anal canal is first undermined using scissor dissection. The vascular tissue of the external plexus is exposed in this way. The two limbs of the incision meet at the mucocutaneous junction and then split again shortly above this point in a V-shaped fashion.

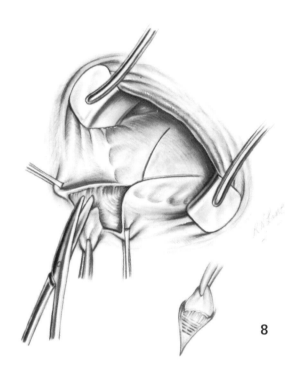

8

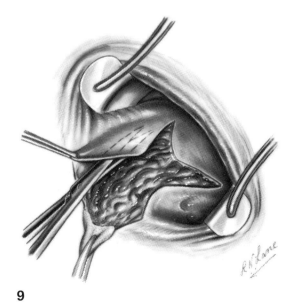

9

9

Lifting the mucosa off the haemorrhoidal vessels

The next step is to lift the mucosa off the haemorrhoidal vessels. This is accomplished with scissor dissection commencing at the mucocutaneous junction. Here the attachment of the mucosa to the muscle must be divided before the haemorrhoid itself can be uncovered. The lower border of the incision is first freed and a flap of epithelium created which stretches from the skin of the anal verge, through the mucocutaneous junction, up into the lowest point of the rectum. It is carried sufficiently far laterally to include any secondary haemorrhoids which may be present. The upper limit of the dissection should be about 4 cm above the mucocutaneous junction. It is wise not to grasp the upper mucosa with forceps as it is very friable; it can be controlled by traction on the anal skin. Scissor dissection is performed by viewing the blades through the translucent mucosa; this is the only way to keep in the correct plane between the haemorrhoidal vessels and the epithelial surface.

10a

The sphincter dissection

The submucosa of the external haemorrhoidal area is dissected free with any veins it may contain. The lower border of the internal sphincter is then identified and the submucosa is carefully dissected off its surface with sharp scissor dissection. Traction applied to the haemorrhoidal tissue distorts the upper part of the internal sphincter, causing it to be drawn into the pedicle in the shape of a V.

The muscle and connective tissue strands linking the muscle and the submucosa must be severed and the muscle bundles pushed outwards on to the anal wall. Above a point about 3 cm from the muco-cutaneous junction this adherence ceases; once the dissection has passed this level, the vascular haemorrhoidal tissue suddenly becomes free and can be drawn out of the anal canal.

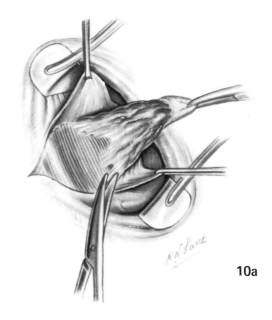

10a

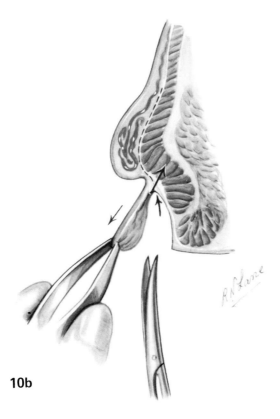

10b

10b

A lateral view of the dissection

This view is shown here to demonstrate the ease with which the internal sphincter can be distorted. It is apparent that dissection could be unwittingly performed into the substance of the internal sphincter itself, resulting in excision of part of it.

11

The dissection complete

The haemorrhoidal submucosa has been stripped off the internal sphincter to an adequate level. The mucosal flaps are clearly demonstrated.

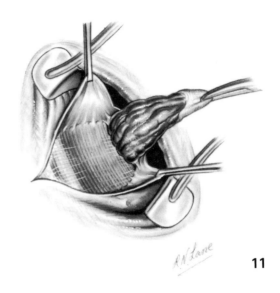

11

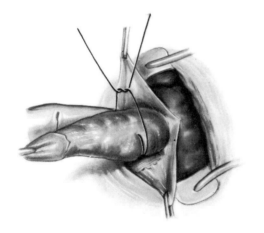

12

12

Transfixion of the pedicle

A transfixion stitch of No. 0 chromic catgut is placed through the upper limit of the pedicle, which contains columnar mucosa on its surface and the submucosa; the pedicle is not bulky and the ligature does not bunch up the tissues of the anal wall. Non-absorbable suture material must not be used, as it will form a granuloma under the mucosa. This procedure is applied to each haemorrhoidal area in turn. The anterior and posterior commissures of the anal canal are carefully inspected for the presence of accessory haemorrhoids which may require to be removed separately.

13

Excision completed

The haemorrhoid has been ligated and removed. The floor of the wound is seen to be composed of the internal sphincter and the conservation of squamous mucosa is demonstrated. Each wound is carefully inspected prior to the plastic reconstruction, care being taken to stop all bleeding points with diathermy coagulation. Contrary to common belief, it is quite frequent to find numerous small arteries perforating the internal sphincter to join the haemorrhoidal tissue. It is these which have to be secured before the next stage is commenced.

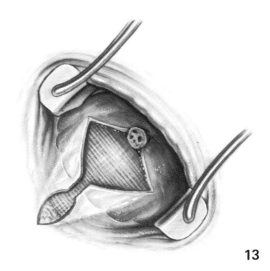

13

14

Reconstruction of the mucosa

The result of the operation is to produce a large wound with internal sphincter in its floor. Rather than allow this to heal by secondary intention, it is covered with the two flaps of squamous mucosa previously prepared. A suture of 2/0 plain catgut is passed through the mucosa of one flap, is then passed under a bundle of the internal sphincter at the top of the wound and finally through the mucocutaneous junction of the other flap. In this way both flaps are firmly secured to the top of the wound. The reason for incorporating internal sphincter is to prevent dislodgement of the flaps during the postoperative phase. Two further stitches can be placed between the upper part of each flap and the lower margin of the rectal mucosa.

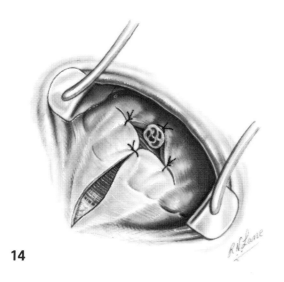

14

15

Final inspection of wounds

Each wound is inspected in turn and any cutaneous bleeding point is coagulated. If there is redundancy of skin at the anal margin, it is trimmed to prevent tag formation. No drain or dressings are applied in the anal canal itself; only a moistened gauze is applied externally.

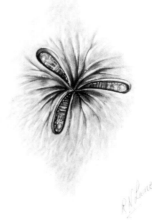

15

POSTOPERATIVE CARE

Bowel action

In the immediate period following operation the amount of pain is variable but is, on the average, less than that following standard techniques. If pain is severe, pethidine is given; usually only one dose is required. Morphine is avoided altogether because it results in prolonged postoperative constipation and also dulls the awareness of a full bladder. Many patients require nothing more than an oral analgesic for discomfort; paracetamol is a good drug for this purpose because it has no tendency to cause constipation. Male patients may stand to micturate on the night of operation, which prevents them getting an overloaded bladder.

No attempt is made to inhibit bowel action. It is far better for a patient to pass a soft stool on the second or third postoperative day than to traumatize the anal canal with a large, hard faecal scybalus on the fifth or sixth day. Liquid paraffin is given for the first 2–3 days after operation and is then replaced with a hydrophilic laxative. The early establishment of normal bowel habits helps in preventing anal stenosis. It is far better that the patient should dilate his anal canal by normal bowel function than by instrumental stretching. He can only do this if there is little pain and no spasm. Other forms of anal dilatation are not used following this operation; because of the conservation of mucosa, anal stenosis is rare. Some pain is experienced with the first bowel movement, otherwise the patient usually complains only of soreness. This ceases after the fifth or sixth day and thereafter he is free of discomfort. On the first day after operation the patient has a bath and this is repeated once or twice daily for the remainder of the stay in hospital. A bath relieves the discomfort of an anal wound better than any other measure.

Wound dressing and examination

The wounds require no treatment at all and the nursing staff is thereby relieved of much time-consuming treatment. The only dressing used is a piece of flat gauze to protect the clothing. A finger is passed on the fifth or sixth day to determine the state of the wounds and to detect any spasm of the internal sphincter. Rectal examination is repeated weekly until the wounds are healed in 3–4 weeks' time. Healing occurs quickly, and once healed the anal canal is suppler than after other operations.

Late care

It is well known that recurrent symptoms can follow haemorrhoidectomy; the true incidence is not known as they can occur many years later. Examination of such cases suggests that most of them have in fact mucosal prolapse of the lower rectal wall rather than true haemorrhoids. Many have lax sphincters such as occurs in the descending perineum syndrome (Parks, Porter and Hardcastle, 1966). It must be explained to all patients after any haemorrhoidal operation that recurrent symptoms are usually due to defaecation straining with development of mucosal prolapse. If symptoms occur, they are relieved by a simple injection and correction of faulty bowel habits. It is very rare for a further operative procedure to be necessary.

References

Allingham, W. (1871). *Fistula, Haemorrhoids, Painful Ulcer, Stricture, Prolapsus and other Diseases of the Rectum, their Diagnosis and Treatment,* pp. 86–97. London: Churchill
Duthie, H. L. and Gairns, F. W. (1960). *Br. J. Surg.* 47, 585
Milligan, E. T. C., Morgan, C. N., Jones, L. E. and Officer, R. (1937). *Lancet* 2, 1119
Parks, A. G., Porter, N. H. and Hardcastle, J. (1966). *Proc. R. Soc. Med.* 59, 477
Petit, J. L. (1774). *Traite des Maladies Chirurgicales et des Operations qui leur Conviennent, Paris,* Vol. 2, p. 137
Watts, J. McK., Bennett, R. C., Duthie, H. L. and Goligher, J. C. (1964). *Br. J. Surg.* 51, 808

[*The illustrations for this Chapter on Haemorrhoidectomy were drawn by Mr. R. N. Lane.*]

Fissure-in-Ano. Lateral Subcutaneous Internal Anal Sphincterotomy

M. J. Notaras, F.R.C.S., F.R.C.S. (Ed.)
Consultant Surgeon, Barnet General Hospital;
Honorary Senior Lecturer and Consultant Surgeon,
University College Hospital, London

INTRODUCTION

Examination of the lower half of the anal canal by separation of the buttocks to open up the peri-anal region will reveal the presence of any simple anal fissure as it is located below the dentate line and is always confined to the anoderm in the mid-posterior position (90 per cent) or the mid-anterior position (10 per cent). The anoderm is that part of the anal skin which lies between the dentate line and the anal verge and is the squamous lining of the anal canal. The acute fissure is a superficial splitting of the anoderm and may heal with conservative management. Once the fissure is recurrent or chronic, operation is required for a permanent cure. The chronic fissure is recognized by the presence of transverse fibres of the internal sphincter in its floor. A late stage in the development of the chronic fissure is the formation of a large fibrous polyp from the anal papilla on the dentate line at the upper end of the fissure. Infection of the sentinel pile which develops at the lower end of the fissure at the anal verge may lead to the formation of a superficial fistula.

Fissures which are multiple or extend above the dentate line should be viewed with suspicion as the simple fissure-in-ano never extends above the dentate line. These complex fissures are usually signs of more serious diseases such as ulcerative colitis, Crohn's disease, tuberculosis or syphilis. When associated with large rubbery inguinal lymph nodes they may indicate a primary syphilitic infection and smears from the anal canal should be taken for dark ground illumination before digital or endoscopic examination spoils the field with lubricant.

A biopsy should always be taken from any suspicious fissure or ulcer.

Treatment of fissure-in-ano

Lateral subcutaneous internal anal sphincterotomy has been shown to have many advantages over other forms of treatment such as anal dilatation and the mid-posterior internal sphincterotomy performed through the floor of the fissure. It has rapidly gained acceptance as it may be performed as an out-patient procedure under local or general anaesthesia. Its main advantages are that it avoids an open intra-anal wound, the divided internal sphincter is bridged by skin, there is minimal anal wound care, postoperative anal dilatation is unnecessary and relief from symptoms is almost immediate with the fissure becoming painless and healing within 3 weeks.

STAGES OF FISSURE - IN - ANO
(illustrated below)

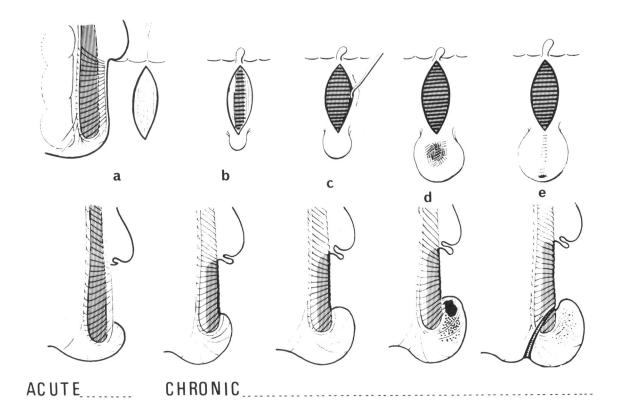

ACUTE ....   CHRONIC ....

TECHNIQUES

CLOSED TECHNIQUE

The lower part of the internal sphincter is divided
subcutaneously in a manner similar to performing
a subcutaneous tenotomy. This method virtually
leaves no wound.

OPEN TECHNIQUE

Through a radial peri-anal incision the internal
sphincter is exposed by subcutaneous dissection
and then incised.

Pre-operative preparation

Both techniques may be performed under local or
general anaesthesia. The author prefers no bowel
preparation so that the urge to defaecate after the
operation is not delayed. The patient may be positioned
in the lithotomy, lateral or 'jack-knife' positions according to the preference of the surgeon. Sigmoidoscopy should be performed on all patients.

THE OPERATIONS

CLOSED TECHNIQUE (lithotomy position)

1&2

A bivalved anal speculum (Parks, Eisenhammer or Goligher) is introduced into the anal canal and opened sufficiently to place the anus on a slight stretch. The internal sphincter is then felt as a tight band around the blades of the speculum. Its lower border is easily palpated and can be demonstrated by gently pressing a pair of forceps into the intersphincteric groove.

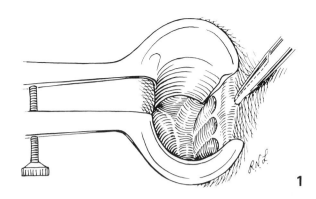

1

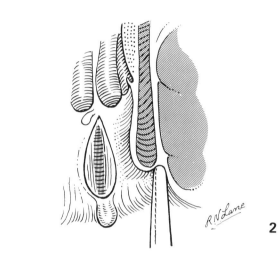

2

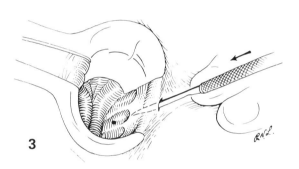

3

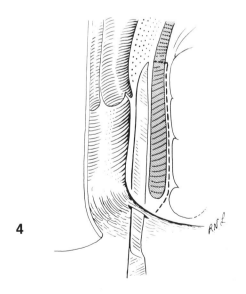

4

3&4

After the internal sphincter has been identified a narrow-bladed scalpel (52L 'Beaver' cataract knife) is introduced through the peri-anal skin at the mid-lateral aspect of the anus (3 o'clock). It is pushed cephalad with the flat of the blade sandwiched between the internal sphincter and anoderm until its point is just above the dentate line.

5 & 6

The sharp edge of the blade is then turned towards the internal sphincter and by incising outwards and laterally the internal sphincterotomy is performed. As the scalpel blade cuts through the internal sphincter there is a characteristic 'gritty' sensation felt and with completion of the division there is a sudden 'give' sensation indicating that the blade has reached the outer surrounding ring of external sphincter muscles.

Another variation of the technique is to introduce the blade between the external and internal sphincter muscles via the intersphincteric groove and then to perform the sphincterotomy by cutting inwards towards the mucocutaneous lining.

Whichever technique is used, the aim is the same, i.e. to preserve a skin bridge over the divided internal sphincter.

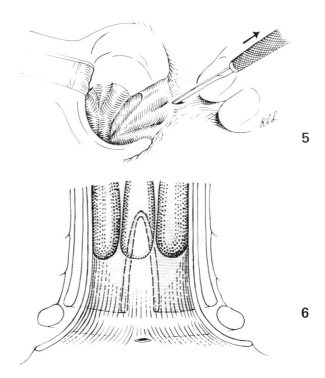

5

6

7

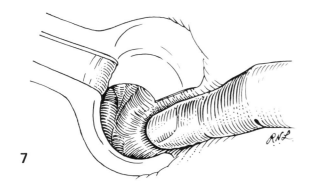

7

Following division of the internal sphincter the completeness of the sphincterotomy may be assessed after withdrawal of the knife by pressure of the finger tip over the site. This will rupture any residual internal sphincter fibres.

Usually there is a slight ooze of blood from the small external wound but this is soon arrested by tamponade as the external sphincters recover and contract around the internal sphincter. The external wound is left open to allow drainage of this blood. A local anaesthetic combined with adrenaline injected into the area prior to performance of the sphincterotomy will help to minimize this blood loss.

8

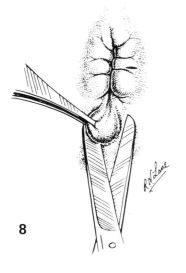

8

If there is a large sentinel pile, it is removed with sharp-pointed scissors without damaging the sphincters and with minimal excision of the peri-anal skin. All overhang is removed.

9 & 10

A fistula in a sentinel pile when present should be laid open. The tract passes through some of the superficial fibres of the lower border of the internal sphincter. It is tempting to perform also a complete internal anal sphincterotomy through the fissure and the rest of the sphincter above the sentinel pile but results are better if the surgeon confines himself to merely laying open the fistula and then performing a lateral subcutaneous sphincterotomy. This avoids the development of a 'key-hole' deformity in the mid-posterior position which may lead to peri-anal soiling.

A dressing is laid on the anal area. Intra-anal dressings are contra-indicated as they cause post-operative pain. Once bleeding has ceased no dressings are required. The patient is encouraged to have a bowel action as soon as the inclination develops.

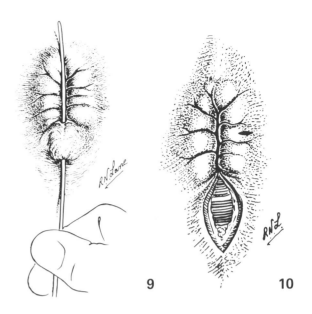

9   10

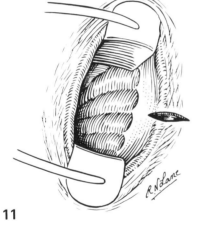

11

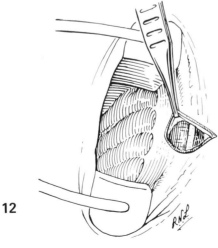

12

OPEN TECHNIQUE

If the surgeon is not happy with the closed technique because of fear of damage to the external sphincter muscle the open method is equally applicable. The author originally practised this technique but with experience found the closed technique more simple and expeditious.

11 & 12

A bivalved anal speculum is inserted into the anus to place the internal sphincter on a slight stretch to assist its identification as described in the closed method.

A local anaesthetic with adrenaline is injected into the subcutaneous area selected for the procedure. A radial incision is made into the peri-anal skin just below the inferior border of the internal sphincter. This incision is preferred to the circumferential type as the wound is left unsutured and open for the egress of blood and the edges of the wound will approximate naturally.

13 & 14

The upper end of the incision is grasped with forceps and dissection with narrow-bladed scissors is carried out so as to separate the anoderm from the internal sphincter. The latter is recognized by its white fibres. To facilitate dissection and the sphincterotomy its lower border may be grasped with forceps.

The exposed internal sphincter is then divided by a narrow scalpel blade or scissors.

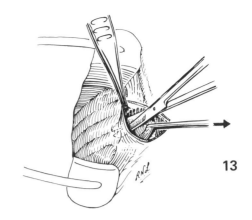

13

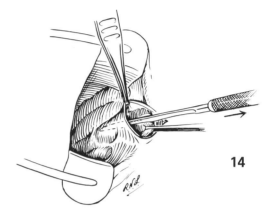

14

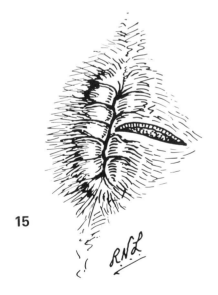

15

15

The wound is left open to allow free drainage. A 'lay-on' dressing of gauze is placed over the anus. Intra-anal dressings should not be used as they cause postoperative pain.

POSTOPERATIVE CARE AND COMPLICATIONS

The patients may be discharged home the same day. Patients who have had the procedure performed under local anaesthesia should be kept at bed rest until the external sphincters have recovered from the effects of the anaesthetic. Very rarely prolapse of internal haemorrhoids has occurred when the patient has assumed the erect position too soon. The patients are given an aperient to ensure early defaecation after the procedure and to keep the stools soft until recovery has been complete. Simple oral analgesics may be necessary in the first 24—48 hr to combat the dull perineal ache which follows the operation.

Complications from the operation are rare. Peri-anal ecchymoses occasionally develop. Persistent haemorrhage from the sphincterotomy wound very rarely occurs but if present may be arrested by direct pressure to the area. Approximately 5 per cent of patients may develop a slight disturbance of anal continence in that they are unable to control flatus as well as prior to operation.

Editorial comment

The editor believes that sometimes the subcutaneous external sphincter overlaps the lower border of the internal sphincter and may be felt so-doing when the finger presses upon the sphincterotomy site (*see Illustration 8*). If so it should be divided to prevent overhang which occasionally makes final healing of the fissure prolonged.

References

Clery, A. P. and O'Riordan, J. B. (1970). *J. R. Coll. Surg. Irel.* **6**, No. 1
Hoffman, D. C. and Goligher, J. C. (1970). *Br. med. J.* **3**, 673
Notaras, M. J. (1966). Annual Report, St. Mark's Hospital
Notaras, M. J. (1969). *Proc. R. Soc. Med.* **62**, 713
Notaras, M. J. (1971). *Br. J. Surg.* **58**, 2
Parks, A. G. (1967). *Hosp. Med.* **1**, 737

[*The illustrations for this Chapter on Fissure-in-Ano. Lateral Subcutaneous Internal Anal Sphincterotomy were drawn by Mr. R. N. Lane.*]

Peri-anal and Ischiorectal Abscess

H. E. Lockhart-Mummery, M.D., M.Chir., F.R.C.S.
Consultant Surgeon, St. Thomas's and St. Mark's Hospitals,
and King Edward VII Hospital for Officers, London

PRE - OPERATIVE

Indications

Infection in an ischiorectal fossa may spread rapidly and extensively in the loose fat that fills these fossae, and any abscess should therefore be opened *without delay*. Diagnosis is often difficult in the early stages when the abscess is small; examination under anaesthesia in the lithotomy position may be necessary before the presence of a suspected abscess can be confirmed.

Chemotherapy and antibiotics are of little value in the treatment of an ischiorectal abscess, and may be harmful if their use leads to delay in surgery.

There are no contra-indications.

Pre-operative preparation

If pain and tenderness allow, the rectum should be emptied by an enema before operation. The anal region should be shaved, but deferred until the patient is anaesthetized.

Pre-operative examination

Before operation, careful examination and assessment of the anatomical site of the abscess are advisable.

An index finger is passed into the rectum and by careful palpation between this finger and a thumb outside, its extent can be determined fairly accurately.

It is essential to be sure whether the abscess to be opened is really in the ischiorectal fossa, and is not supralevator or intersphincteric, for in the latter cases a different approach is necessary.

A proctoscope should be passed to examine the condition of the rectal mucosa and to detect the presence of any anal pathology, such as haemorrhoids, or a visible internal opening of the abscess. It is also advisable to pass a sigmoidoscope in any rectal case before operation.

Anaesthesia

A general anaesthetic should be of such a depth as to avoid complete loss of sphincter tone.

Position of patient

The patient should be in the lithotomy position with the buttocks pulled down over the end of the operating table, the lower flap of which should be removed.

THE OPERATION

1

First incision

With the patient anaesthetized and in the lithotomy position, careful palpation of the swelling is carried out with the index finger of one hand in the rectum and the other hand over the external swelling. The rectum and anal canal should be inspected with a proctoscope.

An index finger steadies the swelling from inside the rectum. A straight incision is made over the most prominent part of the abscess, usually about 3–4 cm from the anal verge. This incision is short to begin with, and is slowly deepened until pus is obtained.

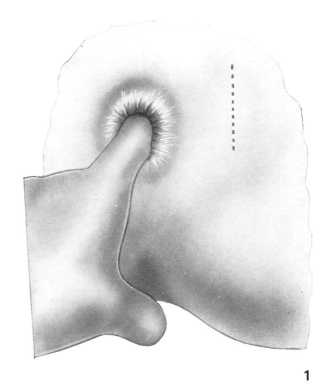

1

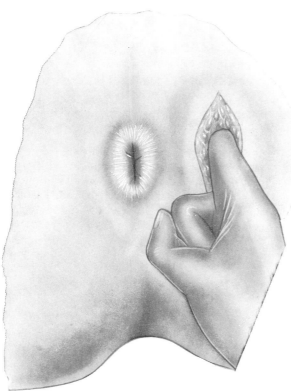

2

2

Exploring the abscess cavity

Pus is allowed to escape, and a specimen is taken for bacteriological examination. A finger is then passed into the abscess cavity, loculi gently broken down, and the extent and direction of the cavity explored.

3

Extension of incision

The incision is extended over the main prolongation of the abscess cavity, and any irregular and over-hanging skin edges are then excised to allow free drainage. Wide excision of skin edges is unnecessary at this stage.

The abscess most commonly extends towards the posterior mid-line, requiring a posteromedial extension of the incision as illustrated.

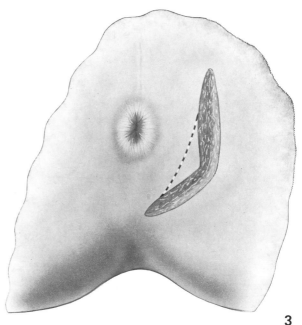

3

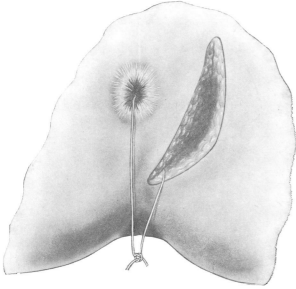

4

4

Final wound: communicating track marked

Should there be an *obvious* communication with the anal canal, a seton may be passed through and loosely tied in order to mark it for a later stage. The relationship of such a track to the anal muscles may be obscured by the oedema and it is usually wiser not to attempt to lay it open in the acute stage.

A flat gauze dressing moistened with Eusol (1:8) or Hibitane (1:2000) is applied, covered with a large cotton-wool pad and held in place with a T-bandage.

POSTOPERATIVE CARE AND COMPLICATIONS

The dressing is changed the next morning, the wound is irrigated with peroxide followed by Hibitane (1:2000) and a fresh dressing of gauze moistened with the same solution is gently placed over the wound keeping the edges apart. The wound should not be packed, and ribbon gauze should *never* be used. On the second day the patient may take a bath and thereafter bathe twice daily.

The bowels should be encouraged to act normally from the second or third day by a full diet and suitable mild aperients. A little olive oil run into the rectum will make the first action easier. A bath, wound irrigation and dressing should follow each bowel action.

After 5–8 days, the patient should again be anaesthetized, placed in the lithotomy position and the wound carefully explored. Particular search should be made for an internal opening into the anal canal (if not previously marked) which, if found, must be laid open.

Extensions in the ischiorectal fossae which may have been overlooked at the first operation are also sought and the wound is extended as necessary to lay these open, skin being now excised where necessary in order to fashion a wound which will heal by granulation without pocketing.

After-care and dressings are continued as before, and are further described in the Chapter on 'Fistula-in-ano' (*see* page 375).

A *persistent fistula* or *recurrent abscess* following drainage of an ischiorectal abscess nearly always signifies that a track or communication with the anal canal has been overlooked or inadequately laid open.

Reference

Morgan, C. N. (1949). 'The surgical anatomy of the ischio-rectal space.' *Proc. R. Soc. Med.* **42**, 189

[*The illustrations for this Chapter on Peri-anal and Ischiorectal Abscess were drawn by Mr. F. Price.*]

Fistula - in - ano

H. E. Lockhart-Mummery, M.D., M.Chir., F.R.C.S.
Consultant Surgeon, St. Thomas's and St. Mark's Hospitals,
and King Edward VII Hospital for Officers, London

and

Ian P. Todd, M.S., M.D. (Tor.), F.R.C.S., D.C.H.
Consultant Surgeon, St. Bartholomew's Hospital, St. Mark's Hospital,
and King Edward VII Hospital for Officers, London

PRE - OPERATIVE

Indications

Spontaneous healing of anal fistulae is very rare. Further, neglected fistulae may cause repeated abscesses and considerable ill-health, and malignant disease may eventually originate in a long-standing fistula. Operation should therefore be advised unless there are definite contra-indications.

Special contra-indications

An anal fistula is sometimes associated with *active pulmonary tuberculosis*, and a radiological examination of the chest should be a routine part of pre-operative investigation. The pulmonary disease must be controlled before the fistula is operated upon.

Any abdominal symptoms, and particularly *diarrhoea*, should be investigated before undertaking operation for anal fistula. Sigmoidoscopy is always necessary to exclude any rectal tumour or inflammatory bowel disease involving the rectum.

Crohn's disease of any part of the gastro-intestinal tract may give rise to an anal fistula. Full radiological investigation of both small and large bowel should be undertaken if there is any factor in the patient's history or examination to suggest the presence of Crohn's disease. Sometimes, but not always, the appearance of a fistula associated with Crohn's disease is characteristic in that it appears indolent and with little induration.

Pre-operative preparation

The lower bowel should be emptied by an enema the night before operation, and a rectal washout given on the morning of operation. The anal region should be widely shaved.

Sterilization of the bowel with sulphonamides or antibiotics is not necessary as a routine measure.

Anaesthesia

General anaesthesia is necessary for all except the most superficial fistulae. Full relaxation should be avoided, as there should be sufficient tone in the muscles to enable the operator to palpate the main parts of the anal sphincters, particularly the anorectal ring.

Position of patient

The patient should be in the lithotomy position, with the buttocks pulled down over the end of the table.

Pre-operative examination

Before starting the operation, the whole anal region should be carefully palpated. With an index finger in the rectum and thumb outside, the induration of a fistulous track can usually be clearly felt, and the probable direction and course of the track estimated. A proctoscope should be passed to detect any anal abnormality, and sometimes the internal opening may be seen.

Pathological examination

A portion of the granulation tissue and fibrous tissue of the fistulous track should always be submitted for microscopic examination.

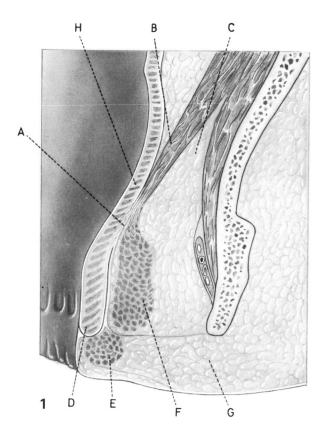

1

THE OPERATION

1

Anatomy

The essential anatomy of the anal region is shown in this diagram. Note that the ischiorectal fossa is a pyramidal space, the apex of which is above the ano-rectal ring. The anorectal ring marks the junction of rectum and anus, and is formed by the puborectalis fibres of levator ani passing round the bowel and blending with the external sphincter. Complete incontinence results if all the anal sphincters, including the anorectal ring are divided; section of muscle below this level may lead to some impairment of control or mucous leak, depending on the amount of muscle divided. The illustration shows (A) anorectal ring; (B) levator ani; (C) ischiorectal fossa; (D) internal sphincter; (E) subcutaneous external sphincter; (F) other parts of external sphincter; (G) peri-anal space; (H) circular muscle of bowel.

2

Classification and types of fistula

It is certain that the majority of anal fistulae result from infection of the anal glands, which arise from the anal crypts and penetrate into and often through the internal sphincter muscle. The infected gland is usually in the mid-line and in 80 per cent of anal fistulae the internal opening will be found in the mid-line, more commonly posteriorly than anteriorly.

Infection in the deeper part of the anal gland leads to a small abscess cavity in the potential space between the internal and external sphincter muscles, i.e. the intersphincteric space. From this focus infection may track in three planes; further radially, vertically up or down, or circumferentially.

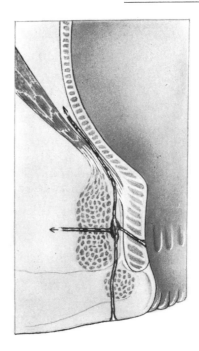

2

3&4

If the track passes through the primary intersphincteric focus downwards to the peri-anal skin, the simplest type of fistula results. However, the infection may track both up and down in that plane, or more rarely upwards only, leading to a rather complex fistula. Nevertheless all such fistula tracks remain in the plane between the internal and external sphincters and are classified as 'intersphincteric'.

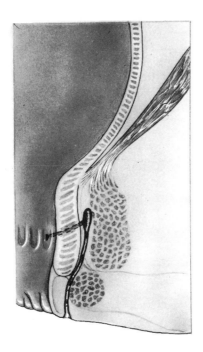

3

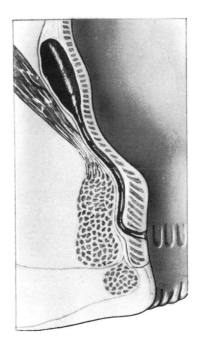

4

5

Further radial extension from the primary inter-sphincteric focus allows infection to pass through the external sphincter into the ischiorectal fossa, from whence also there may be both vertical and circumferential spread. Infection is usually limited above by the levator muscle, so most commonly a fistula follows the under-surface of the levator muscle, with an external opening laterally 2·5 cm or more from the anal verge, but not infrequently with infection in both ischiorectal fossae.

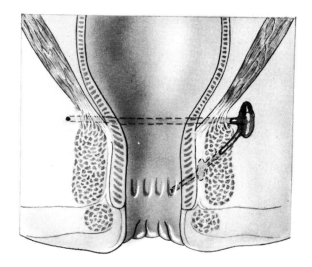

5

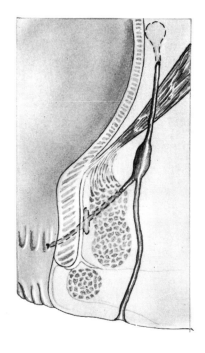

6

6

Rarely, further vertical spread may lead to a track through the levator ani, which even more rarely passes into the *rectum*.

All these fistulae have their main track leading from the primary focus through the *external* sphincter and are therefore classified as 'trans-sphincteric'.

7&8

A very rare type of fistula goes directly from the rectum or intra-abdominal bowel, through the pelvic floor, to open somewhere around the anus. This is not really a fistula-in-ano as there is no origin or connection with the anal canal, and they usually arise from disease within the bowel; i.e. diverticulitis, Crohn's disease or pelvic abscess. Such fistulae may be called 'extrasphincteric' and may be cured by removal of the primary source of infection.

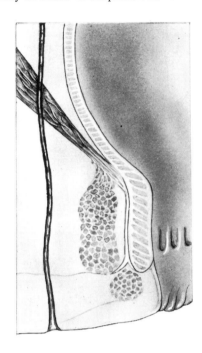

7

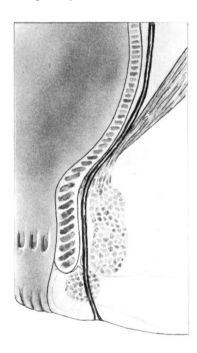

8

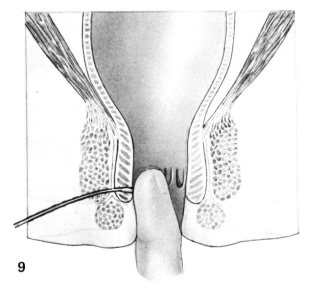

9

LOW ANAL FISTULA

9

Insertion of probe-pointed director

A probe-pointed director is passed from the external opening along the track until its tip emerges into the anal canal through the internal opening. It is helpful to have a finger palpating on to the point of the director, thus steadying the anus, but the director must be worked gently along the track, and should never be forced through the tissues.

A finger passed into the anus checks the level of the internal opening in relation to the anorectal ring, to ensure that division of the muscle superficial to the director will not lead to incontinence.

10

Exit of director through the anus

Once right through the track the tip of the director is angled towards the operator and is then pushed on to the outside of the anus. A curved director (*see* previous illustration) is particularly useful when dealing with rather higher fistulae, or those with a more tortuous track.

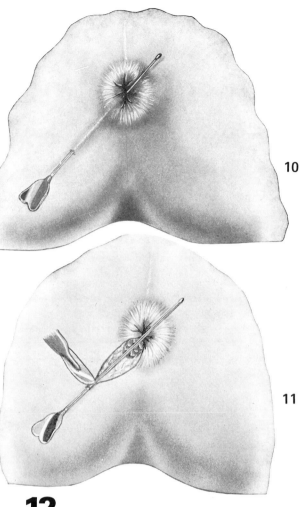

10

11

11

Incision over the director and curettage of granulation tissue

The track is laid open by cutting on to the groove in the director, which is then removed. The edges of the wound are held apart, and the granulation tissue curetted away. Search is made by looking, feeling, and probing for any other track opening out of the main one, and if such a track is found it is also laid open.

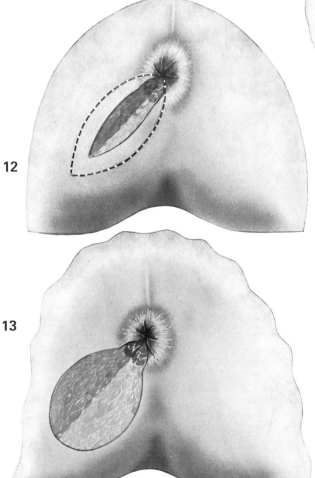

12

13

12

Extension of the wound

The wound is extended outwards for a short distance, and the edges trimmed away so that a shallow open wound can be obtained.

13

Healing of the wound

Such a wound may appear unnecessarily large, but experience has shown that the healing of anal wounds is better and free from complications when there is good external drainage.

A flat gauze dressing moistened with Eusol (1:8) or Hibitane (1 : 2000) is placed over the wound, covered with a cotton-wool pad and held in place with a T-bandage.

Subcutaneous fistulae, and those fistulae with an intermuscular extension, are laid open in a similar way. The size and shape of the external wound varies according to the length and direction of the track and the depth of the internal opening, the surgeon always attempting to get a shallow shelving wound.

HIGH INTERSPHINCTERIC FISTULA

14

Insertion of speculum; probing the fistula

A Sims speculum is passed into the anal canal and held by an assistant. The director is passed into the opening in the anal canal crypt and gently upwards along the track. The point may then come into the rectal lumen if the fistula has tracked back into the rectum, or may be pushed through to make such an opening if none exists.

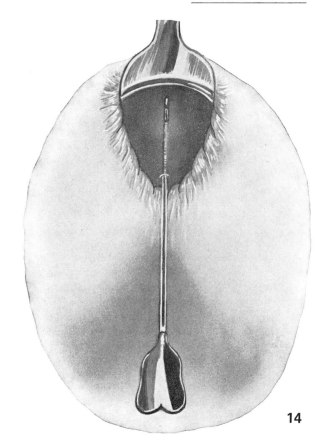

14

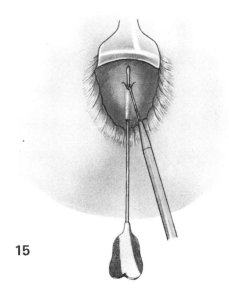

15

15

Laying-open in probe

The mucosa and muscle on the director are then slowly divided with a diathermy needle in order to minimize bleeding. In this way the whole length of the fistula is laid open into the upper anal canal crypt and rectum, the only muscle divided being the upper part of the internal sphincter and some circular muscle of the lower rectum.

FISTULA INVOLVING THE ISCHIORECTAL FOSSA

16

Course of the main track

The main track of an ischiorectal fistula follows the roof of the ischiorectal fossa; that is to say, it lies on the under-surface of the puborectalis muscle. The track is therefore of horse-shoe shape if both sides are involved, with the anterior extension on each side passing deep to the transverse perineal muscle. The communication with the anal canal is most frequently in the mid-line posteriorly, but not invariably so. The track leading to the external opening on the skin is not shown on this diagram, but is usually a vertical track which may descend from any part of the main one (*see Illustrations 5* and *6*, trans-sphincteric fistulae).

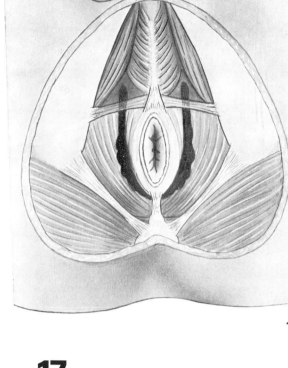

16

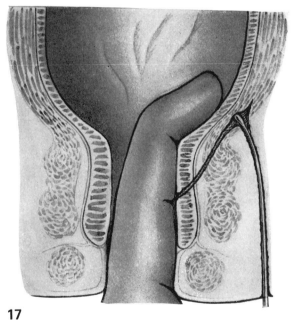

17

17

Insertion of probe to apex

If a probe be passed into the external opening, it will enter deeply, *parallel* to the anal canal, and its tip can often be palpated through the rectal wall at a level above the anorectal ring. It must never be forced through here, as the real internal opening is nearly always below the anorectal ring, still following the under-surface of the puborectalis.

18

First incision

The director is passed up the vertical track, and is held with the groove posteriorly by an assistant. The left index finger steadies and protects the rectum. A scalpel is slid up the groove in the director and cuts out backwards towards the coccyx, thus laying open the posterior part of the track on that side.

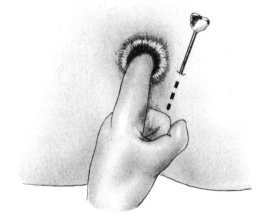

18

19

Exposure of anterior extension

The edges of the wound are held apart and the main bleeding points secured. The anterior extension is sought in the depths of the wound. The director is passed along the track, which is then laid open by dividing the overlying tissues. The posterior part of the perineal membrane and contained muscles may rarely need to be divided in laying open this part.

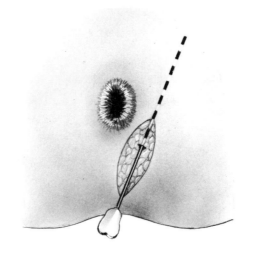

19

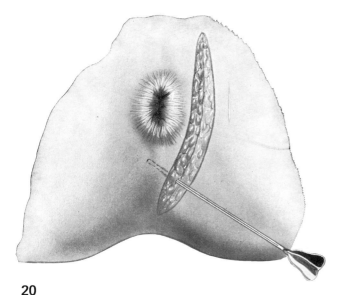

20

20

Extension of track to opposite ischiorectal fossa

Attention is now turned to the posterior end of the wound, where an extension to the opposite ischiorectal fossa is sought in the depths of the wound. Probing must be gentle, but must seek particularly where there are visible granulations or palpable induration.

21

Exposure of extension to opposite ischiorectal fossa

If an extension of the track to the opposite ischiorectal fossa is found, it is laid open for its full length by the division of overlying tissues, as on the other side. The laying open of these deep tracks must be carried out carefully and thoroughly, and many large vessels in the fat may require ligation or coagulation.

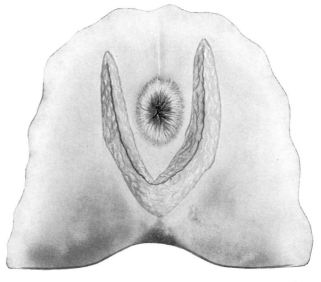

21

22

Search for internal opening

A search is now made for an internal opening, and the area near the mid-line posteriorly should be searched first as this is the most frequent site. The communicating track is often oblique (*see Illustration 16*) and an angled director may be necessary to find it. When found, one must first ensure by careful palpation, and inspection through a proctoscope, that the internal opening is below the anorectal ring.

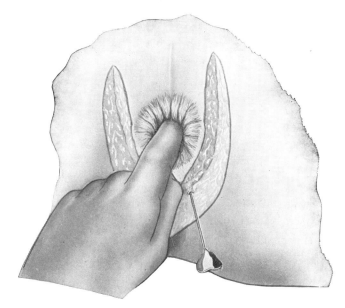

22

23

Division of sphincter muscles

If it is certain that the internal opening is below the anorectal ring, the contained muscles are divided by cutting on the probe. If there is doubt, the superficial muscles only are divided, and a silk suture passed round the deeper part and knotted loosely. Later examination, when the patient is conscious and can actively contract his sphincter muscle, will allow of better assessment of the height of this opening. If findings are favourable, the contained muscles can be divided a few days later.

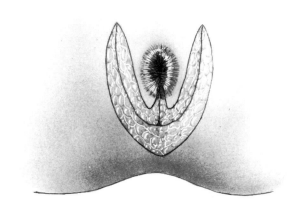

23

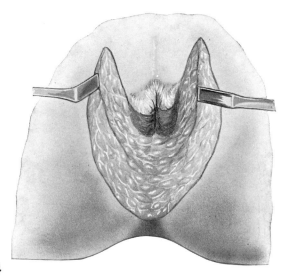

24

24

Extension and trimming of the wound

The wound is trimmed and enlarged by excising some skin edges and redundant fat, and the whole wound fashioned so as to shelve as shallowly as possible. All granulation tissue is meticulously curetted away, and a careful search should ensure that no section of track has been overlooked.

Flat gauze dressings moistened with Eusol (1:8) or Hibitane (1:2000) are applied lightly to keep the edges of the wound apart, covered with a large cotton-wool pad, and held in place with a T-bandage.

25

Healed appearance and sphincteric function

Many weeks later the wound will be almost healed, the final scar being much smaller than the former wound, and the anal appearance may not be grossly altered. Sphincteric function is usually excellent.

Uncommon fistula-in-ano

In a very few of the more complicated fistulae, particularly when there is secondary opening into the rectum above the anorectal ring, a temporary diverting sigmoid colostomy may be advisable. Then the track into the rectum may be dissected out and the wall closed by suturing with fine monofilament steel wire, with a very high chance of success and firm healing. The lower part of such a fistula, including the original anal opening, is dealt with as already described.

SPECIAL POSTOPERATIVE CARE AND COMPLICATIONS

The postoperative care of anal wounds and the attention needed to regulate the bowel action has been fully described in the Chapter on 'Haemorrhoidectomy', page 336. The same regime should be followed in the care of the small and superficial wounds following an operation for fistula.

Larger wounds, and particularly those following operations on ischiorectal fistulae, require rather more detailed attention. The first few dressings will be painful, and a light general anaesthetic may be necessary to allow them to be properly applied, or alternatively an analgesic drug may be given. The bowels should be encouraged to act on the third or fourth postoperative day, and thereafter kept regular and the motions soft with suitable medicines and a full diet.

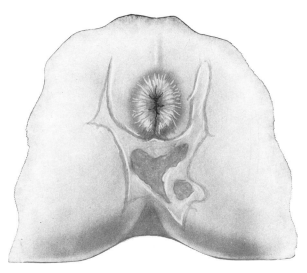

25

After the first few days, a bath, irrigation and dressing should follow each bowel action, and a similar sequence should be adopted each evening. Two experienced nurses are needed for the dressings, and good lighting is essential. After a thorough irrigation, the moist flat gauze is placed gently into the depths of the wound by one nurse while the other holds the wound edges apart.

There is some tendency for large deep wounds to form pockets which delay healing; it is therefore advisable to examine them carefully once weekly throughout the period of healing, with the patient in the lithotomy position in the operating theatre. The first few such examinations should be carried out under anaesthesia. In this way the wound can be trimmed as necessary during the healing process, and any pockets of tracks that have been overlooked, can be laid open. Final healing may take 6–12 weeks, and patience on the part of both surgeon and patient is necessary.

In those cases in which division of the greater part of the anal sphincter has been necessary, the power and function of the remaining portion may be improved by active sphincter exercises throughout the period of healing, and the patient should be instructed to carry them out.

References

Hawley, P.R. (1975). *Clins Gastroent.* **4**, 635
Milligan, E. T. C., Naunton Morgan, C., Lloyd-Davies, O. V. and Thompson, H. R. (1948). 'Fistula in ano.' *British Surgical Practice*, Vol. 4, p. 102. London: Butterworths
Parks, A. G., Gordon, P. H. and Hardcastle, J. D. (1976). 'A classification of fistula-in-ano.' *Br. J. Surg.* **63**, 1

[The illustrations for this Chapter on Fistula-in-ano were drawn by Mr. F. Price.]

Peri-anal and Anal Condylomata Accuminata

James P. S. Thomson, M.S., F.R.C.S.
Consultant Surgeon, St. Mark's Hospital, London

PRE-OPERATIVE

Assessment

The diagnosis of peri-anal condylomata accuminata (viral warts) is usually obvious, but it is important to accurately determine the extent of the disease. Warts may also be present within the anal canal or lower rectum and on the external genitalia. Unless all the lesions are treated recurrence is more liable to occur. Other sexually transmitted diseases must be excluded and, in particular, condylomata lata, which are a manifestation of syphilis.

Treatment

Small numbers of warts confined to the peri-anal region may be treated by the repeated application of 25 per cent podophyllin in tincture benzoin co. However, if there is no response to this treatment, or there is initial involvement of the anal canal then operative treatment under general anaesthesia is required.

Preparation

The lower bowel should, if possible, be free from stool. An enema the evening before operation usually provides adequate preparation.

Anaesthesia

This operation is best performed under general anaesthesia, but a caudal anaesthetic provides adequate relaxation of the anal canal and is very satisfactory.

Principles of treatment

The method described here avoids the use of diathermy or cautery save for its use in controlling persistent bleeding points. A solution of 1:300,000 adrenaline in physiological saline is injected subcutaneously and submucosally. This separates the warts one from another and allows as much healthy skin and mucosa as possible to be preserved when the individual warts are removed with scissors. The resulting small wounds heal rapidly, with minimal discomfort to the patient. In the majority of patients it is possible to remove all the warts on one occasion but if there are too many then the removal may best be done in two stages at an interval of approximately 1 month.

THE OPERATION

1

The solution of 1:300,000 adrenaline in physiological saline is injected subcutaneously. Approximately 50–75 ml of solution are injected into each peri-anal area, and while the injection is being given, the needle of the syringe should be moving so that an intravenous injection may be avoided.

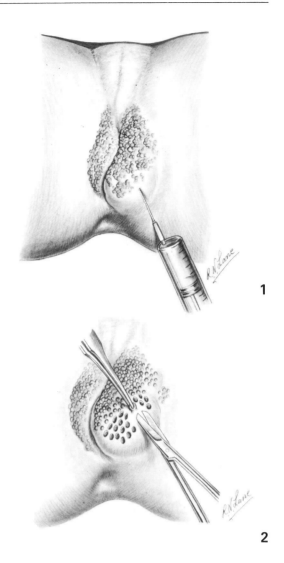

1

2

Excision of warts

Using a pair of fine toothed forceps and fine pointed scissors the warts are individually removed, preserving as much normal skin as possible. There is usually little haemorrhage, but a persistent bleeding point may be controlled with the diathermy.

2

3 & 4

Removal of warts from within the anal canal

With the aid of an anal retractor, such as the Parks retractor, the solution of adrenaline in physiological saline is injected into the submucosa. The warts are removed individually, preserving the mucosa between them. Should a confluent wound be created, this may be sutured, using a 3/0 chromic catgut stitch approximating the mucosa of the lower rectum to the dentate line. When all the warts have been removed, two gauze dressings soaked in diluted hypochlorite solution (e.g. 1:8 Eusol) are inserted into the anal canal and a pressure dressing applied with the aid of a T-bandage.

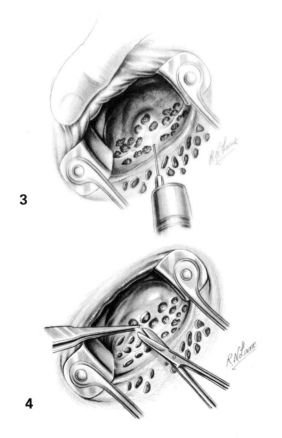

3

4

POSTOPERATIVE CARE

There is usually minimal discomfort after this procedure and the patient usually requires one dose of analgesia only. A normal diet should be started as soon as possible after the operation and the passage of a bulky stool ensured by the taking of a bulk laxative. If extensive warts are removed from the anal canal then an anal dilator (No. 1 St. Mark's dilator) should be passed twice a day with the aid of 1 per cent lignocaine gel.

Recurrence of the warts is always a possibility and patients should be warned of this. If after repeated operations to remove the warts recurrences persist then the use of a chemotherapeutic agent as an ointment, such as 5-fluorouracil (Efudix) may be used. However, the role of this agent in the treatment of condylomata accuminata still requires full evaluation.

There is a well known risk following removal of anal and peri-anal warts of anal stenosis. This is more likely to occur if diathermy is used, but if adequate normal skin and mucosa is left between the wounds then this complication will not occur.

[*The illustrations for this Chapter on Peri-anal and Anal Condylomata Accuminata were drawn by Mr. R. N. Lane.*]

Procedures for Pilonidal Sinus

Douglas M. Millar, M.B., F.R.C.S., F.R.C.S. (Ed.)
Consultant Surgeon, Essex County Hospital,
Colchester

Numerous surgical treatments for pilonidal sinus have been employed; they have varied in their effectiveness and carried significant failure rates. The choice of the procedure has been influenced by changing opinions as to aetiology, significance of recurrence, the presence of infection and secondary sinuses. The expense and availability of operating theatre facilities and in-patient hospital care has influenced the use of the more simple and purely out-patient procedures.

PRE-OPERATIVE

Although the aetiology of pilonidal sinus is a subject of debate the pathology of the established lesion is well recognized; there are one or more mid-line pits in the natal cleft, and deep to these pits is a cavity lined with granulation tissue. The cavity may or may not contain hair. Running cephalad, either in the mid-line or laterally into the buttock from this mid-line cavity there may be one or more tracks which are also lined with granulation tissue which may also contain hair and which discharge on the surface often some distance from the mid-line pits.

SIMPLIFIED PROCEDURE SUITABLE FOR OUT-PATIENTS

Principles

The principle of this technique is to excise the pits, allow free drainage of the mid-line cavity and the lateral tracks and remove all hair. It is important to keep the area carefully shaved to stop hair growing into the operation wound before it has had time to heal. The more extensive and incapacitating operation of wide excision does not give better results than the more limited methods of treatment and it is therefore not generally recommended.

Position of patient

The patient lies on the left side turned slightly face downwards. The right buttock is retracted by an assistant or by adhesive plaster to open up the natal cleft.

Anaesthesia

The procedure may be carried out under local anaesthesia in the form of an injection of 1 per cent lignocaine and 1 : 200,000 adrenaline around the mid-line pits and around the openings of any lateral track.

General anaesthesia is indicated particularly in the presence of a large abscess, local fibrosis, due to previous operative procedures and in cases where tracks extend 6 cm or more from the mid-line epithelial pits or extend into both buttocks.

THE OPERATION

1

Preparation of site

The area immediately around the mid-line pits and the lateral sinuses is meticulously shaved for a distance of 5 cm. Any residual hair that was long enough to enter the operation wound might interfere with healing. After careful shaving mid-line epithelial pits may sometimes show up which were not previously visible.

The elliptical lines indicate the lines of surgical excision. They are closely around the mid-line pits and the lateral sinus openings.

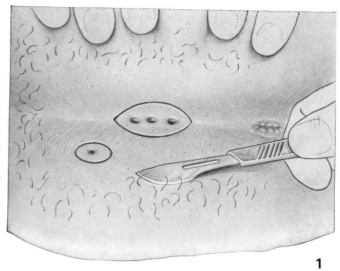

1

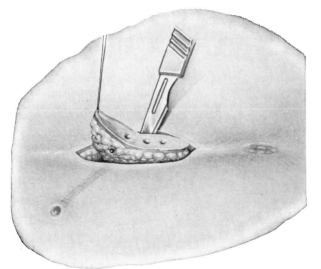

2

2

Excision of mid-line pits

The mid-line epithelial pits are excised in an elliptical fashion removing not more than 0·5 cm of skin on either side. This excision is carried down into the underlying granulomatous cavity from which any hair is carefully removed. No attempt is made to excise the cavity completely.

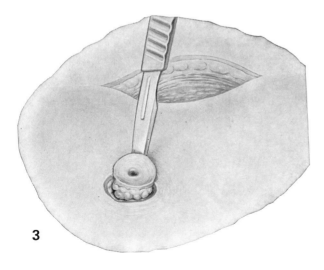

3

3

Excision of lateral sinus opening

Any discharging lateral sinus is probed to show the track which connects it with the mid-line granulomatous cavity. The lateral sinus track is then enlarged with sinus forceps.

The opening of the lateral sinus is excised with a circular incision to gain good access to the connecting track. If there is a lateral abscess this must be unroofed by a similar circular incision to obtain full drainage and the connecting track enlarged with sinus forceps.

4

Debridement of cavity and sinus tracks

All hair must be removed by thorough cleaning of the mid-line cavity and of the lateral sinus tracks.

Following excision of the pits, the mid-line cavity is open to inspection and the hair can be removed with forceps.

The hair in the lateral sinus is removed by inserting successively several small 'bottle' brushes. These are rotated and moved backwards and forwards in the track so that hair is caught up on the bristles. Alternatively, the track may be curetted.

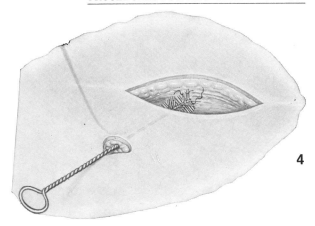

4

Modified simple procedures

Simple incision

Simple incision of the mid-line pits and cavity has been carried out in very severely infected cases.

Marsupialization

Attempts have been made to prevent bridging and to reduce the size of the raw cavity following simple excision of the mid-line pits by suturing the edge of the skin wound all round down to the margin of the opened up sinus. Interrupted chromic catgut or silk sutures have been used. It is claimed to be of some value in very obese patients.

POSTOPERATIVE CARE

Care of the wound

After the simple procedures all that is required is a dry gauze pad for a dressing. On the first postoperative day a bath is taken and the dressing removed. After careful drying of the area the gauze pad is replaced. This procedure is repeated daily.

Subsequent care

Shaving of the area is essential until all the healed scars are quite firm. This may be performed at 2 or 3-weekly intervals according to the rate of growth of the hair in the natal cleft. At this time any bridging of the skin across the deeper cavity can be broken down so that healing takes place from the base towards the surface.

A simple astringent lotion after healing helps to control any intertrigo allowing the scars to become pale and firm. The patient is discharged from surgical care only when this has occurred.

TREATMENT BY EXCISION AND SUTURE

The only advantage of immediate suture after excision is that the prime treatment is continued in hospital if out-patient facilities are not available These methods however, are suitable only for quiescent cases. Badly infected or extensively tracking sinuses carry a high recurrence rate with these methods.

The wound closure can be maintained by direct sutures through the sacral fascia which also holds pressure packs in place.

Suture line breakdown prompted the fashioning of a lateral flap to relieve tension and it is claimed that this is suitable when a lateral sinus has been excised.

An elaboration of plastic surgical methods for closure has been the Z-plasty, but this requires extensive mobilization of buttock tissues and has a recurrence rate comparable to other methods.

MANAGEMENT OF THE ACUTE PILONIDAL ABSCESS

A simple incision over the pointing abscess results in a very high recurrence rate and should be regarded, therefore, as a temporary expedient before definitive surgery. If, however, the sinus pits are excised and the whole cavity laid open and thoroughly cleaned into the lateral tracks, a high percentage of cures result. If the sinus pits are not visible then equally good results are obtained by laying open the whole underlying cavities. In a few cases marsupialization has been employed but it is generally not to be recommended in this situation.

TREATMENT OF RECURRENT PILONIDAL SINUS

A simple excision of the sinus pits and laying open of the underlying cavity with or without marsupialization, is as effective as any other treatment and more simple. *No attempt should be made to totally re-excise a recurrent pilonidal sinus or to close the defect by suture or flaps.*

[The illustrations for this Chapter on Procedures for Pilonidal Sinus were drawn by Mr. R. N. Lane.]

Rectovaginal and other Fistulae between the Intestine and Genital Tract

C. N. Hudson, M.Chir., F.R.C.S., F.R.C.O.G.
Reader in Obstetrics and Gynaecology,
Medical College of St. Bartholomew's Hospital,
London

INTRODUCTION

The principles of repair of rectovaginal fistulae do not differ greatly from those of repair of urinary genital fistulae. Success in treatment depends upon accurate diagnosis, choice of the correct operation and meticulous surgical technique. The latter includes avoidance of tension on suture lines, within individual sutures and within the lumen of the main viscus, together with avoidance of haematoma formation.

PRE-OPERATIVE MANAGEMENT

Diagnosis and choice of operation

Although the presence of an intestinovaginal fistula is usually only too obvious, occasionally the diagnosis can be very elusive. In all cases preliminary examination under anaesthesia is advised, as it is extremely important to identify which loop of bowel is involved. A probe inserted through the vaginal orifice of the fistula may be palpated on digital rectal examination, or may be visible through a sigmoidoscope. If, however, the fistula is in the colon at the apex of the sigmoid loop, the bowel is almost always tethered to the pouch of Douglas with such an acute bend that an ordinary sigmoidoscope cannot reach the intestinal orifice of the fistula although a flexible colonoscope may achieve this. A ureteric catheter should be inserted so that x-ray studies can then be carried out under a viewing screen. It is necessary to inject the medium even as the catheter is being withdrawn as it is very important to determine whether a fistula

is merely a simple communication between bowel and vagina or whether there is an abscess cavity with communications to the bowel and the vagina. This is particularly important when a fistula follows surgery for a primary intestinal disorder such as diverticular disease. If there is an old abscess cavity or a complicated track it is unlikely that a vaginal operation alone will close the fistula permanently.

Endoscopic and x-ray examinations of the bowel are particularly important in order to establish whether there is any associated or underlying disease of the bowel. Even though there is a definite history of trauma the persistence of a fistula can be an indication of underlying asymptomatic and hitherto unsuspected inflammatory disease of the intestine such as Crohn's disease. If there is doubt, biopsy of both the rectum and the wall of the fistula should be carried out.

It is likewise important to establish the local histological condition when there has been a history of radiotherapy for malignant disease, even though the presence of activity does not necessarily rule out the possibility of colpocleisis. Successful colpocleisis in a patient with pelvic malignancy can sometimes relieve the distress or urinary and faecal leakage without the necessity of making an artificial stoma.

When there is neither clinical nor histological evidence of activity of malignant disease, the management of a fistula in those who have been treated with pelvic irradiation is a highly specialized task requiring techniques which are not generally applicable to routine fistula surgery.

TYPES OF OPERATION

Conservative repair operations are usually appropriate to simple traumatic fistulae including those of obstetric origin in which there may have been considerable tissue loss due to pressure necrosis, but only to a selected few inflammatory fistulae in which the disorder remains entirely localized and quiescent.

Radical repair operations, by contrast, will consist of intestinal resection with or without hysterectomy. This type of operation is suitable for ileal fistulae, fistulae involving the uterus, most colovaginal fistulae and a proportion of high rectovaginal fistulae. It will certainly be required for fistulae associated with localized inflammatory disease of the large bowel, and a proportion of fistulae due to pelvic malignant disease, particularly when the primary tumour is in the large intestine. It may occasionally be appropriate for irradiation fistulae but should not be undertaken lightly in these cases unless there is good evidence that healthy bowel can be reached on either side of the irradiated zone. It may also be appropriate for some high obstetric rectal fistulae when there has been complete circumferential loss of a segment of rectum due to pressure necrosis. In all the above circumstances the success of the operation will depend on the availability of an adequate length of healthy distal bowel for anastomosis.

If anastomosis is not feasible, the alternative is rectal excision and colostomy. The anal canal may then be preserved (Hartmann's operation) or removed by combined excision.

In inflammatory intestinal disorders, rectovaginal fistula may be the deciding factor which determines the need for definitive surgery for ulcerative colitis or Crohn's disease. If rectal fistula is a manifestation of actual involvement of the rectum conservative operations are inappropriate and usually doomed to failure. A few inflammatory fistulae will heal with medical treatment of the intestinal disorder, but, if surgery is necessary, then a major extirpation of the large bowel is commonly required and similar arguments may apply to the treatment of rectal strictures and fistulae in lymphopathia venereum as the inherent damage to the anal sphincter mechanism means that subsequent continence may be unsatisfactory even if closure can be obtained.

Permanent colostomy alone should be reserved for patients with fistula due to completely untreatable genital malignancy usually of cervical origin, patients too frail for definitive surgery and patients with an inactive benign condition in which the anal sphincter mechanism has been destroyed. It is emphasized that before resort to permanent colostomy, careful evaluation of the possibility of colpocleisis should be made, because colostomy which has not been made obligatory through rectal excision may cause great distress to the aged and infirm.

CONSERVATIVE REPAIR OPERATIONS

Choice of route

The abdominal route for simple closure is preferred for colonic fistulae, including those which communicate with the uterus. It is also appropriate to some high obstetric rectal fistulae particularly where access *per vaginam* is difficult and where this will be hindered by previous closure of a vesicovaginal fistula. It will be required if tissue loss has caused considerable adhesion to the sacrum. For irradiation fistulae the abdominal route is only advisable when the greater omentum is to be used as a pedicle graft.

The vaginal approach is favoured for the majority of operations. Four operative vaginal techniques will be described:

The per-anal route may be preferred by rectal surgeons and the temporary paralysis of the anal sphincter following stretching by the Parks speculum can be an advantage in preventing subsequent disruption of the suture line by flatus. The techniques employed are identical to those used *per vaginam.*

The transcoccygeal and transperineal approaches are probably only of historic interest but *York Mason's trans-sphincteric approach,* although devised as an approach to the rectoprostatic fistula of the male, has an occasional place in the management of fistulae into the female genital tract.

Pre-operative preparation

The general pre-operative care of all these patients is most important. High obstetric fistulae are almost always associated with a urinary fistula. The urinary fistula should always be treated first and the results of treatment will be improved if faeces are diverted from the vagina before an attempt to close the urinary fistula is made. A transverse colostomy should always be used because it will not embarrass access should a subsequent abdominal approach prove to be necessary to deal with the high rectal fistula. Preliminary colostomy is not generally regarded as essential prior to the preliminary repair of a straightforward rectovaginal fistula.

Apart from associated urinary fistula there may be other sequels to obstructed labour which require attention, such as pelvic inflammatory disease, haematometra, obstructive uropathy and nerve palsies. The patient's morale may be extremely low and this aspect should not be neglected. During an extended pre-operative period anaemia, malnutrition and all infections and infestations should be treated.

Once the general condition of the patient is satisfactory, pre-operative preparation in hospital should be directed more to mechanical emptying of the bowel than pursuit of bacterial sterility. After preliminary colostomy, it may be difficult to empty the distal loop by wash-out, particularly if there is any stricture formation but this is to be regarded as very important. Leak back through the fistula may be stemmed by packing the vagina beforehand. Although the benefit is questionable it is usual to prescribe phthalylsulphathiazole, 12 g daily for 5 days immediately before operation in patients without a colostomy, and the chance of anaerobic infections may be reduced by metronidazole. Some surgeons like to irrigate a distal loop or vagina with a sulphonamide preparation or noxythioline. In a postmenopausal patient oral oestrogen therapy may improve the quality of the vaginal epithelium.

Special contra-indications

No conservative repair should be attempted within 3 months of the causative event or of a previous attempt at repair. No repair should be carried out simultaneously with or prior to repair of a vesical fistula.

THE OPERATIONS

CONVERSION TO THIRD DEGREE TEAR

1

Many small low rectovaginal fistulae represent incompletely healed complete (third degree) perineal lacerations. The best procedure is to divide the bridge of skin and scar tissue and repair the defect as a classical third degree laceration.

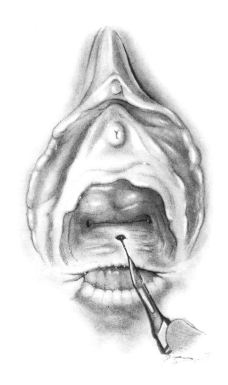

1

2&3

The fistula track should be excised so that there are fresh edges for repair. The vaginal wall must be dissected off the remnants of the perineal body until they can be exposed.

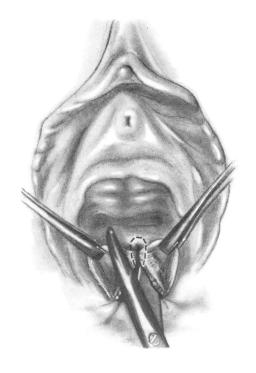

2

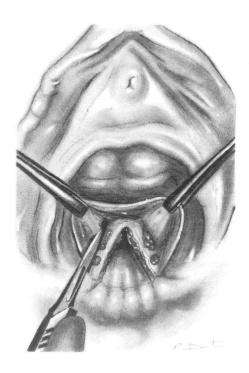

3

4,5&6

The epithelium of the anal canal is repaired with fine extra chromic 2/0 catgut or polyglycollic acid sutures; traditionally the knots are made to lie within the lumen of the anal canal.

The external sphincter is freed where it has retracted into its tunnel on either side of the anus. The internal sphincter muscle of the anal canal may be reconstructed with a series of Lembert sutures. The blood supply is usually not precarious and therefore a continuous suture is permissible.

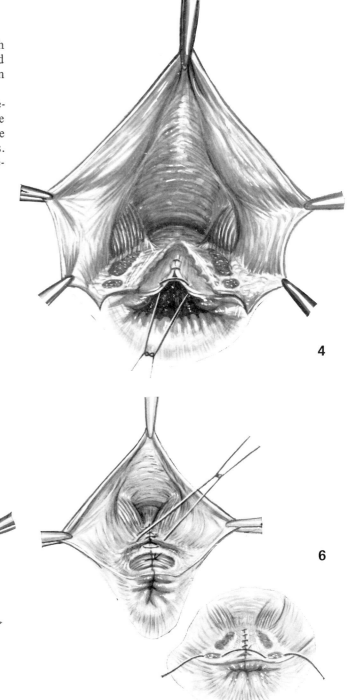

7,8&9

The remnants of the perineal body must be re-united in front of the anal canal with interrupted sutures. Attention to symmetry is important and this may be obtained if each bite of the suture be inserted from within outwards.

The vaginal epithelium is closed with a fine catgut suture and it is best to leave the navicular fossa unsutured, as a small gap allows any collection of blood and serum to discharge thus avoiding haematoma formation.

The skin over the perineum is closed with interrupted or subcuticular sutures.

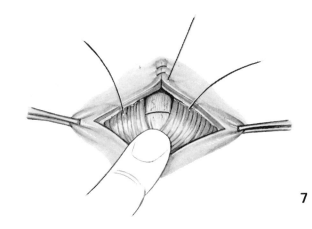

7

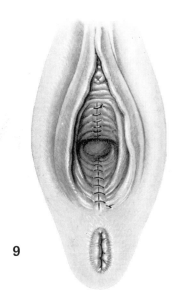

9

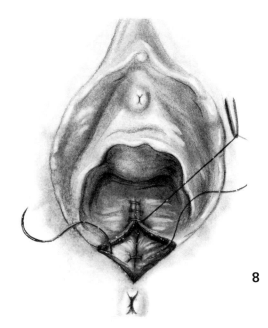

8

PURSE-STRING AND INVERSION

10

If the perineal body is reasonably intact, a small fistula may be dealt with by circumcision and inversion through a purse-string suture using a straight aneurysm needle.

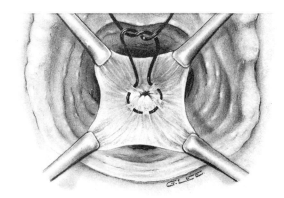

10

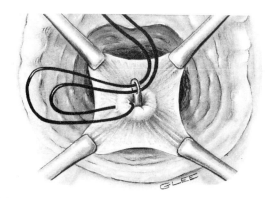

11

Such a fistula is best displayed by the surgeon or his assistant operating with an index finger in the rectum pressing the fistula area forward. When the tract has been dissected free, a purse-string suture is inserted around the base of the fistulous tract and a 'stay' suture through the neck of the fistula is then threaded through the aneurysm needle and withdrawn.

12

Traction on this stay suture inverts the fistula tract into the anal canal through the purse-string which can then be closed. Two or three interrupted sutures provide a second layer of muscle stitches in front of the repair. This will also serve to obliterate dead space. The vaginal epithelium is finally closed with interrupted chromic catgut sutures.

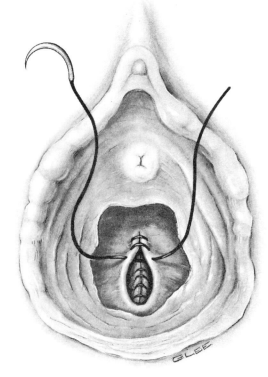

12

FLAP REPAIR

This method is suitable for moderately high fistulae. If there is reasonable access, this procedure is in fact suitable for the repair of surgical fistulae arising after hysterectomy. In post-hysterectomy cases the elevation of vaginal flaps denudes a small area of upper vagina which is closed off (upper partial colpocleisis).

The technique of flap repair is virtually identical to that of repair of bladder fistulae and a Schuchardt incision may likewise be necessary. The operator should beware of extending this incision into the fistula as it may interfere with vaginal closure at the end of the procedure. Exposure of the fistula may be achieved by the use of traction sutures or digital elevation via the rectum.

13&14

A knife is used to elevate flaps around the fistula. The hole in the rectum should be repaired by interrupted sutures.

It is important that the mucous membrane should be excluded from the depths of the wound and therefore it is probably better to avoid including it in the sutures. The direction of the suture line should be determined by the ease in which the walls of the defect can be brought together. There is very little risk of producing rectal stenosis from the repair of fistulae of this sort.

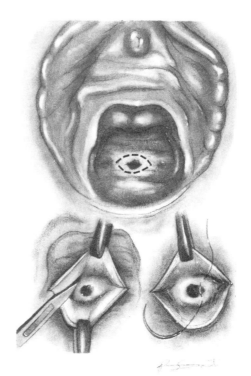

13

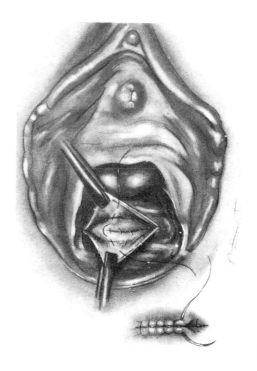

14

MAJOR HIGH FISTULA REPAIR

15,16 & 17

When there has been a major injury of the posterior vaginal wall due to obstetric pressure necrosis it may not be possible to produce sufficient mobility by ordinary flap dissection. In such cases it is desirable to open the pouch of Douglas and bring down the anterior rectal wall with its serous coat. This allows the rectal defect to be closed without tension.

There is insufficient vaginal epithelium to close the defect: it is therefore tacked to the peritoneal covering of the anterior rectal wall which may also be fixed to the back of the cervical stump.

Sometimes the entire vaginal wall is lost (third degree septal loss). *Illustration 16* shows why such a lesion can only be closed with a vertical suture line. There may be considerable reduction in the lumen of the rectum and in such cases it is advisable to cover the repair by preliminary transverse colostomy.

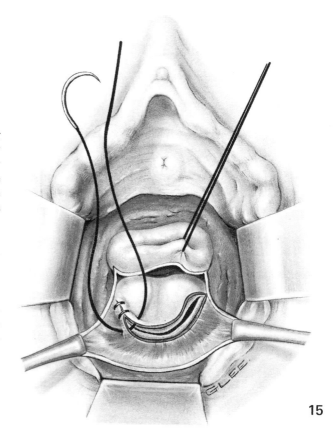

15

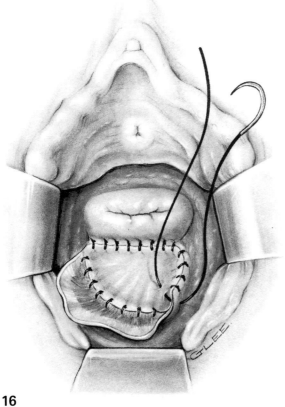

16

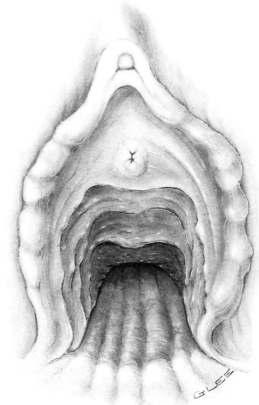

17

TRANSANAL REPAIR

18

This repair is best carried out with the patient in the 'jack-knife' position.

The anal canal dilated by a Parks speculum gives a good exposure of the fistula.

The technique is identical to that used for repair *per vaginam* except that sutures made of stainless steel wire may be used to close the anorectal defect.

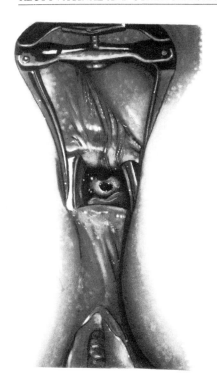

18

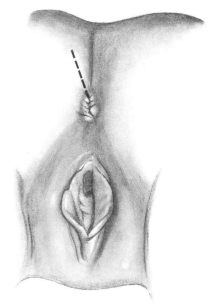

19

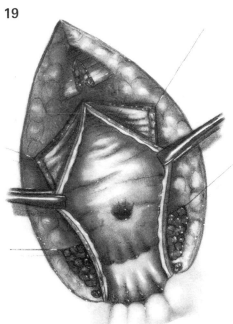

TRANS-SPHINCTERIC REPAIR

19

The patient should be placed in the 'jack-knife' position.

(*1*) An incision is made through the skin radially from the posterior aspect of the anal orifice.

(*2*) As this is deepened muscle layers are identified and marked with silk sutures to aid reconstruction at the end of the procedure.

(*3*) When the anal canal and rectum have been fully opened an excellent exposure of the anterior rectal wall is obtained.

(*4*) Closure of the fistula proceeds as in the previous section.

(*5*) Closure of the incision of access should be carried out in layers with catgut or polyglycollic acid.

COLPOCLEISIS

This has an occasional place.

POSTOPERATIVE CARE AND COMPLICATIONS

Dissection of a rectovaginal fistula may on occasions provoke brisk arterial haemorrhage. The question of vaginal pack following repair has thus to be considered on its merits. In general if a pack is necessary to achieve haemostasis the risk of haematoma formation and breakdown of repair is high. Suction drainage through a perineal stab incision should be considered if there is any significant dead space.

The traditional management of such patients by confining the bowels for 5 days is outmoded. Nothing can be worse for a delicate stitch line at its weakest moment than for it to be stretched by a mass of descending faecal concretions. Early resort to oral laxatives is indicated avoiding those containing liquid paraffin.

The surgeon should insist that no digital rectal examinations or insertion of suppositories or enemas be performed by anyone other than himself. Failure to give this instruction may involve the administration of routine anal medication with disastrous results.

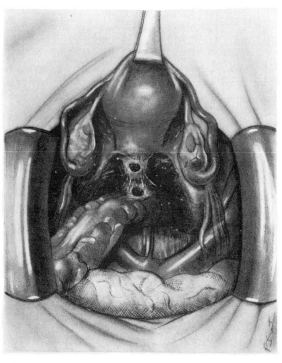

20

ABDOMINAL OPERATIONS

In some instances a preliminary right transverse colostomy will have been made. The operation is most conveniently performed in the lithotomy-Trendelenburg position using Lloyd-Davies' stirrups.

SIMPLE REPAIR

20&21a,b&c

The abdomen should be opened through a left paramedian incision to allow full mobilization of the left colon if required.

The fistulous loop should be freed all round by dissection from the posterior fornix or uterus and the fistula tract divided.

The opening in the rectosigmoid should be excised as a transverse ellipse so that all granulations and unhealthy tissue are removed.

The defect is repaired in two layers using a standard technique for anastomosis. Preferably this suture line should lie separated from the vaginal aperture which need not then be closed.

Any raw area in the pelvis should be covered with absorbable gauze which also helps to keep the affected loop away from the vagina. If necessary the greater omentum can be used for interposition.

The abdomen should be closed in routine fashion with a stab drain through the left flank down to the site of the suture line. If there is troublesome oozing from the pelvis, a suction drain may be passed out through the vaginal fistula. After the operation the anus should be dilated to admit four fingers.

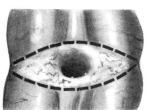

21a

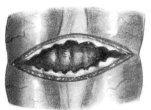

21b

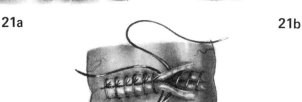

21c

HYSTERECTOMY AND REPAIR

It has long been recognized that hysterectomy may facilitate abdominal repair of a high rectal fistula by improving access to the inferior margin of the fistula. In obstetric cases where there has been gross pelvic infection associated with slough injuries, the pouch of Douglas is often obliterated and the pelvic floor rock hard with scar tissue. The uterus is commonly fixed and adherent in the hollow of the sacrum and this is the cause of the difficulty of access from below.

Subtotal hysterectomy with conservation of the ovaries should be carried out. The cervical stump remnant is firmly fixed in the scar tissue and the anatomy on either side is grossly distorted.

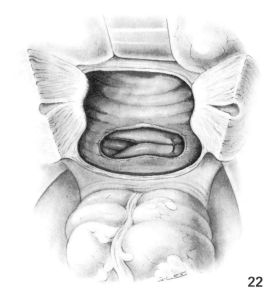

22

22 & 23

A mid-line sagittal split of the cervical stump allows access to the fistula in the posterior fornix when the two halves of the cervix are separated.

The inferior aspect of the fistula may be freed by sharp dissection in the ordinary way. This manoeuvre avoids inadvertent inferior extension of the fistula.

Following conventional repair of the rectal aperture the vaginal opening may also be closed and the cervical stump re-united in front as additional protection. Suction drainage is indicated.

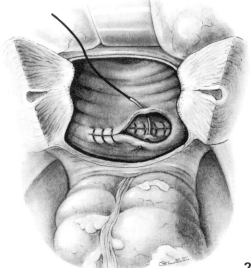

23

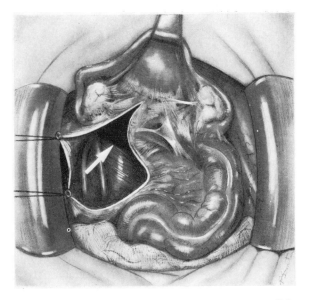

24

RETRORECTAL MOBILIZATION

24 & 25

Dissection behind the rectum may be used to approach a high obstetric fistula. It involves a mobilization of the rectum from the hollow of the sacrum. It is not applicable when this space is grossly distorted by scar tissue.

The rectosigmoid is first mobilized by incision of the white line and the reflection of the sigmoid mesentery.

Access to the rectorectal space allows the adherent vagina and rectum to be freed from the hollow of the sacrum and a tissue plane may be developed below the fistula between the posterior vaginal wall by blunt dissection. The fistula track may then be opened, trimmed and closed as described. Drainage is recommended.

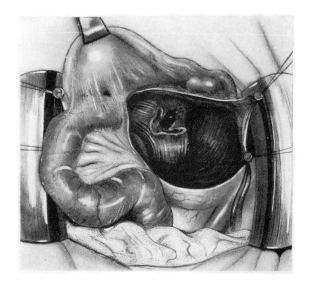

25

POSTOPERATIVE CARE AND COMPLICATIONS

The routine postoperative care of patients who have had intestinal surgery is instituted. An infected pelvic haematoma will almost certainly cause failure and there should be no hesitation in prescribing anti-biotics. The stab drain through the flank should be left in place for 5 days or until the bowels move, whichever be the later. The administration of laxatives should be encouraged as soon as ileus has subsided but this, of course, is not important if a preliminary colostomy has been carried out. Successful closure of the fistula should be confirmed by the instillation of a large volume of blue dye down the distal loop of the colostomy before its closure is contemplated, normally about 3 weeks from operation. Rectal stenosis is not usually a problem provided there is sufficient lumen to admit a finger tip.

Conclusion

The number of potential surgical approaches indicates that difficult fistulae are a major surgical problem. There is a premium on successful closure at the first attempt, and the experienced operator achieves significantly better results than those with little direct experience.

[*The illustrations for this Chapter on Rectovaginal and other Fistulae between the Intestine and Genital Tract were drawn by Mr. P. Darton and Miss G. Lee.*]

Rectoprostatic Fistula

A. York Mason, B.Sc., F.R.C.S. (Ed.), F.R.C.S. (Eng.)
Surgeon, St. Anthony's Hospital (Medical, Educational and
Research Trust); Honorary Consulting Surgeon,
St. Helier Hospital and Associated Hospitals; Late
Honorary Consultant Surgeon, Royal Marsden
Hospital, London

INTRODUCTION

The rectum may be perforated during the course of surgery for benign prostatic obstruction. If this complication is recognized at the time of operation it should be treated immediately by the establishment of a completely defunctioning iliac colostomy and efficient drainage of the bladder. If the perforation is not recognized, or if it is treated by an incompletely defunctioning loop colostomy, the consequences may be serious, with pelvic sepsis, abscess formation between bladder and rectum and rapid deterioration of the patient's general condition. Fistulation may also occur several days after what was thought to be an uncomplicated prostatectomy due to late necrosis caused by deeply-placed sutures in the posterior capsule, or by diathermy. In these patients there is less danger of spreading pelvic sepsis because of surrounding adhesions. Usually there is no difficulty in diagnosis. However, if the fistula is a small one, recognition may be delayed, episodes of pyrexia and urinary infection being treated by antibiotics. Surprisingly, some patients have accepted watery diarrhoea without complaint for several years. It is possible, therefore, that the incidence of rectoprostatic fistula may be somewhat higher than is generally thought.

Pre-operative preparation

It is essential to separate the faecal and urinary streams. No attempt should be made to repair the fistula until all sepsis has been cleared up and the patient restored to good general condition. The first step, therefore, is to establish a completely defunctioning colostomy, and experience has shown that a left iliac end colostomy is the best one. This should be carried out as a planned formal procedure so as to produce a correctly sited stoma. Attention to detail is important because, although this is a temporary colostomy, it may have to be maintained, in some cases, for several months before conditions are favourable for repair of the fistula. Patients will accept this necessary delay if they have a comfortable colostomy which they can manage easily.

THE OPERATION

1

A right paramedian incision, well clear of the transverse suprapubic wound commonly used for retropubic prostatectomy, provides good exposure for the necessary laparotomy. A correctly sited circular opening, through all layers of the abdominal wall, is prepared to receive the end colostomy to the left of the mid-line. A small skin incision is made for a catheter in the right iliac region.

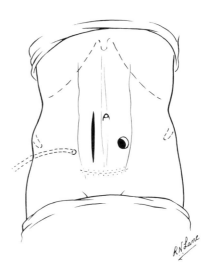

2

A short length of mid-sigmoid is selected, freed from its mesentery and transected between clamps. A Foley catheter introduced through the small skin incision is placed in the distal limb (*a*). A purse-string suture (*b*) followed by an invaginating stitch (*c*) will keep the catheter safely in position.

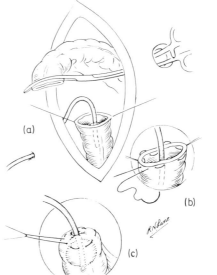

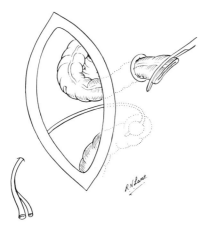

3

The proximal limb is drawn out of the abdomen. The closed distal limb is left lying in the peritoneal cavity, abutting peritoneum, adjacent to the proximal limb.

4

The length of intraperitoneal catheter is adjusted to avoid looping. The laparotomy wound is closed before trimming away the clamped colon and suturing its edges to the circular skin opening.

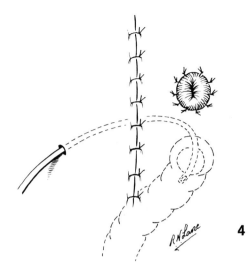

4

5

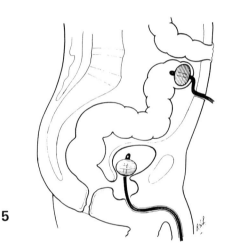

5

The situation at this stage is illustrated diagrammatically. Faeces are completely diverted by the end colostomy. A urethral catheter passed across the prostatic cavity into the bladder provides the best dependent drainage of urine. It is important to check that the inflated balloon is correctly sited in the bladder. The Foley catheter in the blind sigmoid limb decompresses the bowel and is used to irrigate and cleanse the rectum. It is removed on the tenth postoperative day and the mucus fistula closes spontaneously. The urethral catheter is removed on the twelfth postoperative day. If the fistula is a small one the patient may void most of his urine normally, but if it is large, urine drains freely into the rectum, and the patient learns to void most of his urine via the anus, quickly acquiring adequate control.

Formal repair of the fistula is delayed until all infection has cleared up, and for some patients a period at home is advised.

Panendoscopy is essential to exclude any distal urethral obstruction and the urethral catheter is re-introduced immediately before proceeding to repair of the fistula.

TRANS-SPHINCTERIC EXPOSURE

Complete division of the anal sphincters provides the ideal exposure for repair of a rectoprostatic fistula and, contrary to long established teaching, there is no danger of incontinence. Experience has shown that if normal anatomy is restored by accurate suture, the divided sphincters always heal well and patients regain normal defaecation with full anal control.

Anaesthesia

General anaesthesia is preferred, with an endotracheal tube and a muscle relaxant given intravenously.

The patient is positioned prone, with arms extended and hands crossed over above the head. It is important that the pelvis and chest should be raised and supported so as to leave the anterior abdominal wall free to move with respiration.

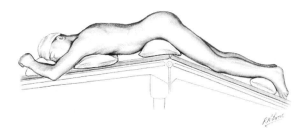

6

7

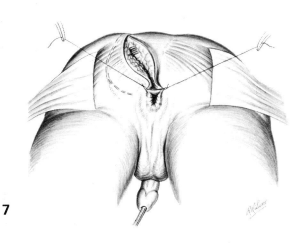

7

The buttocks are strapped apart with waterproof adhesive strapping. The anal verge is marked in the mid-line posteriorly by a pair of stay sutures. The incision starts from a point just to the left of the sacrococcygeal junction and ends up between the two anal verge marking sutures.

As the incision is deepened, the lower fibres of the gluteus maximus will be recognized near the upper end of the incision and, at the lower end, the superficial fibres of the external sphincter come into view. Between these upper and lower muscular landmarks the incision is deepened through the ischiorectal fat to expose the levator ani. There is no danger of injury to the main nerve coming down from the fourth sacral outflow to supply the somatic sphincter, as its course lies well lateral to the line of incision.

8

In order to open up the anal canal and lower rectum, there are essentially only two conical muscular tubes to be divided in the line of the skin incision. The outer somatic tube, as illustrated, is made up of the levator ani, expanded at its lower end to form the puborectalis sling and, below this, the external sphincter complex. It is important to mark each component, as shown, by paired identifying sutures before division between these paired marking stitches.

The muscle coats of the rectum constitute the inner visceral tube, expanded at the lower end to form the internal sphincter, shown in this illustration marked by a pair of identifying sutures.

Throughout the length of the anal canal these two tubes are closely apposed with fibres from the longitudinal coat passing outwards between bundles of external sphincter. Above the level of the puborectalis sling the tubes are separated by a variable layer of pararectal fat.

Deep to these two muscular tubes is the epithelial lining of the rectum and anal canal.

Below the pectinate line the anoderm is closely applied to the internal sphincter, tacked down by fibres from the longitudinal layer which pass inwards between circular muscle coat bundles.

Above the level of the pectinate line there is a vascular cushion and, above this, a loose connective tissue plane separating mucosa from circular muscle coat.

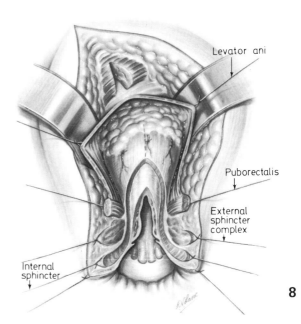

8

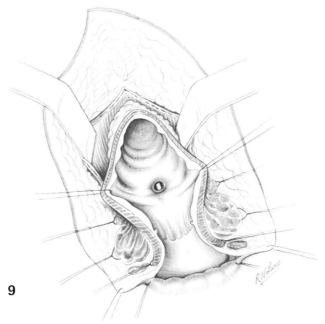

9

9

This illustrates the excellent exposure of the rectal end of a rectoprostatic fistula. In this patient the edges of the fistula are sclerosed and all inflammatory oedema has now disappeared following diversion of the faecal and urinary streams. The Foley catheter can be seen crossing the prostatic cavity from urethra to base of bladder.

The fistulous track is about 1 cm in length and, in well established cases, the fibrous wall will have acquired an epithelial lining. The track needs to be dissected away.

10

A specially designed three-bladed retractor is inserted to maintain the wide trans-sphincteric exposure throughout the repair. Four stay sutures are placed in healthy rectal mucosa and two are placed within this outer ring nearer the fibrosed edge of the fistula. A transverse elliptical incision is made through rectal mucosa between the outer and inner stay sutures, using a small-bladed scalpel.

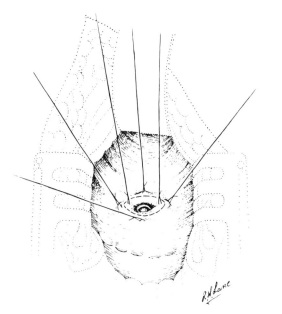

10

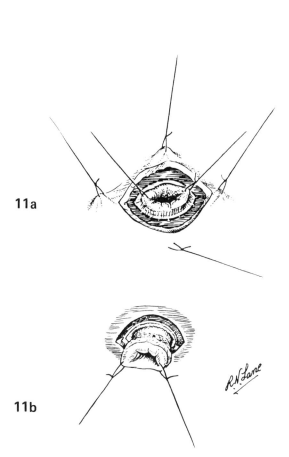

11a

11b

11a & b

Healthy rectal mucosa is dissected back a few millimetres to expose muscle coat of the rectum and a second elliptical incision is made through fibrosed muscle surrounding the track, to expose the capsule of the prostate.

Gentle traction on the fistulous track brings the prostatic capsule clearly into view and an elliptical incision through prostatic capsule frees the track completely.

12a & b

The defect is closed in three layers, using interrupted sutures of 4/0 chromic catgut. First the prostatic capsule (*a*), then the muscular coats of the rectum (*b*) and then, finally, the mucosa of the rectum.

13

Illustrates this three-layer closure diagrammatically in sagittal section.

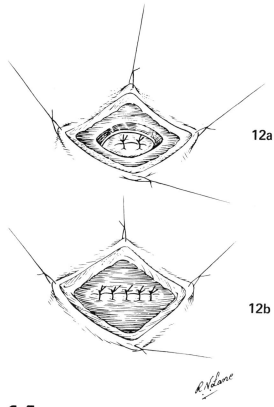

12a

12b

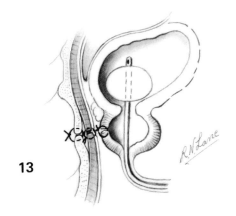

13

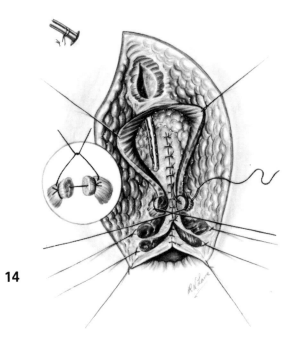

14

14

The trans-sphincteric exposure wound is now closed in layers using chromic catgut throughout. First, a continuous layer of 4/0 for the mucosa, then interrupted sutures of 3/0 for the muscle of the rectal wall and internal sphincter.

A Shirley sump drain is placed to drain the para-rectal space. The value of the identifying sutures will be appreciated at this stage. The pair marking the cut ends of the puborectalis are shown drawn up and crossed over to facilitate accurate end-to-end suture. If these marking sutures are cut short (*see* inset) but left tied, they prevent cutting through of the sutures. Ampicillin powder is sprinkled into the wound before the space in the ischiorectal fat is obliterated by fine subcutaneous sutures. The peri-anal skin is sutured with catgut. The upper part of the wound is sutured with silk or nylon.

POSTOPERATIVE

No special postoperative nursing care is required and patients are allowed out of bed early. It is, of course, important to check that there is free drainage of urine from the urethral catheter until it is removed on the twelfth postoperative day.

The best test that the fistula has been cured is normal passage of urine via the penis.

CLOSURE OF COLOSTOMY

Formal intraperitoneal closure of this end colostomy presents no technical difficulties but, because it is an innovation, the basic steps may need to be described. The proximal colon is cleansed by saline purgation and irrigation and a wide-spectrum antibiotic is given intravenously at the time of operation.

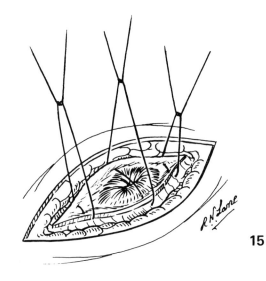

15

An elliptical skin incision is made through subcutaneous fat down to the anterior rectus sheath. Three or more sutures are placed in the peristomal skin and when these are tied they seal off the stoma.

16

A similar elliptical incision is made through anterior rectus sheath and through rectus muscle to expose posterior rectus sheath and peritoneum. A finger passed into the peritoneal cavity will find and free the blind end of the sigmoid. The freed distal limb follows the proximal as this is drawn out by traction on the skin sutures. Both ends are trimmed.

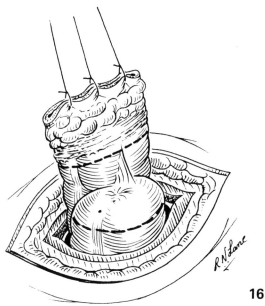

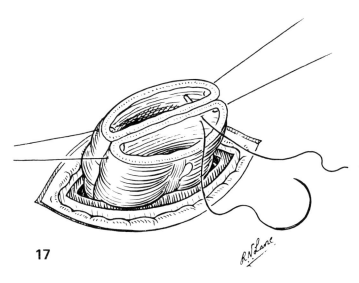

17

Continuity is restored by end-to-end anastomosis, using a single layer of interrupted vertical mattress sutures of 2/0 chromic catgut.

18

The anastomosed bowel is returned to the peritoneal cavity. The wound is closed in layers, using interrupted sutures. Two drains are used, one for the space between cut ends of rectus muscle and the second for the subcutaneous space.

Defaecation after closure of the colostomy occurs normally and no patient has experienced any impairment of normal defaecation, or of anal control after trans-sphincteric exposure for repair of a prostato-rectal fistula.

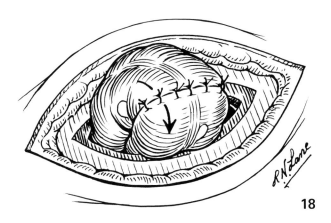

18

[*The illustrations for this Chapter on Rectoprostatic Fistula were drawn by Mr. R. N. Lane.*]

Index